Table of Contents

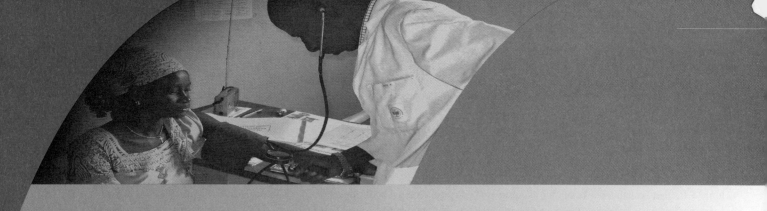

Essentials of
Global Community Health

Jaime Gofin, MD, MPH
Professor
Department of Health Promotion, Social, and Behavioral Health
College of Public Health
University of Nebraska Medical Center
Omaha, Nebraska, USA
Professorial Lecturer Prevention and Community Health
School of Public Health and Health Services
The George Washington University
Washington, DC, USA

Rosa Gofin, MD, MPH
Associate Professor of Social Medicine
Hebrew University-Hadassah School of Public Health and Community Medicine
Jerusalem, Israel
Professor
Department of Health Promotion, Social, and Behavioral Health
College of Public Health
University of Nebraska Medical Center
Omaha, Nebraska, USA
Adjunct Professor
Department of Prevention and Community Health
School of Public Health and Health Services
The George Washington University
Washington, DC, USA

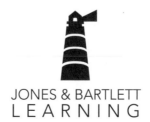

JONES & BARTLETT
LEARNING

World Headquarters

Jones & Bartlett Learning
40 Tall Pine Drive
Sudbury, MA 01776
978-443-5000
info@jblearning.com
www.jblearning.com

Jones & Bartlett Learning Canada
6339 Ormindale Way
Mississauga, Ontario L5V 1J2
Canada

Jones & Bartlett Learning
 International
Barb House, Barb Mews
London W6 7PA
United Kingdom

Jones & Bartlett Learning books and products are available through most bookstores and online booksellers. To contact Jones & Bartlett Learning directly, call 800-832-0034, fax 978-443-8000, or visit our website, www.jblearning.com.

Substantial discounts on bulk quantities of Jones & Bartlett Learning publications are available to corporations, professional associations, and other qualified organizations. For details and specific discount information, contact the special sales department at Jones & Bartlett Learning via the above contact information or send an email to specialsales@jblearning.com.

Production Credits

Publisher: Michael Brown
Editorial Assistant: Catie Heverling
Editorial Assistant: Teresa Reilly
Production Manager: Tracey Chapman
Senior Marketing Manager: Sophie Fleck
Manufacturing and Inventory Control Supervisor: Amy Bacus
Composition: Auburn Associates, Inc.
Image Credit: © Mahesh Patil/ShutterStock, Inc.
Cover Design: Kristin E. Parker
Cover Image: Top to bottom, left to right: Eye Exam: © USAID; Blood Pressure: © Solene Edouard-Binkl/CCF;
  Handing Out Pills: © George Tsereteli/USAID; Medical Aid: © Sue McIntyre/USAID
Printing and Binding: Malloy, Inc.
Cover Printing: John Pow Company

Library of Congress Cataloging-in-Publication Data
Gofin, Jaime.
  Essentials of global community health / Jaime Gofin, Rosa Gofin.
    p. ; cm.
  Includes bibliographical references and index.
  ISBN-13: 978-0-7637-7329-8 (pbk.)
  ISBN-10: 0-7637-7329-8 (pbk.)
  1. World health. 2. Community health services. I. Gofin, Rosa. II. Title.
  [DNLM: 1. Community Health Services—methods. 2. Primary Health Care—methods. 3. World Health. WA 546.1 G612e 2010]
  RA441.G64 2010
  362.12—dc22
                                        2010000293

6048
Printed in the United States of America
14 13 12 11 10   10 9 8 7 6 5 4 3 2 1

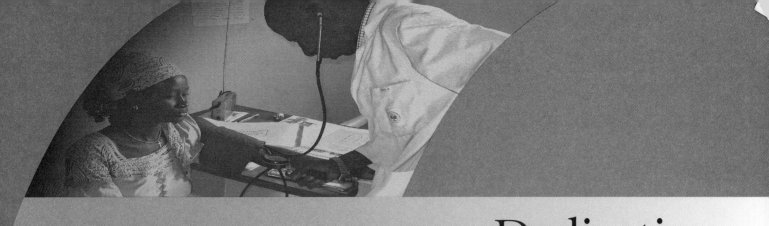

Dedication

To our parents

and

To our children, Oren, Ronit, and Yoel, and their families

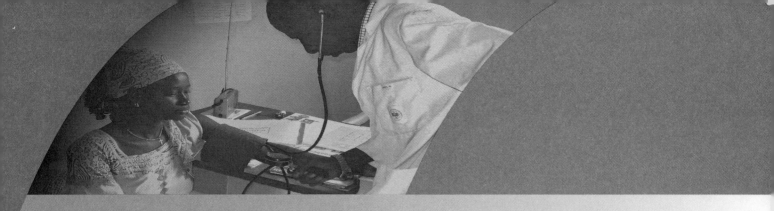

The *Essential Public Health* Series

Log on to www.essentialpublichealth.com for the most current information on availability.

ABOUT THE EDITOR:

Richard K. Riegelman, MD, MPH, PhD, is Professor of Epidemiology-Biostatistics, Medicine, and Health Policy, and Founding Dean of The George Washington University School of Public Health and Health Services in Washington, DC. He has taken a lead role in developing the Educated Citizen and Public Health initiative which has brought together arts and sciences and public health education associations to implement the Institute of Medicine of the National Academies' recommendation that ". . . all undergraduates should have access to education in public health." Dr. Riegelman also led the development of George Washington's undergraduate major and minor and currently teaches "Public Health 101" and "Epidemiology 101" to undergraduates.

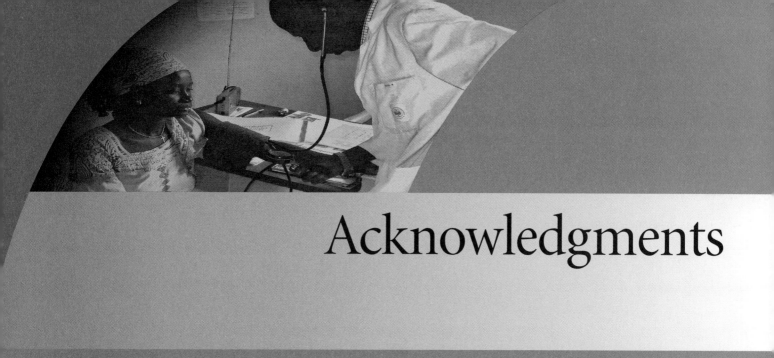

Acknowledgments

We are indebted to our mentors, teachers, colleagues, students, and graduates who have contributed to our understanding and mastering of community health and health care and have stimulated continuous learning.

Sidney L. Kark (deceased in 1998) and J. H. Abramson from the Department of Social Medicine of the School of Public Health and Community Medicine of the Hebrew University and Hadassah played a central role in our professional development. We were privileged to be their students and then their humble colleagues, enjoying not only their wisdom but also a personal relationship throughout the years. J. H. Abramson wrote Chapter 8, "Epidemiology as a Tool for Community Health Care."

Our heartfelt thanks go to each of our colleagues from the Department of Social Medicine and its Hadassah Community Health Center with whom we worked for many years; they shared with us their experience and contributed to our own.

The uniqueness of the integration of the academic framework of the Department of Social Medicine with the practice at the Community Health Center provided the opportunity for service-oriented research in COPC and for the study of health and disease and their determinants.

Special thanks to Professor Ayman El Mohandes, dean of the College of Public Health of the University of Nebraska Medical Center and the former head of the Department of Prevention and Community Health of the School of Public Health and Health Services (SPHHS) of the George Washington University. Professor El Mohandes provided us with an academic home in Washington, DC and wholeheartedly supported, and continues to support, the teaching and practice of COPC.

Professor Richard Riegelman, the founding dean of the SPHHS and the editor of the *Essential Public Health* series, supported the teaching of COPC in the school as the director of the Public Health Program. Our thanks for his initiative, advice, and support throughout the preparation of the manuscript.

We would like to acknowledge the following individuals for their assistance in reviewing, editing, and providing comments and insights at various stages of this manuscript: Elvira Beracochea, MD, MPH; Suzanne Cashman, ScD; Ayman El-Mohandes, MBBCh, MD, MPH; Becca Feldman, PhD; Joan Klevens, MD, MPH; Cara Lichtenstein, MD; Itzhak Levav, MD, MSc; Heather Pitorak, MPH; and Delia Sanchez, MD, MPH. Our acknowledgments also go to Karyn Pomerantz, MLS, MPH for providing the sources of data in Chapter 2.

To all the authors of the case studies, our sincere thanks for your contribution to enriching this book with your experiences.

We extend thanks to our children, who struggled in their young age to explain to their friends what kind of physicians their parents are, working in social medicine. Before long, they were not only able to explain but also to become supporters of our experience with COPC.

Traditionally, authors end their acknowledgments by saluting their spouses. In our case . . . the two together enjoyed this tango.

—Jaime Gofin and Rosa Gofin

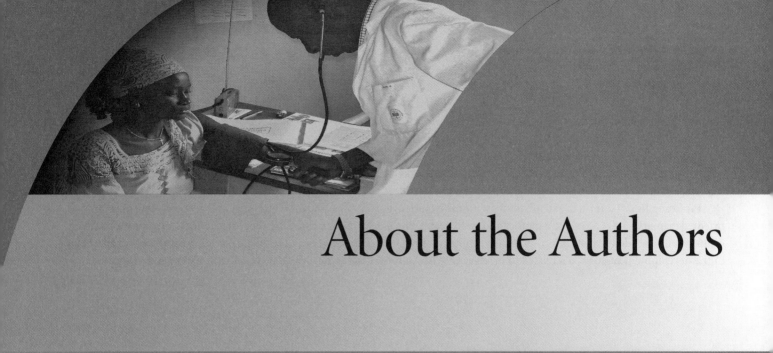

About the Authors

Jaime Gofin, born in Uruguay, got his MD from the Universidad de la República of Uruguay and his MPH from the Hebrew University-Hadassah School of Public Health and Community Medicine in Jerusalem, Israel. He is a public health expert in community health and epidemiology.

Dr. Gofin is a professor of the College of Public Health at the University of Nebraska Medical Center. During the time this book was written, he was visiting professor at the Department of Prevention and Community Health of the School of Public Health and Health Services of the George Washington University as the director of the MPH Community-Oriented Primary Care (COPC) Program.

During 1975–2003, Professor Gofin was a member of the Department of Social Medicine of the Hebrew University-Hadassah School of Public Health and Community Medicine in Jerusalem, academic director of the MPH Program, director of the Hadassah Community Health Center and director of the COPC Teaching Programs. He co-directed the 1-year International Certificate Distance Learning Program on COPC (a joint program of the George Washington University and the Jerusalem School).

Professor Jaime Gofin has developed COPC capacity programs in Portugal; Spain; Turkey; United Kingdom; Washington, DC; Argentina; Costa Rica; Ecuador; Uruguay; South Africa; and Vietnam. He is a consultant and advisor for international organizations, academic institutions, and governments, including the PAHO/WHO; the Catalonian Health Department; the Medical School of the Universesed de la República in Montevideo; and the Ministry of Health of Uruguay. He is a founding member of the COPC Working Group of the Catalan Society of Family and Community Medicine in Catalonia. He is also the chairman of the task force on Integrating Medicine and Public Health of The Network: Towards Unity for Health. Dr. Gofin has delivered lectures on COPC at International Health Organizations and published articles about the practice, teaching and evaluation of COPC.

Professor Jaime Gofin was the recipient of the 2007 Gordon Wyon Award of the International Health Section of the American Public Health Association (APHA) for his "outstanding leadership and contribution to Community-Oriented Primary Health Care."

Rosa Gofin, born in Uruguay, got her MD from the Universidad de la República of Uruguay and her MPH from the Hebrew University-Hadassah School of Public Health and Community Medicine in Jerusalem, Israel. She is an expert in public health in the areas of mother and child health, community health, and epidemiology.

She is an associate professor of social medicine in the Hebrew University-Hadassah School of Public Health and Community Medicine, where she was in charge of the Mother and Child Health Unit, and the MCH clinic at the Hadassah Community Health Center. She is a professor in the College of Public Health of the University of Nebraska

Medical Center in Omaha, NE. She is also an adjunct professor in the Department of Prevention and Community Health of the School of Public Health and Health Services of George Washington University.

Professor Rosa Gofin has published on the subjects of community program development and evaluation, mainly in the areas of mother and child health care, the conceptual frameworks of community health and its teaching, the evaluation of health services, and injury and violence in childhood and adolescence.

Professor Rosa Gofin has extensive international experience in service, capacity building, and research on community-oriented primary care (COPC) and mother and child health. She has served as a consultant for international organizations, governments, and academic institutions in the development of school health services and strategic planning for injury control and in the development of curricula related to primary care in schools of medicine and family medicine residency programs.

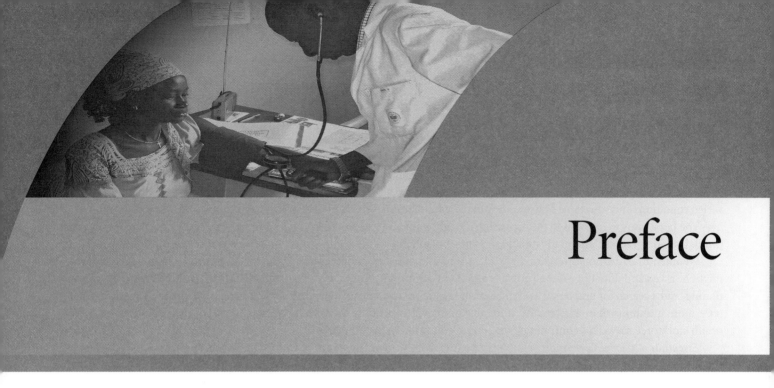

Preface

COMMUNITY HEALTH AND THE COMMUNITY-ORIENTED PRIMARY CARE (COPC) APPROACH

Health and disease are the concerns of individuals, families, and health services. When the health–illness continuum is examined, it becomes clear that beyond individuals and families, there is another dimension related to both, that of the community. The community dimension provides an understanding of the context in which health and disease are expressed. Yet this expression cannot be understood without examining the determinants of health and disease, not only at the individual and family levels, but at other levels as well. The interaction of individual, familial, community, societal, and global determinants shape the community's health.

It is this aspect of health that we develop in this book. As a natural corollary, we approach community health care by addressing the health of individuals and families in the context of their communities, stressing interventions that are intended to promote health and prevent disease at the community level.

A special feature of this book is the presentation of the history, principles, and practical steps in the development of Community-Oriented Primary Care (COPC), an approach in the delivery of community health care through primary care.

The book consists of two main sections. Section I is composed of eight chapters, and Section II is composed of 16 case studies on community health across the globe.

The first chapter elaborates on the concept of community health and its different levels of determinants. In the second chapter, community interventions are addressed, giving an overall picture of methods and types of interventions and guiding the reader through the process of developing a community intervention. Chapters 3 and 4 are specific to health interventions in primary care, addressing the principles and methods of the community-oriented primary care (COPC) approach. Chapter 3 also presents the history and origin of COPC in South Africa and follows it through its development in Jerusalem and beyond, in different countries. These two chapters have special significance because they present an approach in the delivery of care that started in the 1940s in a rural deprived area but has relevance today, considering the widespread disparities in health and inequities in the delivery of health care in many populations. Chapter 4 details the steps in the process of developing COPC programs.

Chapter 5 develops a new concept, that of community-oriented public health (COPH), which applies population health principles in the context of the community's health. It includes a comparison of traditional public health and COPH, and it highlights how COPH differs from COPC.

Chapters 6 and 7 deal with basic features of community health. In Chapter 6, community participation in health care is presented, related to the maintenance and improvement of individual and community health. A framework for the development of community participation in community health care, together with a monitoring framework, is suggested. Chapter 7 analyzes the fragmentation of health services, its negative effects, and the factors responsible for its prevailing situation in different health systems. Various approaches of integration and a framework for integration in community health care are suggested. Chapter 8 deals with epidemiology as a tool in community health and community health care from needs assessment to evaluation and for assessing health information.

Section II describes the global experience of community health and community health care. The 16 case studies examine varied conditions and situations from a variety of places and health systems in developing, transitional, and developed countries.

The book aims to respond to the increasing interest and manifested need to learn and teach public health and community health to undergraduate and graduate students who, potentially, will form the future professional cadre in community health.

We intend for the book to spark the reader's interest, and although it does not provide all the answers to questions that might be asked and does not cover all possible aspects of community health, we hope that it will stimulate further reading, questioning, and a search for answers. The challenges of health services reform and addressing health disparities and inequities may pose more questions than answers. We hope this book will contribute to addressing these issues and to training the public health workforce, as well as contributing to citizens' education in health matters.

Essentials of Global Community Health is an expression of the many years of work, experience, teaching, and learning by the authors, starting in Uruguay, then continuing in Jerusalem and many other parts of the world.

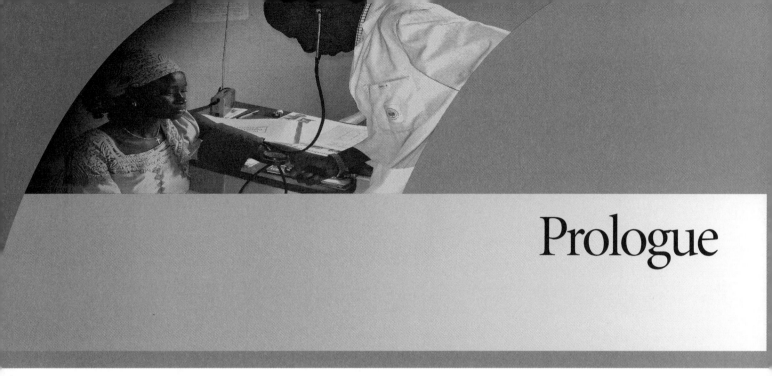

Prologue

Essentials of Global Community Health is a landmark textbook providing health professional students, health professionals, and undergraduates with a practical framework for putting community health into practice. The book is based upon principles of community-oriented primary care (COPC), a step-by-step approach to address health problems in the community. The text provides an abundance of examples of efforts from around the world to apply COPC principles.

Essentials of Global Community Health was written by two of the world's leaders in community health, Jaime and Rosa Gofin. For nearly 40 years the Gofins have been in the forefront of efforts to educate health professionals and citizens about implementing the COPC approach. They themselves have been active in efforts to establish model COPC practices. They have established what is today undoubtedly the largest network of COPC practitioners, including practitioners from every corner of the Earth.

The book is divided into two basic sections. The first is an overview of the content of community health and the COPC approach. The second is a series of structured case studies illustrating the approach in a wide array of settings. The overview is carefully organized to provide the reader with necessary content, complete with illustrative examples, summary tables, plus discussion and review questions to reinforce the material.

The book is ideal as a textbook for health professionals, including clinicians, public health professionals, and administrators. It is also an extremely useful book for future health professionals who want to understand how their future careers might serve communities as well as individuals.

This approach to community health is based upon the COPC principles so well developed by the Gofins and their mentors and colleagues over more than a half century. The book also introduces a recent expansion of these concepts to include a wider focus on the population as a whole through community-oriented public health. The Gofins do a wonderful job of summarizing what has been learned over the last half century and look forward to what needs to be done in the years to come.

I'm delighted that *Essentials of Global Community Health* is now part of our *Essential Public Health* Series. Take a look; I'm convinced you will be equally pleased.

Richard Riegelman, MD, MPH, PhD
Series Editor, *Essential Public Health* Series

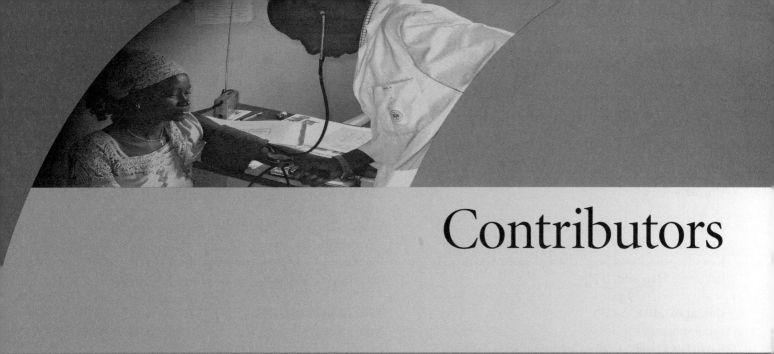

Contributors

J. H. Abramson
Emeritus Professor of Social Medicine
School of Public Health and Community Medicine
Hadassah and Hebrew University
Jerusalem, Israel

Nancy Acosta, MD
Administración de Servicios de Salud del Estado-ASSE—
    Ministry of Public Health
Uruguay

Serafín Alonso, MD
Administración de Servicios de Salud del Estado-ASSE—
    Ministry of Public Health
Uruguay

Ricardo Alvarado, MD, MPH
Centro de Investigaciones Ciencias de la Salud (CICS)
Departamento de Salud Pública y Gestión en Salud
Universidad del Rosario
Escuela de Medicina y Ciencias de la Salud
Bogotá, Colombia

Ron Anderson, MD, MACP
President and CEO
Parkland Health & Hospital System
Dallas, Texas, USA

Mónica Arroyo, Licenciada en Psicologia
Administración de Servicios de Salud del Estado-ASSE—
    Ministry of Public Health
Uruguay

Jeffrey J. Bachar, MPH
Principal Investigator
Cherokee Choices/REACH 2010
Cherokee, North Carolina, USA

Paul Boumbulian, PhD, MPH
Consultant, National Center for Primary Care
Morehouse School of Medicine
Atlanta, Georgia, USA

Geof Bowman
Health Advisor, World Relief
Cambodia

Larry Casazza, MD, MPH
Director, ACAM-African Communities Against Malaria
Washington, DC, USA

Suzanne B. Cashman, ScD
Department of Family Medicine and Community Health
University of Massachusetts Medical School
Worcester, Massachusetts, USA

Ramiro Draper, MD
Coordinator Primary Care, Canelones
Administración de Servicios de Salud del Estado-ASSE—
  Ministry of Public Health
Uruguay

Anbarasi Edward, PhD, MPH, MBA
Assistant Scientist
Johns Hopkins Bloomberg School of Public Health
Baltimore, Maryland, USA

Gonçal Foz, MD
Family Physician
Raval, Nord Health Center (Institut Català de la Salut)
Member of the COPC working group (Catalan Society of
  Family and Community Medicine)
Barcelona, Spain

Emma Garcia, MD, MPH
Vivere's Technical Advisor
Switzerland

Irina Giacosa, SW
Administración de Servicios de Salud del Estado-ASSE—
  Ministry of Public Health
Uruguay

Alfonso González, MD
Former Delegate of the Terre des hommes Foundation
Bénin—Togo

Kay Hansen, RN, MPH
Formerly of World Relief
Cambodia

Patrik Johansson, MD, MPH
Associate Professor
Director, Rural Health Education Network
College of Public Health
University of Nebraska Medical Center
Omaha, Nebraska, USA

Kathleen Kahn, MBBCh, MPH, PhD
MRC/Wits Rural Public Health and Health Transitions
  Research Unit (Agincourt)
School of Public Health, University of the Witwatersrand
Johannesburg, South Africa
and

Epidemiology and Global Health
Public Health and Clinical Medicine
Umeå University
Sweden

Arthur Kaufman, MD
Professor, Department of Family and Community Medicine
University of New Mexico
Vice President for Community Health
Albuquerque, New Mexico, USA

Melissa Klein, MD, MPH
Primary Care Provider
Unity Health Care ReEntry Health Center
Washington, DC, USA

Emilie Kpadonou, MD
Psychiatrist
Professor
University Abomey
Bénin

Claudia López, RN
Administración de Servicios de Salud del Estado-ASSE—
  Ministry of Public Health
Uruguay

Elena Mereacre
Social Educator
President of the local NGO Compasiune
Moldova

Melanie Morrow, MPH
Director of Maternal and Child Health Programs
World Relief
Cambodia

Josep Lluís de Peray, MD
Family Physician
Coordinator for the Creation of the Public Health Agency of
  Catalonia
Direcció General de Salut Pública Department of Health
Generalitat de Catalunya
Barcelona, Spain

Henry Perry, MD, MPH, PhD
Professor
Future Generations Graduate School

Collins A. Pfaff, MBBCh, MMed (Fam Med), DCh, DA, Dip HIV Man
Division of Rural Health, Department of Family Medicine
University of the Witwatersrand
Johannesburg, South Africa

Sharon Phillips, RN, MBA
Senior Vice President, Community Medicine
Parkland Health and Hospital System
Dallas, Texas, USA

Sue Pickens, M.Ed
Director, Strategic Planning and Population Medicine
Parkland Health & Hospital System
Dallas, Texas, USA

Elizabeth Ponce, MD, MPH
Former Program Coordinator
Delegate and Technical Assistant and Consultant in Planning
Swiss NGO Vivere in Moldova
HIV/AIDS, Violence and Gender for international organizations (TSF and RST/UNAIDS/WCA;WHO-Eqg.)

Patricia Rambao, MD
Administración de Servicios de Salud del Estado-ASSE—
Ministry of Public Health
Uruguay

Saverio Sava, MD
Medical Director, First Choice Community Healthcare
Associate Professor, Department of Family and Community Medicine
University of New Mexico
Albuquerque, New Mexico, USA

Clara Savage, EdD
Department of Family Medicine and Community Health
University of Massachusetts Medical School
Worcester, Massachusetts, USA

Silvia Sica, Licenciada en Psicologia
Administración de Servicios de Salud del Estado-ASSE—
Ministry of Public Health
Uruguay

Oun Sivan
Project Director
Light for Life Child Survival
Cambodia

Karina Sosa, MD
Administración de Servicios de Salud del Estado-ASSE—
Ministry of Public Health
Uruguay

Stephen M. Tollman, MBBCh, MPH, MA, MMed, PhD
MRC/Wits Rural Public Health and Health Transitions Research Unit (Agincourt)
School of Public Health, University of the Witwatersrand
Johannesburg, South Africa
and
Epidemiology and Global Health
Public Health and Clinical Medicine
Umeå University
Sweden

Jennifer Tsai, MPH
Senior Associate
AcademyHealth
Washington, DC, USA

Camilo Valderrama, MD, MPH, PHD
Senior Health Advisor
International Rescue Committee (IRC)
A. Muang Chiang Mai, Thailand

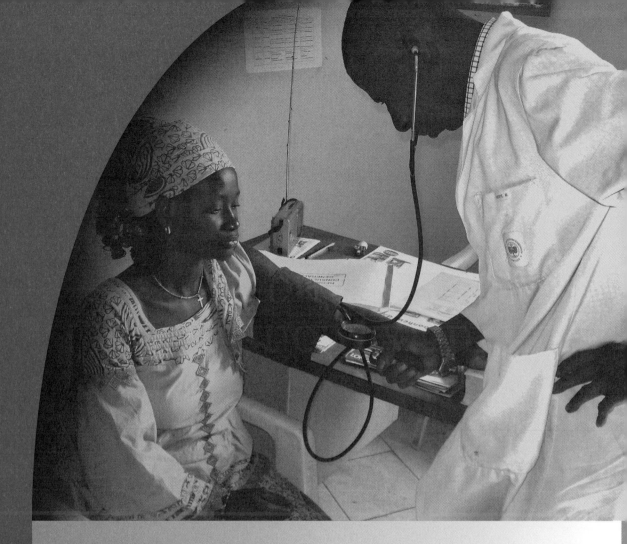

SECTION I

Principles of Global Community Health

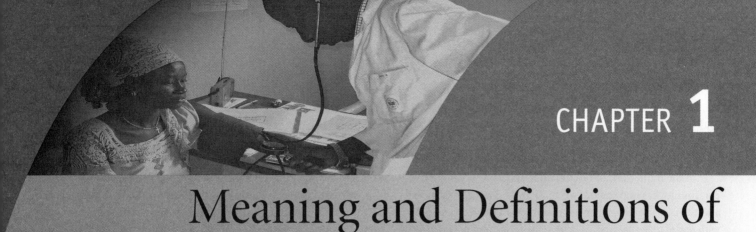

CHAPTER **1**

Meaning and Definitions of Community Health

KEY TERMS

community	community healthcare practice
community health	determinants of community health
community health	health
measurements	

INTRODUCTION

Community health encompasses the health of groups within a certain place and extends beyond the aggregate of the individuals' health. Conceptualizing community health implies recognizing what is meant by community, health, and the relationships among them. The attempts to develop an agreed-upon definition of community and health have been elusive, and to date there is no universal or accepted definition of either term. Similarly, community health is more understood than defined, but this understanding may vary according to context, place, or culture. Moreover, it may vary according to its given purpose and who does the defining (individuals, institutions, organizations, etc.).

In the framework of health and health care, a definition of community has implications for both the community members and the care providers. For the members themselves, especially with regard to health care, the definition of community may determine whether they have access to care or, for example, whether they are included in community health programs. In parallel, providers need to understand the community for which they are responsible for the delivery of care, for examining its quality, and to whom the development and evaluation of prevention, promo-

tion, treatment, and rehabilitative activities are geared. For both the healthcare providers and the community members, the identification of or with a community may be necessary to facilitate the establishment of internal and external collaborations and networks, as well as the involvement of the population in its own care.

In this chapter we will present definitions and concepts pertaining to community health and its determinants, indicators of community health, sources of information, and data gathering. The authors expect that this discussion will stimulate additional thinking about community health and the different factors that affect the health of the community, not only generally but more particularly within specific communities with which the learner may be involved.

Box 1-1 Case study: Community health and community health determinants

The populations of Alabama, Louisiana, and Mississippi are predominantly African American, and these states have poverty rates of 20%, 22%, and 23%, respectively. These areas are characterized by unmet needs in healthcare services. The uninsured populations in about 2005 were high: 22% in Louisiana, 19% in Mississippi, and 15% in Alabama.

On August 29, 2005, Hurricane Katrina made landfall on the US Gulf Coast. New Orleans was significantly affected. Approximately 1.1 million individuals in the city were forced to leave their homes. Hurricane Katrina caused massive intrastate displacement and migration to 27 states. The capacity of healthcare and other services in the city were severely affected, as were services in the areas to which people were displaced because of the influx of large numbers of persons.

Emergency and trauma care capacities were severely compromised or destroyed. Primary care providers who served populations with very low socioeconomic status (SES) in the directly affected areas were nearly eliminated. The National Association of Community Health Centers estimated that more than 100 healthcare centers were affected by Hurricane Katrina, and at least seven centers and affiliated sites were completely destroyed. In addition, the capacity of hospitals to deliver inpatient, outpatient, and emergency services was compromised at a time when the need for the services greatly increased. The damage was not limited to healthcare facilities; patients also lost access to routine medications, diabetic supplies, medical equipment, etc.

The public infrastructure, including electric power, communication networks, roads, and water treatment plants, was severely damaged. As a result of the flooding and damage to drinking water and sanitation systems, new public health threats developed after the hurricane. Public health efforts to prevent the spread of communicable diseases, such as HIV, were put on hold. Psychological stress and trauma related to the destruction, loss of jobs, loss of homes, separation of families, and death had an impact on the mental health of community members. Those who previously suffered from mental illnesses requiring medication lost access to their prescriptions. Elderly and disabled individuals, whether displaced by the hurricane or not, lost their homes, family, and community support, and the need for nursing home care greatly increased.

Sources: Centers for Disease Control and Prevention. Surveillance for illness and injury after Hurricane Katrina—three counties, Mississippi, September 5–October 11, 2005. *MMWR Weekly.* 2006;55(09):231–234. http://www.cdc.gov/mmwr/preview/mmwrhtml/mm5509a2.htm. Accessed April 15, 2009.

Eisenman D, Cordasco K, Asch S, Golden J, Gilk D. Disaster planning and risk communication with vulnerable communities: lessons learned from Hurricane Katrina. *AJPH.* 2007;97(suppl 1):S109–S115. http://ajph.aphapublications.org/content/vol97/Supplement_1/. Accessed April 15, 2009.

Kaiser Commission on Medicaid and the Uninsured. *Addressing the Health Care Impact of Hurricane Katrina.* Washington, DC: Kaiser Family Foundation; 2005. http://www.kff.org/uninsured/upload/7387-2.pdf. Accessed April 13, 2009.

Kaiser Family Foundation. Assessing the number of people with HIV/AIDS in areas affected by Hurricane Katrina. http://www.kff.org/katrina/upload/7407.pdf. Published September 2005. Accessed April 13, 2009.

Ridenour ML, Cummings KJ, Sinclair JR, Bixler D. Displacement of the underserved: medical needs of Hurricane Katrina evacuees in West Virginia. *J Health Care Poor Underserved.* 2007;18:369–381.

DEFINITIONS

Defining *community* and *health* is a challenging task. Scholars are not in consensus regarding the definition of the terms or the main components of the definitions. Moreover, although conceptual definitions are offered, translating them into operational terms tends to be difficult. The following sections present concepts that are inherent to community health.

Family

A family is defined as two or more people who are related by emotional ties, marriage, blood, or adoption. Marriage, however, is a dynamic process that has cultural, spiritual, and social definitions of gender roles, the presence or absence of children (biological, adopted, or foster), and common-law relations. As divorced and single parenthood rates increase, it becomes increasingly challenging to define a family unit.[a,1,2]

Regarding family health and health care, families are the most important and complex units for the communication, reception, and transmission of health information.[3] Families are also determinants of their own health because shared behaviors and practices act synergistically in the unit. Family resources (economic, social, knowledge, skills) and health behavior history are of importance in determining the pathways of each member's own health practices. Family dynamics also can determine, positively or negatively, the events leading to the occurrence of disease and its transmission and severity. Families can also be defined as a setting for health promotion.[4] It is through the family life cycle that continuity of care can be applied—from family formation, to birth until adulthood, and until death.

Community

According to Etzioni, communities have two characteristics: (1) affect-laden relationships among a group of individuals that reinforce one another, and (2) a commitment to shared values, norms, and meanings, as well as shared history and identity.[5] Brown defines community primarily in relation to environmental health and justice. He emphasizes that place, in an ecological sense, has a greater influence on health issues than individual characteristics.[6]

There is growing evidence in the literature about the influence of the community context on health and disease. The measurement of such contextual characteristics has been proposed, including 12 dimensions to define a community contextual profile: economics, employment, education, politics, environment, housing, medicine, government, public health, psychology, behavior, and transportation.[7] A qualitative study that examined community participation in vaccine trials for people living with AIDS[8] identified different dimensions of community: (1) a sense of place (defined by geography or where people gather); (2) sharing common interests, perspectives, and values; (3) joint action and a sense of coherence and identity; (4) social ties; and (5) diversity (the social complexity of a given community).

Although not all population groups have the characteristics proposed by Etzioni, they might nevertheless be the target for the provision of care by a certain provider or providers. Certain groups may have some of the previously mentioned characteristics, which might facilitate the organization of care.

Geographic Definition and Its Alternatives

Communities are often defined in geographic terms. This often provides a clear boundary and description. From healthcare providers' viewpoint, the geographic definition of community may have different meanings and encompass various levels when referring to a neighborhood, county, district, or state, with all of them demarcated by geographic boundaries. A neighborhood may provide a sense of community to its members and close proximity to a healthcare service (both in geographic terms and in a feeling of intimacy and belonging). This proximity facilitates access to care, outreach activities, and knowledge and understanding of community networks and organizations. A larger geographic division can be considered by decision makers for policy purposes in the development and provision of community-based programs.

Even within a geographic area or transcending the geographic boundaries, other shared characteristics can be found. These include belonging to a racial, ethnic, or religious group or possessing other features, such as being homeless or having a disease (e.g., diabetes, HIV). Additionally, within those boundaries a school or group of schools would be the defined community for school healthcare services, or employees of a company or factory might be the community for a certain service. Thus, members of a certain geographic community may belong to other communities, such as schools or ethnic or religious groups.

In urban populations, identifying well-defined geographic communities is becoming increasingly complex. A healthcare service provider may face difficulties in defining a specific population as the community under its care. People living in the same geographic area might go to different providers within or outside those boundaries. Conversely, a service may take care of people who come from different locations. Thus, an alternative identification should be considered in terms of the geographic definition of the community.

---

[a]The US Census Bureau defines a family as "two people or more (one of whom is the householder) related by birth, marriage or adoption residing together." The American Academy of Family Physicians defines it as a group of individuals with legal, genetic, or emotional relationships.

Modern technology may help in developing this alternative definition, which might have some elements of the geographic boundaries but does not always coincide with a statistical area or a county and may even transcend states. Geographic information systems (GIS) can help locate the users of a healthcare practice according to their addresses.[9]

The implications of clearly defining a community in relation to health and health care cannot be overemphasized. For service providers, it will identify the target population for action. For community members, it will identify the availability and access to services. This applies to not only curative care (which can be limited to people who are insured in a certain plan), but also to prevention and promotion activities. Health departments or other healthcare organizations provide services and programs encompassing larger populations that may include several communities. A clearly defined community allows the healthcare services, community organizations, and community leaders and members to recognize and assess their resources, establish networks, identify health needs, determine priorities, and implement programs.

Virtual Communities The advances in communication technology and the penetration of the Internet[10] have enabled the building of virtual communities and opened a new venue for communication, especially about health-related matters.[11] Popular social networking sites that allow new acquaintances to be made or old ones to be maintained virtually, such as Facebook or MySpace, may constitute new ways in which health-related matters are shared. Also, support groups for specific conditions or special interest groups offer new venues for sharing and disseminating knowledge about new developments in health care. This might be particularly important for people who are confined to their homes because of health conditions or limited mobility.

Concerns may arise regarding these virtual communities because of possible divisions among different groups of the population, given the differential access to information technology or the reading abilities of the audience.[12] Moreover, the abundance of information and its sources, which includes unsubstantiated facts and opinions, may pose problems of reliability and accuracy that the audience cannot always discriminate.

Because of the anonymity usually involved in these communities, virtual communications can also have a negative health impact, such as in the case of cyber bullying, which has been shown to affect the mental health and well-being of youngsters.[13,14]

Health

The World Health Organization (WHO) adopted a definition of health in June 1946 at the International Health Conference in New York, and it was entered into use in April 1948. WHO defines health as "a state of complete physical, mental and social well-being and not merely the absence of disease or infirmity."[15] The definition offers a good conceptual framework, although operationally it is difficult to appraise. The definition has been criticized over the years, but it is nevertheless widely used and has not been amended since its inception. Today there is no universally accepted definition.

In 1976, Ivan Illich, a philosopher and Catholic priest of Austrian origin, published *Limits to Medicine: Medical Nemesis, the Expropriation of Health.*[16] He forcefully argued against medical care as a commodity and overmedicalization, especially in the case of life events such as birth and death. He proposed a more dynamic view of health, referring to the ability to adapt to changing environments and to the different stages of the life course.

In his 1974 report, Marc Lalonde, then the Minister of Health and Welfare of Canada, did not define the concept of health, but he proposed the *health field* concept.[b,17] The Lalonde report is credited with setting off some new initiatives regarding the health of populations,[18] including the WHO's 1978 Health for All initiative in the International Conference on Primary Health Care in Alma-Ata, Kazakhstan (a former Soviet republic).[19] The goals of the Health for All initiative were scheduled to be achieved by 2000. The 22-year time frame was too short to achieve all that was set forth, especially without radical changes in the determinants of health and the organization of healthcare services. However, Health for All acknowledged great inequalities in health between and within countries and created targets for the most important aspects of health. In the Declaration of Alma-Ata, health is considered to be "a fundamental human right and the attainment of the highest possible level of health is a most important world-wide social goal whose realization requires the action of many other social and economic sectors in addition to the health sector."

In the European Region of the WHO, the targets were redefined for the 21st century as Health 21.[c,20] Efforts to achieve the Health for All goals were continued, and in 1986, in the first International Conference on Health Promotion in Ottawa,

---

[b]It encompassed (1) the environment—both physical and social, or all that is external to the human body; (2) human biology—all aspects of physical and mental health as the result of its organic makeup; (3) lifestyle—the aggregation of personal decisions; and (4) the healthcare organization—the type and relationship with the service provision.
[c]The targets addressed outcomes through the life course, such as specific conditions (communicable and noncommunicable diseases, injury, and violence), the determinants of health, and the settings for healthcare and healthcare services organizations. There was specific reference to an integrated healthcare sector that offers accessible and quality care through family and community-oriented primary health care.

Ontario, a charter for action was created.[21] The Ottawa Charter, although it did not provide a new definition of health, described health as "a positive concept emphasizing social and personal resources, as well as physical capacities." It introduced the prerequisites for health as the basic elements of peace, shelter, education, food, income, a stable ecosystem, sustainable resources, and the values of social justice and equity.

In addition to the health goals developed by the WHO and their redefinition in Health 21, the Millennium Development Goals (MDGs) are a new endeavor led by the United Nations to be achieved by 2015.[22] The MDGs are drawn from the Millennium Declaration that was adopted by 189 nations and signed by 147 heads of state and governments during the United Nations Millennium Summit in September 2000. Three of the goals (goals 4, 5, and 6) were specifically related to health; four goals referred to the MDGs' determinants and their need to be achieved if changes in health are to be expected (goals 1, 2, 3, and 7). The eighth goal expects the global community to act together for development.[d]

In the United States, Healthy People 2010 delineates the health objectives for the nation.[23] The two main goals of Healthy People 2010 are (1) to increase quality and years of healthy life and (2) eliminate health disparities. The goals focus on 28 health areas, and 10 leading indicators were selected to measure the nation's health. They were selected on the basis of their importance in public health, their ability to promote action, and the availability of data to measure progress.[e]

Health As a Dynamic State Through the Life Course

Health is a dynamic state—a continuum between health and disease—and there are not clear cut-off points determining the limit between one and the other. Health through the life course is another continuum of importance. Typically, each life stage has its own particular health and disease characteristics. For example, infectious diseases and injuries are prevalent during childhood; risk behaviors, such as substance abuse, are developed during adolescence; and chronic conditions, such as cardiovascular diseases and cancer, are more prevalent during adulthood.

However, the origins of these adult diseases are determined earlier in life. There are some conditions that appear in childhood and have long-term consequences. For example, rheumatic heart disease starts as a streptococcal infection that, if left untreated, will damage the heart in the long term. Health-compromising behaviors in adolescence, such as poor eating habits and dieting, lack of physical activity, and smoking, have long-term effects if they are not modified. Today we know about the fetal origins of adult diseases. An unfavorable environment in utero has long-term consequences. The nutritional, hormonal, and metabolic environment in utero programs the physiology and pathology of the offspring.[24] Thus, low birth weight was found to be associated with coronary heart disease, diabetes, and hypertension in later life.

The knowledge about health through the life course has been facilitated by cohort studies, such as the UK National Survey of Health and Development (NSHD) study.[f,25] These studies have emphasized the effects of social factors and inequalities through the life course, such as the affects of consistent lifetime exposure to poor socioeconomic conditions on low cognitive ability in childhood and higher adult mortality; the association of poor maternal care with higher risk of maternal postpartum depression; and the association of poor maternal care and parental divorce with a child's poorer cognitive development and faster decline in mental concentration in midlife.

COMMUNITY HEALTH AND ITS DETERMINANTS

Community health, like individual health, encompasses a continuum from well-being to disease. There is not a universally accepted definition of community health. Frequently, community health is equated with care in the community or community-based care but community health goes beyond the location of health care. In any community context, and for any working definition of community, the health of its individuals will contribute to the collective expression of health. This collective expression of health can be of a physical nature, as well as a mental and social one.

Moreover, community health is an expression of its varied determinants. These determinants act at different levels, from the personal to the familial to the physical and the sociocultural environment levels. Beyond these levels, the influence of global processes is increasingly felt not only at the national level, but it also permeates to the community level.

---

[d]The MDGs are (1) eradicate extreme poverty and hunger; (2) achieve universal primary education; (3) promote gender equality and empower women; (4) reduce child mortality; (5) improve maternal health; (6) combat HIV/AIDS, malaria, and other diseases; (7) ensure environmental stability; and (8) develop a global partnership for development.

[e]Five of the indicators refer to healthy lifestyle—physical activity, overweight and obesity, tobacco use, substance abuse, and responsible sexual behavior. Three of the indicators refer to priority health issues—mental health, violence and injuries, and immunization for preventable diseases. One indicator relates to healthcare access, and lastly, one indicator refers to environmental quality.

---

[f]This study was based on 16,500 births in England, Wales, and Scotland that took place during one week in March 1946. The follow-up included a sample of 5362 participants that were examined 21 times; the most recent was when the sample participants were 51 years old.

Thus, community health is influenced by determinants acting and interacting at different levels and degrees of complexity, from the molecular level to intricate organizational social and service structures. Health and health-related services, while not always determining the state of health of the community, contribute to its expression.

Determinants are those factors that act together in complex webs of causation and interactions to affect the health of the community. Figure 1-1 describes determinants of community health according to different levels of influence. More distal as a health determinant is the global level, although the increasing understanding of how it affects health makes it a crucial level to deal with. The relationships between the different levels may vary in different populations and communities. Complex webs of causation and interactions between the levels and community health may be elaborated accordingly. Their understanding is needed for improving community health and its health care.

Personal and Family Level

This is the micro level, in which the socio-demographic, biological, and behavioral characteristics are expressed.

Socioeconomic Status

An individual's socioeconomic status has been demonstrated to affect morbidity and mortality. Although there is no agreed-upon

> ### Box 1-2
> ### Community health
>
> Community health is the collective expression of the health of individuals and groups in a defined community. It is determined by the interaction of personal and family characteristics, the social, cultural, and physical environments, as well as health services and the influence of societal, political, and globalization factors.

FIGURE 1-1 Determinants of Community Health.

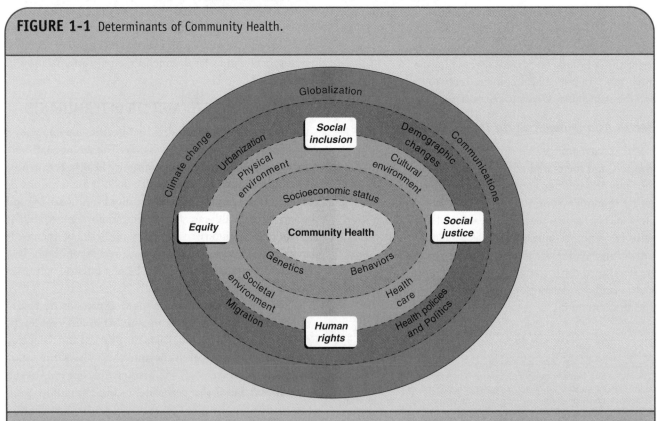

Source: Data from: Commission on Social Determinants of Health. *Closing the Gap in a Generation: Health Equity Through Action on the Social Determinants of Health.* Geneva, Switzerland: World Health Organization; 2008. http://www.who.int/social_determinants/thecommission/finalreport/en/index.html. Accessed February 2009; Dahlgren G, Whitehead, M. *Policies and strategies to promote social equity in health.* Stockholm: Institute of Futures Studies; 1991; Institute of Medicine. *The Future of the Public's Health in the 21st Century.* The National Academy Press. Washington DC, 46–95; 2003.

measure, education, employment or occupation, and income have been used separately or in conjunction in different populations and in different countries to assess socioeconomic status.

Lower socioeconomic status, measured by mothers' education, has been found to be associated with poor health status, disease, and delayed child development in different populations in different countries. Low education was found to be associated with increased cesarean section rates,[26] fetal and infant mortality,[27] cerebral palsy independent of perinatal complications,[28] and delayed child development.[29] School dropouts have consequently higher rates of smoking and drug use than those who complete school.[30] During the 1990s in the Russian Federation, a country in economic transition, life expectancy decreased markedly, particularly among men and women with low education, and it increased among those with university education, resulting in an increased mortality gap between those groups.[31]

The association between long-term lower social status and poor health has been demonstrated in different populations. The report of musculoskeletal pain among 45 year olds who were followed since birth in the NSHD study was higher among those with lower social status in childhood and adulthood than among those with higher social status.[32] The metabolic syndrome among 60- to 79-year-old men in the United Kingdom was found to be associated with childhood and adult social class, the latter acting mainly through its association with poor health behaviors.[33] Mortality rates have been found to be inversely associated with different measures of SES in Canada[34] and Sweden for overall and cause-specific rates,[35] and several studies of cancer survival in different sites showed persistent socioeconomic gaps.[36] In the United States, an inverse association was found between a measure of lifetime social position (participants and their parents) and body mass index (BMI).[37]

Genetic Endowment

The expression of health is partially due to the genetic endowment people bring with them, which constitutes their genotype. The physical expression constitutes their phenotype. Although there is a gene–environment interaction, the actual proportions may differ for different conditions, which would determine the probability that a certain health condition will actually manifest.

With the completion of the Human Genome Project (HGP) in 2003,[38] the sequencing of the human genome was achieved, and a map of human genetic variation was produced.[g]

By 2008, the HGP contributed to the development of about 1500 new genetic tests, mainly for common diseases, thus contributing further to the possibility not only of early diagnosis, but also to understanding and identifying susceptibility to drug treatment (pharmacogenomics). However, not all the genetic tests are readily applicable, and specific criteria have been suggested to determine their suitability in clinical practice.[h,39]

There is concern that genetic test information might be misused by insurance companies or employers. For the former, there is a risk that test results will prompt denying eligibility or increasing premiums for a certain plan or requesting that a person undergo a certain genetic test. For employers, the risk is that genetic information may preclude hiring a person or cause the layoff of a worker. These concerns prompted the passing of a federal law in the United States, the Genetic Information Nondiscrimination Act (GINA).[40] The new possibilities that the HGP offers for genetic screening have generated debate about its use in health care. Translational research that will apply the new genetic discoveries into medical practice is not occurring at the same pace as the discoveries are occurring.[41,42] The community appears to be an appropriate setting for carrying out the translational research, and practice-based research has been suggested[39] through existing networks where this rigorous research can be applied.[43] The dissemination of the tests may bring some potential for inequities in the population if they are not offered and financed for the total population. Moreover, tailored individual care, with screening for diseases that may not develop or prenatal testing for the delivery of perfect babies, may pose not only clinical dilemmas but also ethical dilemmas at the individual and professional levels.

Health Behaviors

Individual and community health is impacted by human behavior. Health behaviors are defined as those that are practiced by people to maintain and improve their health or prevent diseases. Conversely, behaviors can also be negative and have harmful health effects. The health behaviors of individuals together form part of collective health behavior, and as such they affect the health of communities. When these behaviors are consistently performed over a period of time, they

---

[g]The HGP is a joint endeavor of the US Department of Energy and National Institutes of Health, the Wellcome Trust of the United Kingdom, and other countries such as Japan, France, Germany, and China.

[h]The criteria determine (1) the evaluation focus (the definition of the disorder, test clinical scenario, or intended use); (2) analytic validity (whether it measures what it is supposed to measure—reliability and robustness); (3) clinical validity (whether it measures the disease it is supposed to measure); (4) clinical utility (whether it improves outcome, feasibility of implementation, costs, and safety); and (5) ethical, legal, and social issues (confidentiality, discrimination, privacy, and access).

become a lifestyle. The determinants of health behaviors are complex and are associated with biological, social, economic, and cultural factors.

For some societies, the decrease in the prevalence of diseases caused by poor environmental conditions has highlighted the importance of behaviors as determinants of health status. For societies in which sanitation and poor water supply are still the determinants of diseases, mostly of an infectious nature, positive health behaviors in the absence of appropriate changes in environmental conditions are not enough to curb the prevalence of those diseases.

Smoking and poor nutritional and sedentary habits have been implicated in the development of chronic diseases, such as cardiovascular conditions and cancer.[44–47] Sexual behaviors, such as multiple sex partners and limited use of contraception, have been related to sexually transmitted diseases (STDs) and teenage pregnancy.[48,49] Some of these behaviors can be considered risk factors if they have a causal relationship with a specific outcome (smoking and lung cancer, for example), or they can be considered risk markers if the association is not causal.

Risk factors for cardiovascular diseases were first identified by the Framingham Heart Study, which began in 1949.[50] This study found high blood pressure, hypercholesterolemia, obesity, sedentary habits, and smoking to be associated with the prevalence and incidence of cardiovascular diseases. These risk factors are associated with poor health behaviors in addition to the biological component.

Other types of health behaviors, such as the use of protective gear (seat belts, car seats, and bicycle or motorcycle helmets), are associated with a decrease in injury incidents in case of an accident.[51] The use of healthcare services can be considered a health-related behavior, which is influenced not only by personal factors, but also by the availability and accessibility of the services (location, hours of functioning, insurance, cost, and transportation). Other behaviors might be more influenced by social and cultural norms of the community, such as family formation and rearing practices.

Often health behaviors have a long-term health effect or will be manifested later in life or may affect the offspring. This is specifically relevant for pregnant women or mothers. For example, breastfeeding is associated with lower cholesterol in adulthood,[52] and smoking during pregnancy is one of the main factors associated with lower birth weight.[53]

Health behaviors are amenable to change. Several behavioral change theories have been developed and implemented in community interventions. Examples of these are the Health Belief Model, Social Cognitive Theory, Theory of Reasoned Action, and the Transtheoretical Model (see Chapter 2).

Community Level

In this level of community health determinants, the societal, cultural and physical environments are discussed. Health care, including promotion, prevention, treatment, and rehabilitation, is also considered among these determinants.

Societal Environment

The community societal environment, as perceived by its members—their sense of belonging and ownership, as well as the social networks, norms of reciprocity, and trustworthiness that form their social capital[i]—may have repercussions on individual health.[54] This is in addition to the influences of individual and family characteristics and behaviors.[55–60] The community's social capital makes it possible for the community's members and organizations to address the issues affecting their health and cope with health emergencies and crises.

Current evidence suggests that not only is individual socioeconomic status a determinant of health, but the contextual measure of poverty (i.e., the neighborhood's poverty level) is also a health determinant. In the manifestation of obesity in New York City, for example, it was found that there were strong inverse associations between education and BMI in both sexes, as well as between income and BMI among women in richer neighborhoods versus women in lower-income neighborhoods.[61]

Poverty is affecting large segments of the global population. According to the World Bank, in 2005,[62] 1.2 billion people were living on US$1.25 to US$2.00 per day, double the number of people in 1981, and it estimates that the number will remain at around 1 billion until 2015. These income levels persist in some regions of the world, such as sub-Saharan Africa, where 380 million people live on less than US$1.25 per day. In the United States, poverty is defined according to a family's threshold, which takes into account the family size and composition.[j,63] In 2007, 12.5% of the global population (37.3 million individuals) was living below the poverty line, and children younger than age 18 years represented 35.7% of them (13.3 million individuals). Poverty overwhelmingly affects minorities. The implication is that minority groups do not have

---

[i]According to the World Bank, social capital are norms and networks that enable collective action and shape society's interactions. The dimensions of social capital include groups and networks, trust and solidarity, collective action and cooperation, social cohesion and inclusion, and information and communication. The World Bank emphasizes economics and development. Although both are related to health, social capital can impact health directly. (http://web.worldbank.org/WBSITE/EXTERNAL/TOPICS/EXTSOCIAL DEVELOPMENT/EXTTSOCIALCAPITAL/0,,contentMDK:20642703~menu PK:401023~pagePK:148956~piPK:216618~theSitePK:401015,00.html)
[j]The threshold for a family of three, including a child younger than 18 years of age, is a yearly income of $16,689.

equal opportunities to maintain a healthy lifestyle or access medical care. A study in the United Kingdom that assessed the minimum income for healthy living reported that (despite the difficulties in calculations) those earning minimum wages would have greater difficulties than others in maintaining a healthy lifestyle.[64]

The income differences and the distribution of poverty in society are manifestations of equity and social justice or the lack thereof. Equity and social justice denote fairness. Equity has been conceptualized as the absence of socially unjust or unfair health disparities.[65] An operational definition remains elusive because of the different contexts in which equity can be explained, such as via social, political, or cultural spheres. A definition of equity in health has been proposed that alludes to the absence of disparities in health and its determinants, which are systematically associated with social advantage or disadvantage. The definition suggests an "equal opportunity to be healthy for all population groups."[66] In most circumstances these opportunities are not always present.

The WHO Commission on Social Determinants of Health stated, "Inequities in health, avoidable health inequalities, arise because of the circumstances in which people grow, live, work, and age, and the systems put in place to deal with illness. The conditions in which people live and die are, in turn, shaped by political, social, and economic forces."[67] The commission advises the WHO, governments, organizations, and civil society to act on the social determinants of health to achieve health equity.[k]

Notably, the terminology addressing differences in a population's health or health services is not uniform. In the United States the terms *inequalities* or *inequities* are seldom used; instead, the term *disparities* is preferred. Disparities can be considered as a chain of events manifested by "differences in environment, access to, utilization of, and quality of care, health status or a particular health outcome that needs scrutiny." [68] The Institute of Medicine (IOM) describes disparities as "racial or ethnic differences in the quality of health care that are not due to access-related factors or clinical needs, preferences and appropriateness of intervention."[69] Healthy People 2010 defines disparities as "the differences that occur by gender, race or ethnicity, education or income, disability and geographical location."[23] The first two definitions include health care, but the third does not.

Although health diversity between population groups is expected because of different biological or environmental characteristics, it is the underlying social injustice of these differences and the access to health care that are of concern. An example of these disparities is the incidence of infectious diseases, such as cysticercosis, leptospirosis, and Chagas disease, among the poor populations in the Mississippi Delta and other deprived areas in the South that are unheard of in other US regions.[70]

With regards to maternal and child health, a review of health indicators revealed that among US women aged 18–45 years, 75% (and 65% of pregnant women) eat less than the recommended five servings of fruit and vegetables per day, 14% reported poor mental health, 47% were overweight, 39% were frequent drinkers, 16% did not have health insurance, 30% did not have a dental visit in the past year, and 61% had low or very low social capital. These indicators are lower among women of color and of low socioeconomic status.[71] A 10-year stroke risk among 45 year olds was shown to be higher in blacks than whites in the United States,[72] and a decrease in diabetes mortality from 1989 to 2005 favored those with higher education and whites, widening the diabetes mortality gap with regard to education and race or ethnic group.[73]

Culture and Acculturation

The United Nations Educational, Scientific and Cultural Organization (UNESCO) Universal Declaration on Cultural Diversity of 2001, which was approved by 190 member states, defines culture as "the set of distinctive spiritual, material, intellectual and emotional features of society or a social group. It encompasses in addition to art and literature, lifestyles, ways of living together, value systems, traditions and beliefs."[74] These features are the ones that shape how people behave in general and, more specifically, in relation to health. They influence peoples' understanding of their environment and how they act in and manage their daily lives, including family formation, rearing children, lifestyles, health practices, ill-health manifestations, coping with disease, and healthcare-seeking behavior.

Because cultural characteristics are not static and people move from place to place, adaptations to the new contexts and locations occur, especially with regards to health. The process of acculturation, or cultural modification of an individual, group, or people by adapting to or borrowing traits from another culture or a merging of cultures as a result of prolonged contact, has been shown to influence health status and behaviors and the use of healthcare services.[l]

---

[k]The commission defines three principles of action: (1) improve daily living conditions; (2) tackle the inequitable distribution of power, money, and resources; and (3) measure and understand the problem and assess the impact of action.

[l]Acculturation is measured by the time a person lives in a country other than his or her own, the language used inside or outside the home, the proportion of friends from one's own culture, or pride in ethnic identity when among others.

Acculturation has been found to affect drinking or alcohol dependence in the Unites States among Hispanic adolescents[75] and Hispanics aged 18 years and older but not among all Hispanic nationalities.[76] Levels of physical inactivity were shown to be higher among immigrant Hispanic children in the United States than among natives, but the differences decreased with acculturation.[77] Higher acculturation was shown to be associated with depression during pregnancy among Latina women.[78] Among Vietnamese families in the United States, children whose parents used authoritarian parenting styles, as in Vietnam, showed higher rates of low self-esteem and depression than others.[79] Spanish-speaking Hispanics reported worse health status and access to health care and receiving less preventive care than English-speaking Hispanics.[80] However, higher levels of acculturation had a positive effect on the use of screening tests by Latina women in New York.[81] Practices such as female genital mutilation, which are prevalent in some African countries, are continued after moving to industrialized countries,[82,83] mostly among those with less integration into the local culture.[84]

Physical Environment

Poor water quality, sanitation, waste disposal, and hygienic conditions, as well as indoor pollution (due to combustion from biomass fuels and coal used for cooking and heating), outdoor air pollution (due to traffic and industrial activity), and chemical hazards (such as lead in paint, mercury in fish, smoking, and pesticides) all affect the health of individuals and cause premature mortality.[85] According to the WHO, environmental risk factors cause 85 of the 102 major diseases and injuries, and about 24% of the total global burden of disease and 23% of all deaths can be attributed to environmental exposure. The impact of environmental risks is higher for children than adults, due to their physical and behavioral characteristics and special vulnerability, contributing to 34% of the disease burden and 36% of overall mortality among 0 to 14 year olds.[86] The diseases that are considered to have the largest environmental contribution are diarrhea, respiratory infections, and injuries.

Health Care

The health care of a community includes functions of promotion, prevention, early diagnosis, treatment, and rehabilitation. These functions can mostly be provided at the first level of care.[m] Secondary and tertiary levels of care are mostly in-

dividual and disease oriented. The distinctions among the levels of care become obscured when specialists, such as internists, pediatricians, or obstetricians, provide primary care or when highly specialized professionals, such as cardiologists or neurologists, care for the chronically ill. Moreover, hospitals occasionally take responsibility for the health of communities and extend their services outside the hospital walls.

The IOM defines primary care as "the provision of integrated, accessible health care services by clinicians who are accountable for addressing a large majority of personal health care needs, developing a sustained partnership with patients, and practicing in the context of family and community."[87] At a meeting of experts in 2002, the WHO defined primary care as "a span or an assembly of first-contact health care services directly accessible to the public."[88]

Starfield regards primary care as the foundation of a healthcare system and defines it as the point of entrance to the system. It is characterized by provision of care to a defined population; delivering long-term, person-focused, and comprehensive services to assure continuity of care and coordination with other services; and being accessible.[89,90]

Primary health care was defined at the 1978 WHO meeting in Alma-Ata[19] as "the essential health care made universally accessible to individuals and families in the community by means acceptable to them, through their full participation and at a cost that the community and country can afford. It forms an integral part both of the country's health system of which it is the nucleus and of the overall social and economic development of the community."

Within the various definitions of primary care, some common elements can be identified—first contact, practiced in the context of family and community; accessibility; coordination; continuity; accountability; and comprehensiveness. Although there are common characteristics between primary care and primary health care (accessibility, family and community centered), the main distinction and emphasis for the latter is a holistic view of health and community participation and its relation to social and economic development of the community.

Following the conference on primary health care at Alma-Ata, primary care or primary health care did not have the repercussions or the development that were expected. Fragmentation of services and inequity continue to be a reality in most countries, and in some cases, primary care is considered to be a service that provides poor care to poor people.[91] Hospitals and hospital care consume most of the resources of a healthcare system, mostly because of the increasing development and cost of medical technologies and the cost of pharmaceutical products and administration. Primary health care receives the least amount of resources, but it is where most of the problems present and are solved.

---

[m]This first level of care is denominated primary care. Secondary care is provided by community hospitals or by specialists in community clinics, and tertiary care is provided in hospitals that have highly specialized care and diagnostic technologies (oncology, neurosurgery, trauma, burn unit, plastic surgery, etc.).

The renewal of primary care was first proclaimed in the American Region of the WHO in 2007 by the Pan American Health Organization (PAHO).[92] This renewal was further promoted when primary health care was highlighted as the central theme of the 2008 World Health Report.[93] The report proposed four types of reforms: (1) universal coverage, which will foster equity in health and social justice; (2) services that will be reorganized to answer the needs and expectations of the population; (3) healthy public policies that will integrate public health and primary care; and (4) leadership that will be more participative and will pursue the involvement of the relevant stakeholders in health care.

Societal Level

At this level, policies and politics influence community health and may collide with communities' priorities; populations movements, including migration and urbanization, an increasing phenomenon by which people look for better life opportunities, have an influence in their own health and that of the absorbing community; demographic changes in developed, transitional and developing countries also imply an epidemiological transition, changing the burden of disease in different populations

Policies and Politics

Health promotion and prevention activities can be determined by government policies. Politics have an impact on health policies and affect the continuum of health and disease. For example, policies related to the use of guns, smoking in public places, the use of drugs and needle exchanges, sexuality, reproductive health, and family formation might be determined by the ideological background or philosophical approach of those who are in charge or in positions of power. These factors may also influence the allocation of resources to certain organizations or programs, as well as the regulation of institutions and the availability of medicines and services. Areas of research, and their financing, that will affect the individual's and community's health might be influenced by the same factors.

In the beginning of the 21st century, the government of South Africa, a country with a severe AIDS epidemic that affected nearly 20% of the adult population in 2005, maintained that the disease was not caused by the human immunodeficiency virus (HIV), and consequently antiretroviral (ARV) drugs were of no use. It was maintained that poverty, bad nourishment, and general ill health were the causes of the disease. From 2000 to 2005, this caused an estimated loss of 330,000 lives, and 35,000 babies were born with HIV because of a lack of mother-to-child transmission prophylaxis.[94] Since then the situation has improved, and also the government has changed, but the major impact of the government policies is irreversible.

The consideration of health and health care as either a right or a commodity will shape the coverage and affordability of care for community members, as well as the set of health-related regulations and recommendations that are decided at local or national levels or by an insurance agency or healthcare organization. Considering health to be a human right means that there is a need to respect (assure that no policy, program, or action will violate that right and that healthcare services will be equitable), protect (regulate the healthcare industry, including the private sector, pharmaceutical companies, and national and multinational enterprises), and fulfill that right (put into practice health and health-related policies to assure human rights promotion and protection, with special focus on vulnerable populations).[95]

The increasing influence of multinational companies and supranational funds are also shaping the health agenda of governments, but in the words of Garret, "most funds come with strings attached and must be spent according to donors' priorities, politics, and values."[96] In other words, they do not always consider the local needs and priorities.

The influence of politics on health was acknowledged by Virchow, a German cellular pathologist born in 1821. In addition to being a pioneer in his field, he expanded his activities to public health. Studying an epidemic of typhus in Silesia, he concluded that the epidemic was essentially a social and political phenomenon associated with famine due to crop failure that affected the poor and uneducated. The elimination of social inequality would therefore be associated with the prevention of the condition. He asserted that "medicine is a social science, and politics nothing but medicine at a larger scale."[97]

Population Movements

Population movements, such as migration and urbanization, are increasing across the globe. Migration, whether within or among countries, affects physical and mental health and has an impact on the environment. Furthermore, internal displacement due to war or natural disasters affects the social and economic fabric of a community, the family structure, and individuals' physical and mental health. The migration of rural community members looking for better opportunities in the city is another increasingly common phenomenon.

In 2005, 49% of the world population (3.15 billion individuals) lived in cities, compared to 29% of the population in the mid-20th century. The United Nations predicts that by 2030, 60% of the global population (4.91 billion individuals) will live in urban areas. Also in 2005, the proportion of urban dwellers in developed regions of the world accounted for 74% of the population; in less-developed regions, urban dwellers accounted for 43% of the population. New York–Newark was third among the 20 megacities in the world, after Tokyo and Mexico City, with 18.7 million inhabitants.[98]

The mostly unplanned movement of the population causes the sprawling of settlements around cities, which do not have the appropriate infrastructure, such as water, sewage systems, appropriate healthcare facilities, and other services. Crowded and insufficient housing facilitates the spread of communicable diseases, increased injuries, violence, and poor health habits.[99,100] Also, the physical and mental health of educated migrants is affected, especially if their employment circumstances do not match their education and skills.[101]

Demographic Transition

In developed countries, decreasing or stable death rates are coupled with decreasing fertility and birth rates.[102] In some of these countries, like Spain, the mortality rate (10/1000 population) is equal to the birth rate. In 2008, Russia, a country in transition, experienced an increasing mortality rate (16/1000 population) that was higher than the birth rate in the same year (11/1000 population). These trends are associated with an aging population[n] and the consequent increase in the burden of chronic diseases. Most developing countries present high birth rates (for example, 38/1000 in Kenya and 26/1000 in El Salvador) and low mortality rates (10/1000 in Kenya and 6/1000 in El Salvador); these countries, in epidemiological transition, are enduring a double burden of disease which combines communicable and noncommunicable conditions.[103]

The WHO's 2008 report on the burden of disease shows that the top 10 causes of death worldwide include four noncommunicable diseases (ischemic heart disease; cerebrovascular disease; chronic obstructive pulmonary disease [COPD]; and trachea, bronchus, and lung cancers).[104] These four conditions rank among the top five causes of death in high-income and middle-income countries. In low-income countries,[o] two of these conditions share those rankings, but the rest are lower respiratory infections (first), diarrheal diseases (third), and HIV/AIDS (fourth). The leading disease burden as measured by disability-adjusted life years (DALYs) for low-income countries is lower respiratory infections, and ischemic heart disease ranks ninth. Unipolar depression disorders, followed by ischemic heart disease, are the leading disease burdens in middle- and high-income countries. Although these rankings attest to global changes, they are also reflected at the community level. Healthcare service organizations need to have the workforce, expertise, and resources to care for a changing population and a changing pattern in disease burden.

Global Level

At this level, climate change creates environmental changes, and consequently affects health directly or indirectly; globalization, which is blurring borders not only economically but health-wise as well; communications and the new information technologies that are transforming health interventions and personal contacts.

Climate Change

Climate changes are associated with some of the basic elements to sustain life—food, air, and water. Climate changes are occurring across the globe, most likely because of human activity. The use of fossil fuel and changes in land use and agriculture (mainly through deforestation) have increased the emission of CO_2 methane and nitrous oxide.[105] These greenhouse gases remain in the atmosphere for extensive periods of time and help trap heat near the Earth's surface. Different scenarios project that for the next two decades, there will be a warming of 0.2°C per decade, which is twice as large as the previous century.[105]

Food security is threatened by climate change, especially in the least developed regions of the world. Air quality is expected to change, with consequential effects in lung diseases, such as asthma. Floods and the contamination of water are associated with infectious diseases. Climate change has been associated with vector- and rodentborne and other infectious diseases, as well as water- and foodborne diseases.[106,107]

Changing patterns of rainfall and temperature bring draught, storms, heat and cold waves, the raising of sea levels, floods, and melting of snow and ice, and they have an affect on physical and mental health. The heat wave that affected Europe in 2003 was associated with excess mortality of approximately 60% in France,[108] 40% in Portugal,[109] and 17% in England and Wales.[110,111] The health systems in those countries were ill prepared for such an event. International organizations have suggested adaptation and mitigation strategies to deal with global warming.[p,105,107,112]

Globalization

Globalization[q,113] influences all spheres of life. Although globalization is not a new phenomenon, its impact is becoming more apparent and recognized, especially with respect to

---

[n]An increase in the number and proportion of elderly persons in the population.
[o]Low-income countries include the categories of low income (US$825 or less), low-middle income (US$826–3255), upper-middle income (US$3256–10,065), and high income (US$10,066 or more), according to 2004 gross national income (GNI) per capita.

[p]Adaptation has been defined as "adjustment in natural or human systems in response to climate changes, which can be initiated either by individuals or organizations in the population (autonomous), or implemented by governments (planned)." Mitigation is "an intervention aimed at reducing the severity of climate change by controlling emissions of greenhouse gases and/or enhancing carbon sinks."
[q]Globalization is the development of an increasingly integrated global economy marked especially by free trade, free flow of capital, and the tapping of cheaper foreign labor markets.

health, and it compounds the conceptualization of community health. Globalization influences the transference of risks, for example, tobacco and illicit drugs and the spread of new diseases and epidemics throughout the world, such as AIDS, severe acute respiratory syndrome (SARS), and swine flu. Multidrug-resistant and extensively-drug-resistant tuberculosis is a threat for the control of the disease in some countries.[114] Travel and migration have the potential for spreading this condition.

Globalization has also been implicated in the obesity epidemic through the diffusion of mass media networks that propagate and promote the use of consumer products, food, and beverage brands that have a powerful influence on eating behaviors across different countries and cultures.[115,116] The financial crisis affecting the Organisation for Economic Co-operation and Development (OECD) countries at the end of the first decade of the 21st century had repercussions on developing countries and countries in transition. Economic recession[r] has implications for the physical and mental health of populations, especially vulnerable people, both on a country and global level. Health care is also impacted by financial crises, and during these times an adjustment of the provision of healthcare services is needed, although governments do not always prioritize healthcare budgets. The WHO suggests that crises can stimulate healthcare services reform, emphasizing primary health care with the aim of universal coverage, and address the social and economic determinants of health.[117]

Communications

Communications, whether at the individual or community level, have an influence on health. The first contact that an individual may have regarding a health problem or a health behavior might be with family members. Communication with physicians or nurses through face-to-face contacts or group discussions may influence compliance with treatment, following advice, or acquiring skills for self-management of a disease.

At the community level, communication takes a different form. The use of mass media and information technologies are shaping health and health care. Mass media has been shown to influence body image, sexual behaviors, violence, and substance abuse among teenagers.[118] The obesity epidemic is linked to TV advertisement.[119] New technologies like text messaging are being used for health interventions on varied topics, such as sexual health,[120] smoking cessation,[121] and diabetes management.[122] The new technologies appear to have promising results.[123]

According to Internet World Stats,[124] in 2008 the Internet was being used by increasing numbers of people across the globe. The use of the Internet ranges from 73.1% in North America to 5.6% in Africa. The use of the Internet for health purposes in seven European countries who participated in the WHO/European eHealth Consumer Trends Survey was 52.2% in 2007.[125,126] Most Internet users reportedly used it for health information (52%) and whether to see a doctor (46%).[127]

The widespread use of the Internet for health and healthcare purposes has led to a new term: eHealth. A review of the literature revealed 51 different definitions of the term.[128] The varied definitions had some common themes; although all of them included the word *health*, it was most commonly used for healthcare services delivery or their outcomes in terms of efficiency, suggesting that the term is more commonly used for service than for health status.

The wide use of the media and new information technologies for health matters has raised some questions regarding the accuracy and understanding of the information obtained. Issues of media literacy[129] and media health literacy[s,130] are of concern.

There is also the potential for a digital divide to occur. This can be intergenerational because youngsters may be more savvy in the new technologies than their parents and educators. Most importantly this divide might be due to unequal access to the new forms of health and medical information, which may increase disparities among community and population groups.

COMMUNITY HEALTHCARE PRACTICE

Community health care is population based and deals with the natural history of a disease, from its origins to its manifestation to its outcome. It integrates preventive and health promotion activities in conjunction with the care of the sick and their rehabilitation. The two main approaches of delivering community health care are community-oriented primary care and community-oriented public health.

Community-Oriented Primary Care

Community-oriented primary care (COPC) was defined by Kark in 1983 as "a way of practicing medicine and nursing, or of providing primary care, which is focused on care of the individual who is well or sick, or at risk for illness or disease, while also focusing on promoting the health of the community as a whole or any of its subgroups."[131] COPC is based on the following principles: (1) responsibility for a defined population;

---

[r]An economic recession is two successive quarters of negative growth in gross domestic product.

[s]Media literacy is the critical understanding of the nature and techniques of mass media and its impact. Media health literacy is the ability to identify, recognize, and analyze health-related content in the media and its influence on health behavior.

(2) care based on identified health needs; (3) prioritization; (4) intervention covering the natural history of a disease, involving prevention, promotion, treatment, and rehabilitation; and (5) community involvement. COPC is presented in Chapters 3 and 4.

Community-Oriented Public Health

Community-oriented public health (COPH) blends population health principles in the context of the community's health. It deals with the identification and analysis of health and its determinants in a specific community or communities, followed by different interventions that are needed to promote and maintain this state of health. Usually, COPH programs are the domain of public health authorities, health maintenance organizations, or other community institutions that act either together or in their own spheres of action. COPH is presented in Chapter 5.

MEASUREMENT OF COMMUNITY HEALTH

Although health is a positive attribute, its measurement often encompasses morbidity and mortality. Additionally, health is expressed by measures of health behaviors and well-being.

Health Indicators

Health indicators are measurements that reflect a community's state of health. Indicators such as infant mortality and maternal mortality reflect not only the health status of a specific group, but also of the total population. Health indicators draw attention to overall socioeconomic conditions and the community's quality of and access to medical care.

Health indicators have been used to measure targets that a country or region strives to achieve, such as targets for Healthy People 2010[23] or the Millennium Development Goals.[22] For example, Healthy People 2010 was set up to measure changes in immunization coverage (the proportion of children aged 19–35 months who received all recommended vaccines, the proportion of noninstitutionalized adults aged 65 years and older who received an influenza vaccine in the past 12 months, and the proportion of those adults who ever received a pneumococcal vaccine). The Millennium target number four on reducing child mortality was set up to reduce by two-thirds, between 1990 and 2015, the under-five, and infant mortality rates, and also the proportion of children aged 12–23 months who received at least one dose of measles vaccine. These health indicators are the benchmarks by which it is possible to monitor a program's progress in attaining its targets and achieving its target deadlines.

Health indicators are also the way in which the health status of communities and populations or their subgroups are compared with one another, and they are used for international comparisons. For example, the infant mortality (IM) rate in Washington, DC for the years 2003 to 2005 was 12.2/1000 live births, the highest in the country and nearly two times the average infant mortality rate in the United States (6.83/1000 live births).[132] The rates for African Americans were 15.83/1000 live births in Washington, DC (3.5 times higher than for whites) and 13.33/1000 live births in the United States (2.3 times higher than for whites). The US IM rate ranks 29th in the world (Singapore is the lowest with an IM of 2/1000 live births).[133] The IM rate target specified by Healthy People 2010 was 4.5/1000 live births by 2010.[23]

The expressions of these community health measurements require a clear definition of the community. This will provide the numerical value for the denominator information for the measurement of rates. The numerator is provided by the number of cases of the specific health issue being measured.

GATHERING INFORMATION ABOUT COMMUNITY HEALTH

As summarized in Table 1-1, the measurement of a community's state of health requires some questions to be answered by those who request the measurements and those who will gather or use the information.

More and more communities are taking center stage in defining their needs and aspirations regarding health, education, the environment, and general development. However, there are those who are dispossessed and communities whose members lack the basic elements to sustain a dignified life, such as education, food, shelter, and health. As one of the basic rights of individuals, health evolves beyond individuals and individual rights to encompass the community and its rights.

SUMMARY

Community health may be considered the collective expression of the health of individuals and groups within a community, which is affected by personal, familial, and community characteristics and societal and global influences. Equity and social justice are values inherent to community health and health care. Community health care is provided by different levels of the healthcare system, mostly primary health care, which is the level where most problems can be resolved. Community health can be measured and expressed through health indicators.

TABLE 1-1 Questions Regarding the Measurement of Community Health

Which community is being studied?	The identification of the population or community under study is essential for the definition and calculation of denominators and numerators. The population can vary in size and level of organization, from members enlisted in a certain health or medical practices to a neighborhood, county, state, or a country as a whole. The population can further be defined according to age groups throughout the life course, such as infants and children, adolescents, or the elderly, or the definition can be gender specific. Additionally, the population can be defined by ethnic or racial groups, or it can address the health of migrants.
What information needs to be gathered?	The information to be gathered needs to be carefully determined. Because health and disease issues and their determinants may be extremely variable in different populations and involve varied types of problems, following a process of consultation and prioritization regarding the information to be collected is critical. A general survey of the health status of a certain community might be considered, but it needs to be done in accordance with the specific place and based on knowledge of the community. Gathering information about issues that are not relevant for the specific place consumes usually scarce resources, and the information may not be pertinent to later analysis.
Are methods and instruments appropriate for the community?	When designing the data collection methods, consideration should be given not only to a sound methodology, but also to the appropriateness of the instruments in terms of language (which language is spoken by the community and which local words are used for different ailments), literacy level, and sensitivity to social norms and cultural issues. The community's clear understanding of what is asked and why, as well as respect for its social and cultural values, are essential for building trust and fostering future cooperation and partnership.
Is there available information, or does new data need to be collected?	Efforts should be made to identify available sources of information regarding the specific community. Local or national agencies, such as departments of health, national centers for health statistics, universities, and non-governmental organizations, may gather information that could be suitable for the needs of a specific community. The appropriateness of this information should be analyzed regarding timeliness (when the data was collected), whether it is targeted (it covers the population of interest), whether the definitions used are the ones that are relevant for the community, and whether pertinent determinants are included.
Are data valid and reliable?	The validity (to what extent it measures what it intended to measure) and reliability (to what extent the information is reproducible) of the data should be analyzed when using already collected information and when planning a study of the community.
For what purpose is this information gathered?	Data are collected for various purposes. They might be collected to identify the needs of a community or of populations that are at risk or in need of special care. Perhaps the data were collected as a baseline for program implementation and evaluation or to assess whether national targets (like Healthy People 2010) or global targets (like Millennium Development Goals) were achieved. Identifying needs and special populations in need of care is a community diagnosis. Similar to individual medical care, it is imperative that the diagnosis be followed by an appropriate intervention that supports promotion of health and addresses the treatment or rehabilitation needs of the community.
Who are the stakeholders?	The stakeholders involved in data gathering might be the community itself or its representatives, community organizations, government organizations, or academic institutions. Issues of partnership, ownership, and the uses of the information have to be clarified and agreed upon from the planning phase.
What are the available resources?	Resources—financial, personnel, infrastructure, and time—have to be carefully planned and organized beforehand so tasks can be completed on time.
Were ethical considerations taken into account?	The gathering of personal and private information is secured by ethical considerations. Informed consent is required for the disclosure of information by institutions, the linkage of records, or the provision of personal information. Informed consent covers topics such as a description of the survey content, what will be done with the information, the right to refuse to participate without jeopardizing medical care, and the right to receive referral information. Internal and external review boards are institutions that examine these issues and provide approval or reject applications for data gathering.

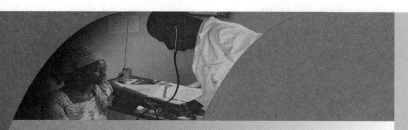

Discussion Questions

- Why is it important to define a community in the framework of community health and community health care?

- Can there be a universal definition of health? Why?

- Are all determinants relevant in different communities in different places?

- Are there universal determinants of community health? What are they?

- Can there be a universal definition of community health? Why?

- Which health determinants did you identify in the case study in Box 1-1?

Review Questions

- How is community defined for the purpose of assessing the community's health and health care?

- What is health?

- What is community health?

- What are the levels of determinants of community health?

- What are community health indicators?

- What are the questions to be asked when measuring community health?

REFERENCES

1. US Census Bureau. Current population survey (CPS)—definitions and explanations. http://www.census.gov/population/www/cps/cpsdef.html. Accessed February 2009.

2. American Academy of Family Physicians. Family, definition of. http://www.aafp.org/online/en/home/policy/policies/f/familydefinitionof.html. Accessed January 2010.

3. Holland J, Mauthner M, Sharpe S. *Family Matters: Communicating Health Messages in the Family*. London, England: Health Education Authority Family Health Research Reports; 1996.

4. Christensen P. The health-promoting family: a conceptual framework for future research. *Soc Sci & Med*. 2004;59:377–388.

5. Etzioni A. Communitarianism. In: Christensen K, Levinson D, eds. *Encyclopedia of Community: From the Village to the Virtual World*. Vol. 1. Thousand Oaks, CA: Sage Publications; 2003:224–228.

6. Brown P. Who is the community? What is the community? http://www.researchethics.org/uploads/pdf/Phil.commun.ss.pdf. Accessed March 5, 2009.

7. Hillemeier MM, Lynch J, Harper S, Casper M. Measuring contextual characteristics for community health. *Health Serv Res*. 2003;38(6, pt 2):1645–1717.

8. MacQueen KM, McLellan E, Metzger DS, et al. What is community? An evidence-based definition for participatory public health. *Am J Public Health*. 2001;91:1929–1938.

9. Geographic Information Systems (GIS) at CDC. http://www.gis.com/. Accessed January 2010.

10. Internet World Stats. Internet usage statistics. http://www.internetworldstats.com/stats.htm. Accessed January 2008.

11. Jadad AR, Enkin MW, Glouberman S, Groff P, Stern A. Are virtual communities good for our health? *Br Med J*. 2006;22:925–926.

12. Walsh TM, Volsko TA. Readability assessment of Internet-based consumer health intervention. *Respir Care*. 2008;53:1310–1315.

13. Ybarra ML, Mitchell KJ, Wolak J, Finkelhor D. Examining characteristics and associated distress related to Internet harassment: findings from the second Youth Internet Safety Survey. *Pediatrics*. 2006;118:e1169–e1177.

14. Juvonen J, Gross EF. Extending the school grounds? Bullying experiences in cyberspace. *J School Health*. 2008;78:496–505.

15. World Health Organization. WHO definition of health. http://www.who.int/about/definition/en/print.html. Accessed February 2009.

16. Illich I. *Limits to Medicine: Medical Nemesis, the Expropriation of Health*. New ed. London, England: Boyars; 1976.

17. Lalonde M. A new perspective on the health of Canadians. http://www.hc-sc.gc.ca/hcs-sss/alt_formats/hpb-dgps/pdf/pubs/1974-lalonde/lalonde-eng.pdf. Published April 1974. Accessed January 2009.

18. Pinder L, Rootman I. A prelude to health for all. *World Health Forum*. 1998:235–238.

19. International Conference on Primary Health Care. Declaration of Alma-Ata. http://www.who.int/hpr/NPH/docs/declaration_almaata.pdf. Published September 1978. Accessed January 2009.

20. World Health Organization. Health 21. Health for all in the 21st century. http://www.euro.who.int/document/EHFA5-E.pdf. Accessed January 2009.

21. World Health Organization. The Ottawa charter for health promotion. http://www.who.int/healthpromotion/conferences/previous/ottawa/en/. Accessed January 2009.

22. United Nations Millennium Development Goals. http://www.un.org/millenniumgoals/. Accessed January 2009.

23. US Department of Health and Human Services. Healthy People 2010. http://www.healthypeople.gov/About/goals.htm. Accessed January 2009.

24. Barker DJP. Fetal origins of coronary heart diseases. *Br Med J*. 1995;311:171–174.

25. Medical Research Council. National Survey of Health and Development: NSHD. http://www.nshd.mrc.ac.uk/. Accessed February 2009.

26. Cesaroni G, Forastierre F, Perucci CA. Are cesarean deliveries more likely for poorly educated parents? A brief report from Italy. *Birth*. 2008;35:241–244.

27. Guillory VJ, Cai J, Hoff GL. Secular trends in excess fetal and infant mortality using perinatal periods of risk analysis. *J Natl Med Assoc*. 2008;100:1450–1456.

28. Hjern A, Thorngren-Jerneck K. Perinatal complications and socio-economic differences in cerebral palsy in Sweden—a national cohort study. *BMC Pediatr*. 2008;8:49.

29. Gofin R, Adler B, Palti H. Time trends of child development in a Jerusalem community. *Paediatr Perinat Epidemiol*. 1996;10:197–206.

30. Aloise-Young PA, Cruickshank C, Chavez EL. Cigarette smoking and perceived health in school dropouts: a comparison of Mexican American and non-Hispanic white adolescents. *J Pediatr Psychol*. 2002;27:497–507.

31. Murphy M, Bobak M, Nicholson A, Rose R, Marmot M. The widening gap in mortality by educational level in the Russian Federation, 1980–2001. *Am J Public Health*. 2006;96:1293–1299.

32. Macfarlane GJ, Norrie G, Atherton K, Power C, Jones GT. The influence of socio-economic status on the reporting of regional and widespread musculoskeletal pain: results from the 1958 British cohort study. *Ann Rheum Dis*. 2009;68:1591–1595.

33. Ramsay SE, Whincup PH, Morris L, Lennon L, Wannamethee SG. Is socioeconomic position related to the prevalence of metabolic syndrome? Influence of social class across the life-course in a population-based study of older men. *Diabetes Care*. 2008;31:2380–2382.

34. Wilkins R, Tjepkema M, Mustard C, Choiniere R. The Canadian census mortality follow-up study, 1991 through 2001. *Health Rep*. 2008;19:25–43.

35. Weires M, Bermejo JL, Sundquist K, Sundquist J, Hemminki K. Socio-economic status and overall and cause-specific mortality in Sweden. *BMC Public Health*. 2008;8:340.

36. Rachet B, Woods LM, Mitry E, et al. Cancer survival in England and Wales at the end of the 20th century. *Br J Cancer*. 2008;99(suppl 1):S2–S10.

37. Clarke P, O'Malley PM, Johnston LD, Schulenvberg JE. Social disparities in BMI trajectories across adulthood by gender, race/ethnicity and life-time socio-economic position: 1986–2004. *Int J Epidemiol*. 2009;38:499–509.

38. US Department of Energy Office of Science, Office of Biological and Environmental Research, Human Genome Program. Human Genome Project information. http://www.ornl.gov/sci/techresources/Human_Genome/home.shtml. Accessed February 2009.

39. Khoury MJ, Berg A, Coates R, Evans J, Teutsch SM, Bradley LA. The evidence dilemma in genomic medicine. *Health Affairs*. 2008;27:1600–1611.

40. Hudson KL, Holohan MK, Collins FS. Keeping pace with the times—the genetic information nondiscriminatory act of 2008. *N Engl J Med*. 2008;358:2661–2663.

41. Hudson K. The health benefits of genomics: out with the old, in with the new. *Health Affairs*. 2008;27:1612–1615.

42. Woodcock J. The human genome and translational research: how much evidence is enough? *Health Affairs*. 2008;27:1616–1618.

43. Westfall JM, Mold J, Fagnan L. Practice-based research—"Blue Highways" on the NIH roadmap. *JAMA*. 2007;297:403–406.

44. Taubert KA, Clarck NG, Smith RA. Patient-centered prevention strategies for cardio-vascular disease, cancer and diabetes. *Nat Clin Pract Cardiovasc Med*. 2007;4:656–666.

45. Renehan AG, Howell A. Preventing cancer, cardiovascular disease, and diabetes. *Lancet*. 2005;365:1449–1451.

46. Beaglehole R, Magnus P. The search for new risk factors for coronary heart disease: occupational therapy for epidemiologists? *Int J Epidemiol*. 2002;31:1117–1122.

47. Ford ES, Bergmann MM, Kroger J, Schienkiewitz A, Weikert C, Boeing H. Healthy living is the best revenge: findings from the European Prospective Investigation into cancer and nutrition. Postdam study. *Arch Int Med*. 2009;10:1355–1362.

48. Kelley SS, Borawski EA, Flocke SA, Keen KJ. The role of sequential and concurrent sexual relationships in the risk of sexually transmitted diseases among adolescents. *J Adolesc Health*. 2003;32:296–305.

49. Lara-Torre E. Update in adolescent contraception. *Obstet Gynecol Clin North Am*. 2009;36:119–128.

50. Framingham Heart Study. History of the Framingham Heart Study. http://www.framinghamheartstudy.org/about/history.html. Accessed February 2009.

51. Agency for Healthcare Research and Quality. US Preventive Services Task Force. http://www.ahrq.gov/clinic/uspstfix.htm. Accessed February 2009.

52. Owen CG, Whincup PH, Kaye SJ, et al. Does initial breastfeeding lead to lower blood cholesterol in adult life? A quantitative review of the evidence. *Am J Clin Nutr*. 2008;88:305–314.

53. Triche EW, Hossain N. Environmental factors implicated in the causation of adverse pregnancy outcome. *Semin Perinatol*. 2007;31:240–242.

54. Kawachi I, Berkman L. Social cohesion, social capital and health. In: Berkman LF, Kawachi I, eds. *Social Epidemiology*. New York, NY: Oxford University Press; 2000:174–190.

55. Sapag JC, Aracena M, Villaroel L, et al. Social capital and self-rated health in urban low income neighborhoods in Chile. *J Epidemiol Comm Health*. 2008;62:790–792.

56. Islam MK, Merlo J, Kawachi I, Lindstrom M, Burstrom K, Gerdtham UG. Does it really matter where you live? A panel data multilevel analysis of Swedish municipality-level social capital on individual health-related quality of life. *Health Econ Policy Law*. 2006;1(pt 3):209–235.

57. Fujiwara T, Kawachi I. A prospective study of individual-level capital and major depression in the United States. *J Epidemiol Comm Health*. 2008; 62:627–633.

58. Stafford M, De Silva M, Stansfeld S, Marmot M. Neighborhood social capital and common mental disorder: testing the link in a general population sample. *Health Place*. 2008;14:394–405.

59. Scheffler RM, Brown TT. Social capital, economics, and health: new evidence. *Health Econ Policy Law*. 2008;3:321–331.

60. Putnam RD. *Bowling Along. The Collapse and Revival of American Community*. New York, NY: Shimon and Schuster; 2000.

61. Rundle A, Field S, Park Y, Freeman L, Weiss CC, Neckerman K. Personal and neighborhood socioeconomic status and indices of neighborhood walk-ability predict body mass index in New York City. *Soc Sci & Med*. 2008;67:1951–1958.

62. Chen S, Ravallion M. The developing world is poorer than we thought, but no less successful in the fight against poverty. http://siteresources.worldbank.org/JAPANINJAPANESEEXT/Resources/515497-1201490097949/080827._The_Developing_World_is_Poorer_than_we_Thought.pdf. World Bank Development Research Group Policy Research Working Paper 4703. Published August 2008. Accessed January 2010.

63. DeNavas-Walt C, Proctor BD, Smith JC. Income, poverty, and health insurance coverage in the United States: 2007. http://www.census.gov/prod/2008pubs/p60-235.pdf. US Census Bureau Current Population Reports, P60-235. Published August 2008. Accessed February 2009.

64. Morris JN, Donkin AJM, Wonderling D, Wilkinson P, Dowler EA. A minimum income for healthy living. *J Epidemiol Comm Health*. 2000;54: 885–889.

65. Whitehead M. The concepts and principles of equity in health. *Int J Health Serv*. 1992;22:429–445.

66. Braveman P, Gruskin S. Defining equity in health. *J Epidemiol Comm Health*. 2003;57:254–258.

67. Commission on Social Determinants of Health. *Closing the Gap in a Generation: Health Equity Through Action on the Social Determinants of Health*. Geneva, Switzerland: World Health Organization; 2008. http://www.who.int/social_determinants/thecommission/finalreport/en/index.html. Accessed February 2009.

68. Carter-Pokras O, Baquet C. What is a "health disparity?" Public Health Reports 2002;117:426-434.

69. Smedley BD, Stith AY, Nelson AR, Institute of Medicine Committee on Understanding and Eliminating Racial and Ethnic Disparities in Health Care. *Unequal Treatment: Confronting Racial and Ethnic Disparities in Health Care*. Washington, DC: National Academies Press; 2002.

70. Hotez PJ. Neglected infections of poverty in the United States of America. *PLoS Negl Trop Dis*. 2008;2(e256):1–11.

71. Ebrahim S, Anderson JE, Correa-de-Araujo R, Posner SF, Atrash HJ. Overcoming social and health inequalities among US women of reproductive age—challenges to the nation's health in the 21st century. *Health Policy*. 2009; 90:196–205.

72. Cushman M, Cantrell RA, McClure LA, et al. Estimated 10-year stroke risk by region and race in the United States: geographic and racial differences in stroke risk. *Ann Neurol*. 2008;64:483–484.

73. Miech RA, Kim J, McConnell C, Hamman RF. A growing disparity in diabetes-related mortality US trends, 1989–2005. *Am J Prev Med*. 2009;36: 126–132.

74. United Nations Educational, Scientific and Cultural Organization. Universal declaration on cultural diversity. http://www.unesco.org/most/lnlaw37.htm. Published November 2001. Accessed February 2009.

75. Wahl AM, Eitle TM. Gender, acculturation and alcohol use among Latina/o adolescents: a multi ethnic comparison [published online ahead of print September 2008]. *J Immigr Minor Health*.

76. Caetano R, Ramisetty-Mikler S, Rodriguez LA. The Hispanic Americans Baseline Alcohol Survey (HABLAS): the association between birthplace, acculturation and alcohol abuse and dependence across Hispanic national groups. *Drug Alcohol Depend*. 2009;99:215–221.

77. Singh GK, Yu SM, Sihapush M, Kogan MD. High levels of physical inactivity and sedentary behaviors among US immigrant children and adolescents. *Arch Pediatr Adolesc Med*. 2008;162:756–763.

78. Davila M, McFall SL, Cheng D. Acculturation and depressive symptoms among pregnant and postpartum Latinas. *Maternal Child Health J*. 2009;13:318–325.

79. Nguyen PV. Perception of Vietnamese father's acculturation levels, parenting styles, and mental health outcomes in Vietnamese American adolescents. *Soc Work*. 2008;53:337–346.

80. DuBard CA, Gizlice Z. Language spoken and difference in health status, access to care, and receipt of preventive services among US Hispanics. *Am J Public Health*. 2008;98:2021–2028.

81. Sussner KM, Thompson HS, Valdimarsdottir HB, Redd WH, Jandorf L. Acculturation and familiarity with, attitudes toward and beliefs about genetic testing for cancer risk within Latinas in East Harlem, New York City. *J Genet Couns*. 2009;18:60–71.

82. American Academy of Pediatrics, Committee on Bioethics. Female genital mutilation. *Pediatrics*. 1998;102:153–156.

83. Kangoum AA, Flodin U, Hammar M, Sydsjo G. Prevalence of female genital mutilation among African women residents in the Swedish county of Ostergötland. *Acta Obstet Gynecol Scand*. 2004;83:187–190.

84. Elgaali M, Strevens H, Mardh PA. Female genital mutilation—an exported medical hazard. *Eur J Contr Repr Health Care*. 2005;10:93–97.

85. World Health Organization. *The World Health Report 2002: Reducing Risks, Promoting Healthy Life*. Geneva, Switzerland: World Health Organization; 2002.

86. Prüss-Üstüm A, Corvalán C. How much disease burden can be prevented by environmental interventions? *Epidemiology*. 2007;18:167–168.

87. Donaldson M, Yordy K, Vanselow N, eds. *Defining Primary Care: An Interim Report*. Washington, DC: Institute of Medicine, National Academies Press; 1994.

88. World Health Organization. Meeting on primary care, family medicine/general practice. Definition and links to other levels of care. Barcelona, Spain, 1–2 November 2002. http://www.euro.who.int/InformationSources/MtgSums/2002/20030506_1. Accessed February 2009.

89. Lee TH, Bodenheimer T, Goroll AH, Starfield B, Treadway K. Perspective roundtable: redesigning primary care [video]. *N Engl J Med*. http://www.nejm.org/perspective/primary-care-video/. Accessed February 2009.

90. Starfield B. Refocusing the system. *N Engl J Med*. 2008;359:2087–2091.

91. Chan M. Commentary. Return to Alma Ata. *Lancet*. 2008;372;865–866.

92. World Health Organization, Pan American Health Organization. *Renewing Primary Health Care in the Americas*. Washington, DC: Pan American Health Organization; 2007.

93. World Health Organization. *The World Health Report 2008. Primary Health Care Now More Than Ever.* Geneva, Switzerland: World Health Organization; 2008.

94. Chigwedere P, Seage GR III, Gruskin S, Lee TH. Estimating the lost benefits of antiretroviral drug use in South Africa. *J Acquir Immune Defic Syndr.* 2008;49:410–415.

95. Tarantola D, Byrnes A, Johnson M, Kemp L, Zwi A, Gruskin S. Human rights, health and development. University of New South Wales Initiative for Health and Human Rights. Technical series paper #08.1. Published 2008. http://www.ihhr.unsw.edu.au/images/Publications/2008_IHHR_Technical_Series_Paper_08v1.pdf. Accessed January 2010.

96. Garrett L. The challenge of global health. *Foreign Affairs.* 2007;86:14–38.

97. Mackenbach JP. Politics is nothing but medicine at a large scale: reflections on public health's biggest idea. J Epidemiol Community Health 2009:63:181-184.

98. United Nations Department of Economic and Social Affairs. World urbanization prospects: the 2005 revision. Data tables 1, 4, and 7. http://www.un.org/esa/population/publications/WUP2005/2005wup.htm. Accessed February 2009.

99. World Health Organization. Housing and health. http://www.euro.who.int/Housing. Accessed February 2009.

100. Centers for Disease Control and Prevention. Healthy homes. http://www.cdc.gov/healthyplaces/newhealthyhomes.htm. Accessed February 2009.

101. Dean JA, Wilson K. "Education? It is irrelevant to my job now. It makes me very depressed . . ." exploring the health impacts of under/unemployment among highly skilled recent immigrants in Canada. *Ethnic Health.* 2009;14:185–204.

102. US Census Bureau. International data base. http://www.census.gov/ipc/www/idb/summaries.html. Accessed February 2009.

103. Tollman SM, Kahn K, Sartorius B, Collinson MA, Clark SJ, Garenne ML. Implications of mortality transition for primary health care in rural South Africa: a population-based surveillance study. *Lancet.* 2008;372:893–901.

104. World Health Organization. *The Global Burden of Disease: 2004 Update.* Geneva, Switzerland: World Health Organization; 2008. http://www.who.int/healthinfo/global_burden_disease/GBD_report_2004update_full.pdf. Accessed February 2009

105. Intergovernmental Panel on Climate Change. Summary for policymakers. In: Solomon S, Qin D, Manning M, et al., eds. *Climate Change 2007: The Physical Science Basis. Contribution of Working Group I to the Fourth Assessment Report of the Intergovernmental Panel on Climate Change.* Cambridge, United Kingdom and New York, NY: Cambridge University Press; 2007. http://www.ipcc.ch/pdf/assessment-report/ar4/wg1/ar4-wg1-spm.pdf. Accessed February 2009.

106. Haines A, Kovats RS, Campbell-Lendrum D, Corvalán C. Climate change and human health: impacts, vulnerability and mitigation. *Lancet.* 2006;367:2101–2109.

107. World Health Organization. Sixty-first World Health Assembly. Climate change and health. . WHA61.19. Published May 24, 2008. http://www.who.int/globalchange/A61_R19_en.pdf. Accessed January 2010.

108. Institut de Veille Sanitaire. Impact sanitaire de la vague de chaleur en France survenue en août 2003. http://www.invs.sante.fr/publications/2003/chaleur_aout_2003/rap_chaleur_290803.pdf. Published August 29, 2003. Accessed February 2009.

109. Botelho J, Caterino J, Calado R, Nogueira PJ, Paixao JM. Onda de calor de Agosto 2003: os seus efeitos sobre a mortalidade da população portuguesa. http://www.onsa.pt/conteu/onda_2003_relatorio.pdf. Published April 2004. Accessed February 2009.

110. London Climate Change Partnership. Adapting to climate change. Lessons for London. Greater London Authority, London. http://www.sfrpc.org/data/ClimateChange/9.pdf. Published July 2006. Accessed February 2009.

111. Johnson H, Kovats RS, McGregor,G et al. The impact of the 2003 heat wave on mortality and hospital admissions in England. *Health Stat Q.* 2005;25:6–11.

112. High level conference on world food security: the challenges of climate change and bioenergy. Rome. June 3–5. Climate change adaptation and mitigation: challenges and opportunities for food security. http://www.fao.org/fileadmin/user_upload/foodclimate/HLCdocs/declaration-E.pdf.Accessed January 2010.

113. Merriam-Webster Online. http://www.merriam-webster.com. Accessed February 2009.

114. Wright A, Zignol M, Van Deun A, et al. Epidemiology of antituberculosis drug resistance 2002–07: an updated analysis of the Global Project on Anti-Tuberculosis Drug Resistance Surveillance. *Lancet.* 2009;373:1861–1873.

115. Labonte R, Schrecker T. Globalization and social determinants of health: introduction and methodological background. *Global Health.* 2007;3:5–14.

116. Bornstein SR, Ehrhart-Bornstein M, Wong ML, Licinio J. Is the worldwide epidemic of obesity a communicable future of globalization? *Exp Clin Endocrinol Diabetes.* 2008;116(suppl 1):S30–S32.

117. World Health Organization. The financial crisis and global health. Report of a high-level consultation. http://www.who.int/mediacentre/events/meetings/2009_financial_crisis_report_en_pdf. Published January 19, 2009. Accessed February 2009.

118. Strasburger VC. Why do adolescent health researchers ignore the impact of media? Commentary. *J Adolesc Health.* 2009;44:203–205.

119. Blass EM, Anderson DR, Kirkorian HL, et al. On the road to obesity: television viewing increases intake of high density foods. *Physiol Behav.* 2006;88:597–604.

120. Levine D, McCright J, Dobkin L, Woodruff AJ, Klausner JD. SEXINFO: a sexual health text messaging service for San Francisco youth. *Am J Public Health.* 2008;98:393–395.

121. Whittaker R, Maddison R, McRobbie H, Bullen C. A multimedia mobile phone-based youth smoking cessation intervention: findings from content development and piloting studies. *J Med Internet Res.* 2008;10:e49.

122. Franklin VL, Greene A, Waller A, Greene SA, Pagliari C. Patients' engagement with "Sweet Talk"—a text messaging support system for young people with diabetes. *J Med Internet Res.* 2008;10:e20.

123. Krishna S, Boren SA, Balas FA. Health care via cell phones: a systematic review. *Telemed J E Health.* 2009;15:231–240.

124. Internet World Stats. Internet usage statistics: the Internet big picture. http://www.internetworldstats.com/stats.htm. February 2009.

125. Norwegian Centre for Telemedicine. WHO/European eHealth Consumer Trends Survey. http://www.telemed.no/index.php?id=275869. Accessed February 2009.

126. Kummervold PE, Chronaki CE, Lausen B, et al. eHealth trends in Europe 2005–2007: a population-based survey. *J Med Internet Res.* 2008;10:e42.

127. Andreassen HK, Bujnowska-Fedak MM, Chronaki CE, et al. European citizens' use of E-health services: a study of seven countries. *BMC Public Health.* 2007;7:53. http://www.biomedcentral.com/1471-2458/7/53. Accessed February 2009.

128. Hans OH, Rizo C, Enking M, Jadad A. What is eHealth (3): a systematic review of published definitions. *J Med Internet Res.* 2005;7:e1.

129. Hobbs R. Literacy for the information age. In: Flood J, Heath SB, Lapp D, International Reading Association, eds. *Handbook of Research on Teaching Literacy Through the Communicative and Visual Arts.* New York, NY: Macmillan Library Reference; 1997:7–14.

130. Levin-Zamir D. *Development and Measurement of the Concept of Media Health Literacy and Its Association with Empowerment and Health Behavior Among Israeli Adolescents* [PhD thesis]. Jerusalem, Israel: Hebrew University of Jerusalem; 2007.

131. Kark SL, Kark E. An alternative strategy in community health care: community-oriented primary health care. *Isr J Med Sci.*1983;19:707–713.

132. Mathews TJ, Marian F, MacDorman MF. Infant mortality statistics from the 2005 period. Linked birth/infant death data set. *Natl Vital Stat Report.* 2008;57(20):1–32.

133. UNICEF. The state of the world's children 2009. http://www.unicef.org/sowc09/. Accessed February 2009.

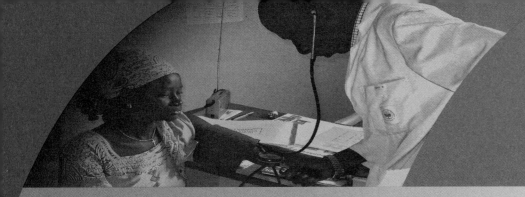

CHAPTER 2

Community Health Interventions: Planning and Methods

KEY TERMS

behavioral change models
community health
  interventions
community intervention
  settings

community involvement
evaluation
needs assessment
planning community
  interventions

Box 2-1 Case study

In the mid-1980s in Israel, studies on children younger than 15 years old and on newborns in their first ride home showed a very low use of car seats. Among those who used them, most used them incorrectly.

New information was emerging from the literature on the effectiveness of car seats on preventing serious injuries and death, the characteristics of appropriate car restraints for different age groups, and the enactment of laws for the use of car restraints. As a result of these facts, a working group for child protection and health matters was created, led by a member of an academic institution in partnership with representatives of the Ministry of Transport and nongovernmental organizations (NGOs). The working group conducted educational activities throughout the country regarding the importance of car seats and their proper use. The target audience included parents, medical students, and healthcare professionals.

In parallel, advocacy activities were carried out, which included writing position papers, increasing car seat accessibility, the establishment of car seat loan schemes, and approaching members of Parliament to draft a law for the use of car seats for children, which was eventually passed.

With the passing of years, standards were adopted, the quality of car seats improved, and the use of car seats increased. Education of parents became routine in the mother and child health clinics, which, as studies showed, were needed to advise parents on the proper use of the restraints. Programs were also developed for the use of car restraints for children with physical handicaps and special needs.

INTRODUCTION

Community health interventions deal with the health–illness continuum through organized and systematic actions directed to maintain, promote, or restore health in a defined community. Interventions should also address health determinants within this continuum, considering their diverse nature, the varied strength of their association with health status, and the complex web of interaction and causation. This might be expressed by the need of different types of interventions according to the context and realities of the specific community and the setting in which they will be developed. Addressing health determinants, not only the health condition, have the potential to diminish inequities and inequalities within the community if there is a differential impact of the intervention for those who need it most.

In this chapter we will address the different types of interventions, the diverse settings in which community health interventions are developed, and the practical steps to develop community health interventions.

TYPES OF COMMUNITY HEALTH INTERVENTIONS

Community health interventions include prevention of diseases and promotion of the community's health; early diagnosis of conditions through screening and further analysis of those at higher risk; treatment with medicines and procedures; reha-

bilitation to restore function; and palliative care for life support and pain relief. Any of these interventions can be carried out at the community level, although treatment, rehabilitation, and palliative care are often directed at the individual level and take place in healthcare settings. The integration of these latter interventions (usually the focus of clinical individual care) with prevention and promotion (usually the focus of public health) is seldom carried out because separate healthcare institutions or organizations are responsible for these different healthcare activities. The integration of clinical care and public health takes place with the community-oriented primary care (COPC) approach, which is the subject of Chapters 3 and 4.

Prevention

Immunizations are a classic example of disease prevention. They are considered among the most effective public health interventions and biomedical achievements.[1,2] Immunizations have made the global elimination of smallpox and the control of polio possible. This has been achieved by suitable immunization coverage of the population.

Although the coverage of immunizations might be high in industrialized countries, other countries are starkly in contrast. As an example, the coverage of measles immunization in 2007 was 93% in the United States, similar to other developed countries, while coverage was 69% in Western and

Central Africa.[3] These percentages represent averages for the countries, but at the community level, lower coverage can be expected, with notable differences between rural and urban areas or among communities with low and high socioeconomic status and where barriers to access of healthcare services exist.[4] Lower coverage results in the emergence of epidemics as herd immunity decreases.[a,5]

Another method of prevention is through the early diagnosis of a condition, such as identifying problems in hearing or vision, testing for anemia, or using mammography to screen for breast cancer and identify it in its early stages. Although early detection does not prevent disease, if followed by treatment it may alter the progression of the condition and avoid deleterious outcomes.

The effectiveness of early diagnosis for given conditions has been analyzed by the US Preventive Services Task Force[6] and the Canadian Task Force on Preventive Health Care.[7] Both have analyzed the evidence of effectiveness and produced recommendations for the performance of screening tests. For example, there are recommendations for cervical cancer screening in women who have been sexually active and for neural tube defects and Rh incompatibility among others. Both task forces provide recommendations as to which procedures or tests should not be performed. Examples of the latter are testing for prostate-specific antigen in men older than 75 years of age for prostatic cancer; testing for syphilis and gonorrhea infection in men and women who are at low risk for infection; screening of asymptomatic adolescents for idiopathic scoliosis; susceptibility gene testing for women whose family history is not associated with an increased risk for deleterious mutations in breast cancer susceptibility gene 1 (BRCA1) or breast cancer susceptibility gene 2 (BRCA2). There are also conditions for which the evidence is not yet available to support or reject the performance of early diagnosis, such as glaucoma in adults or speech and language delay in children younger than 5 years of age. The Cochrane Library,[8] which presents systematic reviews of treatments and procedures, also provides a wide variety of information on screening tests.

Health Promotion

The concept of health promotion has existed for a long time, but it received a strong boost through several meetings held by the World Health Organization (WHO). The Ottawa Charter defines health promotion as "the process of enabling people to increase control over, and to improve their health."[9]

Health promotion may be applied through varied frameworks, such as organizational (policy development and reorientation of healthcare services), contextual (creating supportive environments for health and strengthening community action for health), and individual issues (developing personal skills). Thus, health promotion activities may encompass enacting laws for health protection or injury prevention, such as laws requiring helmet use, advocacy and actions for the creation of separate bicycle paths on urban roads, or interventions through education to increase skills for proper road behavior and use of helmets.

THE SETTINGS FOR COMMUNITY HEALTH INTERVENTIONS

Community health interventions are implemented in a variety of settings. According to the Merriam-Webster dictionary, *setting* is the time, place, and circumstances in which something develops.[10] The WHO Health Promotion glossary defines *setting* as "the place or social context in which people engage in daily activities in which environmental, organizational and personal factors interact to affect health and wellbeing."[9] For the purpose of community health interventions, we will refer to a setting as the site or space where an intervention takes place. This site can be extended to diverse locations depending on the program that is developed and the degree of cooperation among the different organizations that take part in the program.

The setting location and its identification by the community as the place where the intervention is taking place is important because this may contribute to attendance. The setting may attract members of the community who feel closeness in terms of cultural and social characteristics, or, for the same reasons, they may not identify with it. The location may also be important for accessibility. In the case of a healthcare setting, accessibility (whether location, economic, cultural, or other type) must be assured to facilitate the participation of community members who are to benefit from the program.

Types of Settings

The smallest settings for interventions are family units. Family is the social unit where many health promotion activities take place.[11] Institutions and organizations—such as schools, community centers, churches, synagogues, mosques, factories, or other places where the community or its subgroups (adolescents, elderly) gather, study, work, or spend leisure time—are larger settings where prevention and promotion activities can occur. Health clinics are the settings where diagnosis, treatment, and rehabilitation are carried out, but they may also

---

[a]Herd immunity is a group's resistance to a disease that a large proportion of the group members are immune to because of immunization.

incorporate prevention and promotion interventions. Environments where social interactions take place, such as laundromats, have been found to be effective settings for health promotion in selected populations.[12]

Entire communities can be the setting where interventions take place. The development of Safe Communities by the WHO is such an example. The concept, proposed in 1989 during the First World Conference of Accident and Injury Prevention in Sweden, included the formulation of public policy for safety, the creation of supportive environments and strengthening community action for injury prevention, and the incorporation of all services and institutions to strengthen injury prevention. Although Safe Communities have been initiated in many countries, there is insufficient evidence to show the effectiveness of this intervention model.[13] Healthy Communities are another development (following the Ottawa Charter) that address health and health determinants at the community or city level.[14]

With the advancements and widespread use of information technology (IT), the traditional location or setting of the intervention might be challenged. Cyberspace has become another major setting, and the Internet is the channel through which health interventions can be delivered. Using IT as a vehicle for health interventions redefines the meaning of setting. IT interventions can be delivered to heterogeneous and geographically widespread audiences who have a common interest or cause. The target of interventions can be cancer survivors, smokers, drinkers, or pregnant or postpartum women who live in various cities, states, or countries. The target population may also belong to a defined community setting, such as school children who, for example, could receive their intervention through their cellular phones or other electronic devices.[15]

Notably, settings may vary for a specific intervention and could include a combination of settings according to the purpose and type of health intervention or available community resources.

THE ROLE OF THE COMMUNITY IN COMMUNITY HEALTH INTERVENTIONS

In preparation for a community health intervention, it is necessary to contemplate the involvement that the community will have in the development and implementation of the intervention. Community members' involvement may vary from being merely a recipient of the program and participating in the activities to being a full partner in the different stages of the program. This will depend on the community's degree of organization, leadership, and resources, as well as on the focus and goals of the intervention.

Partnership with the community requires having a common vision and goals, joint planning and implementation, and shared accountability. The healthcare team should have an understanding of the community's culture and its capabilities, and mutual respect and trust must exist. To initiate a dialogue for partnership, the community's leadership, organization, and assets need to be identified. The definition of roles and expectations at the outset of the program may facilitate the engagement of stakeholders and their continuous participation and partnership.

There are approaches that involve the community in interventions and related research. One of those approaches is community-based participatory research (CBPR).[b,16] Few evaluations have been conducted of the CBPR approach, and results are not conclusive regarding the outcomes of intervention programs or the degree of participation in all phases of the research or program.[17–20]

For a comprehensive discussion of community participation, see Chapter 6.

THE PROCESS OF COMMUNITY HEALTH INTERVENTIONS

The process of conducting community health interventions requires various steps: (1) conducting an assessment of the community's health status, its determinants, and the resources available, including a process of prioritizing the health conditions that need to be dealt with among all competing problems; (2) selecting an effective and adequate intervention; (3) planning the intervention and its implementation in the community; and (4) evaluating the intervention to assess the process of the program and its effect on the community health status. To effectively address the needs of a community, it is desirable to follow these steps. Knowing what the community health problems are, and deciding on the appropriate programs will aim to improve the community's health status. A bottom–up approach that originates in the community and involves healthcare services, other organizations, and community members who collaborate in the decision-making process about their health may better tailor the program to the needs and priorities of the community.

---

[b]One of the definitions of this approach asserts that CBPR is a "collaborative approach to research that equitably involves all partners in the research process and recognizes the unique strengths that each brings. CBPR begins with a research topic of importance to the community [and] has the aim of combining knowledge with action and achieving social change to improve health outcomes and eliminate health disparities."

Occasionally, decision makers at different levels in the hierarchy of an institution, organization, or government decide on interventions without addressing the specific needs of communities. Although this top–down approach may have some impact on the health status of a certain community, it may not address its actual priorities. Vertical programs address diseases instead of people, support fragmentation of services, often duplicate services, and usually compete for limited resources.

Health Assessment

Healthcare professionals encounter many and varied health problems that affect the whole community or some of its subgroups. Information about these problems and their determinants is needed for planning the intervention. A health assessment analyzes the health status of the population to inform the process of community health interventions. This assessment will identify the community's health needs and will be used as a baseline for evaluation of the intervention program. The health assessment can be based on information already stored in the community, or it may involve the collection of new information, or it may utilize a combination of both.

Gathering Available Data

Gathering available data includes published data such as vital statistics and specific health indicators, available surveys on specific health conditions or behaviors, or other relevant information. Sources may be national health surveys, which might offer the opportunity for comparison with other regions, national figures, or specific studies that were carried out in the community. Hospital discharge data or other clinical data might provide hints of what main health issues require medical care. This, however, only provides information about those who received the service, not about those who were sick but did not seek services because of economic constraints, lack of knowledge, or other reasons.

The use of available health or medical information is based on various existing sources.[c] To utilize these sources, their quality must be examined (uniformity of definitions, standardized methods of data collection, completeness, etc.). Data might have been collected for administrative purposes, and thus their suitability for the specific community has to be scrutinized. Additionally, data might be outdated, not cover the area of interest, or provide only numerator information (number of cases without reference to the population). Moreover, data may not provide information about the determinants of the health situation or identify populations at risk.

Primary Data Collection

When available data does not provide enough information on the community health status and its determinants, it is necessary to gather new information. Two different approaches may be taken: comprehensive health needs assessment or selective health needs assessment.

Comprehensive Health Needs Assessment A comprehensive health needs assessment is used when there is no previous information on the overall health status of the community. This approach consists of a survey or series of surveys that address the multiple aspects of the health of the community. The survey content may include, among other topics, sociodemographic data (age, sex, education, race or ethnicity, and occupation) and questions to assess the prevalence of physical and mental health conditions (cardiovascular disease, anemia, injuries, and depression). It may also include subjects such as health behaviors, cultural practices and lifestyles (smoking and drinking, performance of physical activity), risk factors, social networks, and the support and use of healthcare services. Other topics include somatic and psychological characteristics of the community (cholesterol, child development quotients) and functional capacity and disabilities (activities of daily living, types of disabilities, proportion of bedbound and housebound individuals). Additionally, test results (lipid profiles, ECG), anthropometric measurements (weight and height distribution and body mass index, blood pressure distribution), and detailed nutrition information (24-hour recall, frequency of food consumption) may be included. Information can be gathered for a specific age group, or life course information for men and women (from family formation to aging) can be gathered.

This list of health issues and determinants can be expanded depending on the purpose of collecting the information. However, special consideration must be given to the use of the gathered information and the best use of available resources. The justification of such an extensive health assessment has to be considered by weighing the relevance of the information against the resources and time available for collection and analysis.

The information might be gathered for additional purposes, such as academic use. This has its importance and contributes to generating knowledge on health issues at the time of data collection or studying long-term processes if the data is going to be used as a cohort for future studies. The contribution to science is valuable, but it might not be feasible for the

---

[c]See Appendix 2-1 for a list of potential sources of data from national organizations and federal departments in the United States.

specific community. Ethical considerations, such as consent from participants and confidentiality of the information, need to be ensured.

The information provided by a comprehensive needs assessment can be mapped. When there is information on the participants' addresses, geographic information system (GIS)[21] software can be used to identify the spatial locations of populations where poor health behaviors or health conditions are more prevalent.[22] This is useful to determine priority areas or populations for community health interventions.

In addition, the opinions and perceptions of the community's stakeholders need to be gathered. Healthcare professionals can offer their knowledge, experience, and insights on the health problems they see in their practices, and community members can express their perceived needs and offer insights on the determinants of their health state, as well as their opinions of the healthcare services.

These different sources of data will provide basic information about and quantification of the health problems. Healthcare professionals, as well as the community, may need to decide how to best allocate the usually scarce resources to address these problems. When this is the case, a prioritization process is called for. This process offers healthcare professionals and community members an opportunity to decide on the most compelling health problems that need a systematic intervention.

For a detailed description of the prioritization process, see Chapter 4.

Selective Health Needs Assessment A selective health needs assessment follows the choice of a health problem (or related health problems) after existing data was examined and a prioritization process was followed. As a consequence there is a detailed assessment of the selected condition or a community diagnosis of the selected condition. A selective assessment is more feasible than a comprehensive one, and it makes efficient use of resources.

Because this assessment will be the baseline for the intervention program, the following steps need to be taken:

Reviewing the Literature The literature review will provide knowledge of the state of the art regarding the selected health problem and its measurement at the population level. It will also provide information about best practices regarding intervention. Because the information gathered at this stage will guide the intervention and will serve as the baseline for the evaluation, the literature review will focus on the nature and content of the health assessment. It can also provide useful information on instruments and methodologies to be used.

Formulating Objectives Formulating the objectives specifies the relevant issues that the health assessment will address. This may include the prevalence and severity of the disease; the environmental, behavioral, or biological determinants associated with it; the consequences of this health status; and the use of services. For example, the objectives for the health assessment of a program that will address preterm births in a specific population may include the following:

- study the incidence of preterm births
- determine the factors associated with preterm births—sociodemographic characteristics, obstetric history, social and family support, family violence, and availability of health insurance
- determine maternal and offspring outcomes—postpartum physical and mental conditions, health status of the newborn

Selecting the Target Population In the previous example, because the study will be based on pregnancy outcomes, the target population is clear (pregnant women and women of reproductive age). Yet it may be further segmented, for example, according to specific ethnic or racial groups or a specific age group. If prevention and control of hypertension is the selected issue, the target population could be all adults aged 25 to 64 years in the community. Or, if the program is geared toward the elderly, the target population would be adults aged 65 years and older (or another relevant age limit used in the community).

In addition to defining the target population, a decision needs to be made as to whether information will be collected from all community members. This is seldom feasible because the population is often large. In that case, a sample needs to be selected. A sampling frame (from which the population for the assessment will be selected) and sampling methods need to be chosen. The use of computer programs facilitates the calculation of the sample size.[23]

Defining Variables For a common understanding of the health problem, an operational definition is needed. For example, if the program is about prevention of preterm births, the definition would be babies born at less than 37 weeks of gestation. If the outcome variable is overweight adults, the definition would be a body mass index (BMI)[d] between 25 and 29.9, and obesity is present with a BMI of 30 or greater. For children, overweight is defined as a BMI from the 85th percentile to less than the 95th percentile, and obesity is defined as a BMI equal to or greater than the 95th percentile for children of the same

---

[d]BMI is a reliable indicator of body fat. It is calculated as weight $\div$ height^2.

age and sex. If the outcome variable is a health behavior or family violence, the literature will provide scales and other instruments for their measurement.

Selecting Data Collection Methods The methods of gathering information can be qualitative, quantitative, or a combination of both. Qualitative methods, which are summarized in Table 2-1, are used to get an in-depth knowledge of the determinants of health status and provide the perceptions, attitudes, feelings, and insights of the population regarding the problem under study, the use of healthcare services or traditional healers, and barriers and facilitators for change. They also generate ideas for the development of questions or instruments to be used in gathering quantitative information, as well as the appropriate wording for the questions. Qualitative methods can also be used after a quantitative study to explain its findings. Qualitative methods require a systematic collection of information and sound analysis. When more than one qualitative method is used, triangulation, the use of more than one approach, is needed to corroborate common conclusions.

Quantitative methods are used to determine the frequency of conditions and how they are distributed across variables and determinants of interest. They also provide information on associations between determinants and an outcome or a set of outcomes. This type of information identifies groups at an increased risk of a certain outcome, as well as inequalities or disparities in health conditions or in the use of healthcare services. It can also provide the baseline to evaluate changes after the implementation of the intervention. Several quantitative methods for collecting information are summarized in Table 2-2.

Planning the Analysis The plan of analysis should be prepared beforehand and follow the objectives of the health assessment. It may also include additional analyses when issues of interest to the community or healthcare professionals arise. Thus, in addition to the primary analysis guided by the study objectives, there will be a secondary analysis of the information. Careful consideration should be given to whether the sample size or methods of data collection were adequate for that secondary analysis.

Planning Community Health Intervention Programs

Intervention programs are an organized and integrated set of activities and services that are carried out in a predetermined sequence. They are aimed at preventing diseases or promoting health or to treatment and rehabilitation of community members experiencing a disease or a set of diseases that were identified during the assessment process. The different steps involved in planning and performing the intervention are described in the following sections.

TABLE 2-1 Qualitative Methods

Focus groups	Focus groups involve knowledgeable people from the community who freely exchange their thoughts and discuss specific questions developed by the healthcare team. Participants might have common characteristics (high school students, pregnant adolescents) or include a variety of members in the community. The number of participants varies between 6 and 10, but sometimes there are more.
In-depth interviews	In-depth interviews can be made with community leaders, service providers, or selected community members to provide insights, opinions, and attitudes on health-related issues. The number of subjects recruited for in-depth interviews is more limited than for other qualitative methods.
Observations	Observations provide information on the gaps that might occur in reporting versus the actual activity. The researcher observes events in their natural setting, such as children's activities in playgrounds to determine safety behaviors or parent–child interactions to study verbal communications. Participant observation is the term used when the researcher is a participant to varying degrees in the actual event that is being observed.

TABLE 2-2 Quantitative Methods

Interviews	Interviews are based on questionnaires, which can be structured (the answers are predetermined in categories that are comprehensive and mutually exclusive) or semistructured (with a narrative provided by the participant for some of the questions). These questionnaires can be administered face to face in different settings, such as the household (household survey), a clinic, or any other location. They can also be administered via telephone. Consideration should be given to possible bias where there is an uneven distribution of landline telephones in the community. The increasing use of only cell phones by the younger generation, the absence of a directory that lists cell phone numbers, and the reluctance of people to participate in phone surveys poses increasing constraints to telephone interviewing, especially among the younger generation.[24–26]
Self-administered questionnaires	Self-administered questionnaires are filled out by the person participating in the survey. These questionnaires may be used when sensitive questions are asked or when privacy is needed for the answers. This method is often used when examining the health status and behaviors of school children or the lifestyles of adults. Additionally, questionnaires can be sent by mail to the persons involved. This method usually has a low response rate, even when preaddressed, postage-paid envelopes are provided. Self-administrated questionnaires can also be completed via the Internet, which appears to be a cost-effective alternative.[27,28] Although the wording of the questionnaire is important with any method, it is especially important in self-administered questionnaires. Unambiguous terms and an appropriate reading level have to be used to allow all participants to understand the questions. Equally important, questionnaires have to be culturally sensitive in terms of content, language, and terminology.
Records review	A records review is used to get information on morbidity patterns and use of services, such as clinic visits and their cause, emergency room attendance, hospital discharge diagnosis and length of stay, and causes of mortality. In addition, information on laboratory tests, ECGs, or other relevant information can also be extracted from clinical records. Consideration should be given to the quality of the information gathered (completeness, validity, and reliability), as well as to the ethical issues involved in accessing people's data.
Observations	Observations can also be used in quantitative methods; for example, observations of the use of child car seats or seat belts. This information, as opposed to a report by the parents, provides a more valid and reliable measure of the prevalence of car restraint use and whether the restraint is used correctly.[29,30]

Examining What Has Already Been Done in the Community

It is essential to identify different activities that have been done by healthcare services, health-related organizations, or the community itself regarding the selected health condition. The array of activities may have been done with no specific organization, systematization, or coordination. However, they can provide insights about what worked and what did not, and they may highlight the challenges and barriers for implementation. This information may be incorporated into the planning process to improve the program's organization and implementation.

Defining the Target Population for the Intervention

The health assessment may show that there are vulnerable groups with a greater need for intervention or that are at greater risk for the condition. For example, in the United States there might be a higher incidence of preterm births among Hispanic and African American women than among others;

certain schools in affluent neighborhoods may have experienced an increase in substance abuse and mental health problems, which include suicide attempts; and a section of the community may have a larger proportion of elderly people living alone. Careful consideration should be given to whether selecting a specific group within the community will do more harm than good, however. Selecting a specific subgroup of the population could unintentionally stigmatize that population.

Moreover, the selection of a high-risk approach versus a population approach should be balanced in terms of the expected achievements in the improvement of the community's health.[31] A high-risk approach will have a high impact on those who have the disease, but it will not have much of an effect on the health status of the entire community. Alternatively, a population approach, which will address both those who have the disease and those who are healthy but potentially at risk for the condition, will have an effect on the total community. For example, if the population approach is taken in anemia prevention among infants by promoting the proper foods and adequate iron supplements, the hemoglobin levels curve may shift to the right, more so than by treating only children who suffer from anemia. Both approaches have their advantages and disadvantages and should not compete with each other.

Formulating Goals and Objectives of the Intervention

The overall goal of a program must be determined. The goal provides a general expression of the outcomes the program ultimately intends to achieve. Goals are not always expressed in measurable terms. For example, a goal in a program for pregnant women would be to improve the outcomes of pregnancy; a goal in an injury prevention program could be to improve the safety of children or to develop a culture of safety in the community.

The importance of well-defined objectives cannot be underestimated. Objectives provide the framework for the program activities and are used as the benchmark to assess whether the targets were achieved. Objectives express what the intervention strives to achieve regarding the health problem. They have to be clearly stated and expressed in measurable terms. They should also state a time limit. For example, in a program to decrease corporal punishment of children as a disciplinary measure, the objectives (to be achieved in a stated period of years) may be as follows:

- decrease by X percent the number of parents that use corporal punishment as a disciplinary measure
- increase the knowledge of parents by X percent regarding the long-term effects of corporal punishment and alternative methods of disciplining children

For a program to promote breastfeeding, the objectives may include the following:

- increase the proportion of mothers who exclusively breastfeed at birth, 3 months, and 6 months by X percent in X years
- increase the duration of breastfeeding until 6 months of age by X percent in X years

Objectives have to be achievable in terms of the amount of change proposed within the defined time limit. The feasibility of achieving the goals is based on the information provided by the literature on similar interventions and on the knowledge of the community where the intervention will take place in conjunction with the available resources.

In addition to the objectives in the previous examples, which are related to change in behavior and knowledge, other types of objectives associated with the determinants need to be stated. In the case of the breastfeeding objectives, the determinants may relate to support from the father and other family members, the education level of the mother, and other sociodemographic variables. Objectives may also relate to organizational or contextual issues, such as maternity leave for new mothers or breastfeeding facilities for working mothers.

Examining the State of the Art for Effective Interventions

The scientific literature offers information about the implementation and success of programs, but the quality and comprehensiveness of the information varies. The program description might be presented but lack information about the program's effectiveness. Although it can provide ideas for program activities, the description may not be sufficient enough to know how the program performed.

When reviewing literature for evidence-based interventions, careful attention should be paid to the evaluation methodology. The most rigorous evidence is provided by a randomized controlled trial (RCT) in which two populations were randomly selected. Only one was exposed to the program; the other was not exposed and was used as a control. It is then possible to know whether the effect of the program was due to the intervention because the results were compared before and after the intervention in both populations. RCTs are not always performed; there might be a comparison only before and after the intervention, with no comparison to a nonexposed group. This can provide evidence of changes, but it lacks the certainty that the changes were due to the intervention itself or if the changes occurred because of other factors or activities that were acting in the community at the same time.

Selecting the Appropriate Intervention

The literature offers information about different types of community health interventions. These interventions need to be analyzed and selected based on evidence of effectiveness and appropriateness for the specific community. There are different sources of information, which includes the previously mentioned US Preventive Services Task Force,[6] the Canadian Task Force on Preventive Health Care,[7] and the Cochrane Library.[8] Interventions are analyzed in terms of the benefit to the population and whether they will do more good than harm. Cost is also considered but is not decisive in the recommendations.

The US Preventive Services Task Force[6] recommendations on health interventions are based on the degree of evidence discovered in their review of studies, which is based on strict methodological criteria. The best evidence is provided by randomized controlled trials; followed by well-designed, nonrandomized cohort or case-controlled studies and multiple time series with or without intervention; and lastly by opinions of respected professionals, descriptive studies, case studies, and reports from committees. The evidence is also weighed against the benefits, harm, and costs, and the net benefit is obtained by considering other interventions vis-à-vis allocating resources.

Other sources of information for good practices are provided in the literature, mainly in peer-reviewed journals. The use of Internet search engines is warranted, following keywords in accordance with the planned intervention. Utilizing Internet sites requires a meticulous appraisal to avoid interested parties' opinions, unsubstantiated conclusions, anecdotal evidence, or poorly conducted studies.

What Type of Intervention Is Needed?

Community intervention programs can follow different strategies, such as promoting behavior change, instituting policies and laws, bringing about changes in the environment, performing early diagnosis, and treating and rehabilitating conditions.

Behavioral Change Interventions Table 2-3 provides examples of behavioral change models that guide interventions.

Policies and Enactment of Laws Policy changes are the responsibility of healthcare institutions or governments at the national to local levels. Within a healthcare institution, policies can take the form of enrolling community members in screening programs. Other policies might assist in promoting the health of the wider community and protect individuals from the action of others.

For example, a smoke-free healthcare institution or banning smoking in flights protects not only the employees of the institution from secondhand smoke, but also others within the space (visitors and hospital patients or plane passengers), and it contributes to strengthening a general smoke-free environment.[41] At the national or local government levels, implementing policies that ban smoking in public places protects the general public from secondhand smoke. Health Act 2006 in the United Kingdom dealt with the prohibition of smoking in certain premises, places, and vehicles and amended the minimum age of persons to whom tobacco may be sold.[42] In Uruguay, a smoke-free policy instituted by the government and led by the president, an oncologist by profession, exemplified the increase in the social unacceptability of smoking, and in time there was a decrease in the resistance to the policy.[43] Another example is that the enactment of laws for highway speed limits[44] and the mandatory use of seat belts,[45] child car restraints,[46] and motorcycle helmets[47–49] have been effective in decreasing the incidence of injuries. Finally, policies to use water fluoridation have decreased the incidence of caries in populations.[50]

The enactment of policies, however, poses challenges. In the case of laws and regulations, when there is not strict enforcement, the effect may be limited. There is also a tension between personal freedom of choice and the enactment of laws. The actions of individuals can affect others (such as smoking or drunk driving), or individuals' actions can affect only themselves (such as poor eating habits and the use of motorcycle helmets), even when those actions might have a general impact on the community's health and use of resources. In some instances, this tension had led to laws being repealed; for example, the use of motorcycle helmets. In 2003, Pennsylvania's motorcycle helmet law was repealed. A comparison from 2001 to 2002 and 2004 to 2005 showed a decrease in helmet use from 82% to 58%, an increase in head injury mortality of 66%, and an increase of noninjury mortality of 25%. Hospitalizations increased dramatically.[51] Similarly, water fluoridation has stimulated debate between advocates and detractors.[52,53]

Environmental Changes Addressing environmental changes is another type of intervention to prevent diseases or to promote community health. For example, changes in product design, such as playground surfaces and childproofing medicine bottles, have been shown to reduce injuries and poisonings.[54] Another classic example is the Children Can't Fly program in New York, where window bars became mandatory after analyzing the causes of children's falls.[55] Creating bicycle lanes separate from car traffic is another type of environmental change to improve safety.

These examples of injury prevention led to the conceptualization of safety culture, an environment conducive to injury

TABLE 2-3 Behavioral Change Models and Theories

Health Belief Model[32]	This model was developed by Becker. It proposes that people behave in a certain way according to the individual's beliefs and perception regarding (1) how susceptible they are to the condition (for example, to heart disease, obesity, or being involved in a traffic crash, and whether this will or will not happen to them); (2) how serious the condition is (whether it may cause pain, discomfort, lost work days, disability, or death); (3) the benefits of taking an action, whether preventive or treatment (whether using a bicycle helmet or performing a screening test will avoid a condition or improve the chances of survival, or whether taking medication will improve the situation as weighed against the disadvantages of not following a certain action); and (4) what the costs will be (what expenses are involved and whether they are justified in light of the benefits of taking action).
Social Cognitive Theory[33,34]	This theory proposed by Bandura relates to the interaction among behavior, the environment, and personal factors. This interaction involves beliefs and cognitive competences that are influenced by social factors. A person's behavior and its consequences, and the observation of others' behavior and its consequences, influences the person's future behavior according to personal standards, self-reflection, and analysis. This translates into self-efficacy or the ability to translate a thought into the actual performance of an activity or task. The understanding of these processes makes it possible to identify interventions to change behavior.
Theory of Reasoned Action[35,36]	This theory, developed by Ajzen and Fishbein, proposes that behavior is determined by intentions that are influenced by personal and societal attitudes. These attitudes are formed by the belief that a behavior will have a determined outcome. It is the assessment of this outcome and the assessment of the opinions of relevant groups in society that will motivate a person to behave in a certain manner.
Transtheoretical Model[37–39]	This model, developed by Prochaska and Velicer, proposes six stages in behavioral change: (1) precontemplation—the stage in which there is lack of awareness that life can be improved by a change in behavior; (2) contemplation—there is recognition of the problem coupled with an initial consideration of behavior change and finding out about possible solutions and actions; (3) preparation—reaffirmation of the need and desire to change behavior and the completion of final preaction practices; (4) action—implementation of the practices needed for successful behavior change; (5) maintenance—consolidation of the behaviors initiated during the action stage; and (6) termination—the former problematic behaviors are no longer perceived as desirable.
Social Marketing[40]	Social marketing, as defined in 1971 by the originators of the concept, Kotler and Zaltman, "is the design, implementation, and control of programs calculated to influence the acceptability of social ideas and involving considerations of product planning, pricing, communication, distribution, and marketing research." The techniques of social marketing are considered by the authors to be "the bridging mechanisms between the simple possession of knowledge and the socially useful implementation of what knowledge allows." The approach is based on the *product* (the behavior promoted, such as healthy eating or safety practices; or the service, such as immunizations or a new clinic); *promotion* (the strategy that will make the product known and acceptable, such as advertising, public information, and publicity); *place* (an accessible channel to facilitate the action); and *price* (the social, psychological, time, energy, effort, or monetary cost that must be paid for the product, weighed against its benefit).

prevention and safety. Safety culture has been defined mostly in terms of the work environment, but it can be adapted to a community context. There is no agreement on a definition of safety culture, but one commonly used definition was developed by the UK Health and Safety Commission: "the product of individual and group values, attitudes, perceptions, competencies, and patterns of behavior that determine the commitment to, and the style and proficiency of, an organization's health and safety management."[56]

Another form of environmental change that is conducive to promoting the health of a community is the creation of walking trails in rural communities to promote physical activity.[57] They have been found to be effective, especially for women and those in low socioeconomic brackets who are at risk of physical inactivity. The construction of walking trails has been recommended, along with other strategies, by the CDC's Guide to Community Preventive Services: Promoting Physical Activity.[58] A cost–benefit analysis of physical activity using bike and walking trails in Nebraska showed that for every dollar invested in trails for physical activity, there was a $2.94 direct medical benefit (range $1.65 to $13.40).[59]

Early Diagnosis and Screening Although the previously discussed community intervention approaches are geared toward prevention and health promotion, early diagnosis directly addresses diseases. In the health–illness continuum and the natural history of a disease or health condition, early diagnosis detects the very early stages of a disease when treatment is potentially more effective and the outcome can be modified.

The WHO established criteria for screening that considers the condition, the characteristics of the screening test, the availability and effectiveness of treatment, the cost, and the organizational aspects.[e,60] Early screening is only the first step in the chain of events that leads to the diagnosis of a condition. That is why one of the criterion implies the need for referral and diagnosis and another calls for a clear definition of what constitutes a diagnosis of the condition. In addition, the issue of the reliability and validity of the test is also considered. The validity of the test indicates that there should be a decision on an acceptable proportion of cases that will not be identified (false negatives) or will be wrongly diagnosed (false positives).

The balance in the acceptability of false negatives or false positives will depend on the type of condition that is examined and whether it is acceptable to miss some cases or label a person with a condition the person does not have. The US Preventive Services Task Force[6] and the Canadian Task Force on Preventive Health Care[7] have analyzed screening tests for their validity and have provided recommendations for the performance (or not) of the screening tests.

Treatment and Rehabilitation Treatment and rehabilitation interventions are carried out in clinical settings. Beyond individual care, treatment and rehabilitation can be part of a community intervention program, such as a program for the control of cardiovascular risk factors (hypertension, hyperlipidemia, obesity), injuries, or child growth and development.

Single Approach or Combination of Approaches

Ultimately, a combination of approaches and partnerships among different stakeholders might be needed for an effective community intervention.[61] There are models that potentially encompass multiple approaches, such as the ecological model that the WHO adapted to address violence. The model considers the personal, family, peer, community, and societal factors that are associated with violence.[62] This kind of model can also be applied to other types of conditions because it can address the health determinants that could interact at different levels of complexity and organization.

Another example is the Haddon matrix, which was developed by William Haddon Jr. for traffic injuries but subsequently has been used for other types of injuries.[63–65] The matrix involves the classical factors in the epidemiological triangle (the human factor, the agent or vehicle, and the social and physical environment) as applied to the natural history of a crash (the preevent, the event, and the postevent). It addresses which actions need to be considered in each one of the resulting matrix's cells. For example, in the agent–preevent cell, one considers what needs to be done to modify the agent to prevent an injury (such as the design of playgrounds to prevent injuries if a child falls from a slide).

Planning of Activities and Implementing the Program

Interventions are implemented for different populations and environments. Communities may have different healthcare services (with particular features regarding availability and accessibility) or settings through which the intervention is performed. It is necessary to examine the context of the community intervention, as well as the participants. In other words, the feasibility of adapting an intervention needs to be

---

[e]The criteria are as follows: (1) the condition should be an important health problem; (2) there should be an accepted treatment or useful intervention; (3) the natural history of the disease should be understood; (4) there should be a latent or early symptomatic stage; (5) there should be a suitable and acceptable screening test or examination; (6) facilities for diagnosis and treatment should be available; (7) there should be an agreed-upon policy on whom to treat; (8) early treatment should do more good than harm; (9) the cost–benefit ratio should be acceptable; and (10) the screening should be a continuing process.

assessed. Will an intervention to address obesity that was tested in a Hispanic community be applicable to a predominantly African American population? Will an injury prevention program tested in Sweden be applicable to the United States? Will an intervention for prevention and treatment of hypertension that was tested in males be applicable to females?

Ethnic and cultural diversity in the community has to be assessed to determine whether the intervention can be adapted. Cultural sensitivity—in terms of language used, means of communication, and overall understanding and respect for the community—is an essential element for a successful intervention. When an intervention is designed to change behavior, the knowledge of the community's cultural background and beliefs is essential to understand its practices. If an intervention is planned to change nutritional habits, consideration should be given to the staple diet of the community and how that can be adapted to a healthy diet. Likewise, a family planning program should consider religious and sociocultural factors.

Communication channels to deliver the intervention need to be assessed. In a clinic setting, face-to-face interventions delivered by doctors, nurses, or health-related professionals might be adequate. In addition, audiovisual materials can be provided in this setting. Audiovisual materials are used for community-wide interventions through newspapers, radio, or television. More recently, the Internet and other forms of information technology are often used to communicate with participants.[66–68] All of these means have to be tested for suitability, appropriateness (culturally sensitiveness, language adequacy), and access.

One of the important issues in the implementation of community health interventions is health literacy.[f,69] The WHO asserts that a person must be able to get health information, understand it, and use it to improve one's own health or the health of his or her family or community; also, a person does not need to be literate to get health information and use it.[70]

The planning of program activities requires securing the appropriate human and material resources, which should be in accordance with a planned budget that is realistic and appropriate for the needs of the program. The use of existing human resources should be examined to maximize their potential in terms of time allocated to planned activities and possible role changes because of the program. New personnel with specific skills might be needed to address different program components. Capacity-building activities for all parties involved in the intervention also need to be developed. These activities should be geared toward the acquisition of new knowledge

and skills and for a common understanding of the overall program and specific tasks involved. In addition, while the program is being carried out, the team should have regular meetings for updates and reports and for further acquisition of knowledge and skills. Roles need to be clearly defined for a smooth-running program with regard to organizing, reporting, and updating the responsible parties.

Intersectoral cooperation is needed because the healthcare sector alone may not be able to function effectively with sole responsibility for the health of the community. The complex nature of health problems requires the cooperation and partnership of different agencies and professions, which will complement the knowledge and skills of healthcare professionals and community members. The organization of this cooperation or partnership requires time, skills, and a clear definition of roles to ensure that the program runs smoothly.

Evaluation

The evaluation measures the degree to which the intervention objectives were achieved. It is an integral part of the intervention and should be planned at the outset of the program.

If the plan is to demonstrate the effectiveness of a new community program, it should be planned as a *program trial*. Specifically, the intervention will be carried out in a particular community (the intervention community), and there will be another community that will serve as a comparison (the control community). The control community should be as similar as possible to the intervention community in its sociodemographic characteristics, but it will not undergo the intervention. In that way, when the results are analyzed, the effectiveness of the program can be ascribed to the program itself, not other intervening factors. In some cases more than a community is needed to be able to demonstrate a significant difference in the outcome of the study. The selection of the intervention and control communities can be done randomly (a randomized controlled trial) to obtain the strongest study design for showing evidence of effectiveness.

When deciding on the type of intervention design, ethical questions may arise. Can a community (used as the control) be deprived of an intervention? Because the community intervention was not yet shown to be effective, this issue may not pose an ethical problem. In addition, the community program can be delayed in the control community until after the evaluation. To comply with ethical principles, the organization that plans to implement the intervention may be required to submit the intervention design to its institutional review board (IRB) for approval.

When there is evidence that an intervention is effective (for example, home visits for the prevention of child abuse),

---

[f]According to Healthy People 2010, health literacy is "the degree to which individuals have the capacity to obtain, process, and understand basic health information and services needed to make appropriate health decisions."

another type of evaluation called a *program review* can be conducted. In this case, a before-and-after design will explore the changes in the intervention community; the changes that occurred after the program will be compared with the baseline data. In the absence of a comparison group, there is no certainty that the changes occurred as a consequence of the program (other factors could have influenced the outcome).

According to Abramson,[71] there are several basic questions that need to be answered in an evaluation. These questions are examined in the following sections.

Program Quality

The quality of the program is assessed through the outcome, process, and structure dimensions. These dimensions measure the achievement of the intervention objectives, performance of activities, and use of infrastructure according to the established plan. Additionally, the economic aspect of the program, the satisfaction of those involved, and the differential value of the program in terms of outcomes needs to be analyzed. The elements of a program quality evaluation are presented in Table 2-4.

TABLE 2-4 Evaluation of Program Quality

Outcomes	The achievement of the program outcomes can be assessed by measuring mortality, morbidity, and changes in knowledge, behavior, and attitudes or any other characteristic defined in the objectives. In some cases, the ultimate objective of the program is to decrease mortality or morbidity (for example, to decrease mortality or incidence of cardiovascular conditions). Yet intermediate objectives may also be defined (increase the rate of physical activity or decrease the prevalence of smoking in the population). The latter objectives can themselves be the ultimate objectives of programs that were designed with only that aim.
	The adverse effects of interventions must also be assessed. This is particularly relevant in the case of screening programs, where false positive results may cause harm to individuals who were labeled with a condition they do not have (Hypertension, child, delayed development). It is also pertinent for the adverse effects of prescribed medications, such as postmenopausal hormone replacement therapy (HRT). In the Women's Health Initiative study, an RCT to study the effect of HRT in the form of estrogen alone or with progestin found an increased risk of stroke and blood clots as compared to those using placebo. In addition, for those using the combination of drugs, there was an increase in heart attacks and breast cancer as compared to those using placebo.[72]
Process	The program process is assessed by determining whether activities were performed as proposed. If the activities and their quantities were well defined in the intervention plans, they are the benchmarks that will be used to assess whether the activities were performed as planned (for example, the number of educational sessions or home visits that were carried out). Additionally, it is important to assess the quality of these encounters.
	The coverage of the proposed intervention is another program process measure, such as the proportion of children who were immunized or the number of women who had a mammogram compared to the total number of children or women in the program. The utilization of services and the compliance with medication or advice are also measures of the program process.
Structure	The structure of the program is measured according to the appropriateness of facilities and equipment; the adequacy of the material and human resources (training and performance); the availability and accessibility of the services provided; the organization of the services and coordination with other sectors; financial, language, or other barriers; the accountability system, if any; and community participation.
Efficiency	The efficiency of the program addresses its costs in relation to the results obtained. Measurements such as cost-effectiveness (the relative expenditure for a certain outcome or outcomes of an intervention) and a cost–benefit analysis (the total costs compared to the total benefits of one or more interventions) are key indicators.

Satisfaction

Participant and healthcare team satisfaction are additional evaluation measures because they can contribute to better compliance by community members and contribute to the maintenance of the program. Questions regarding participants' satisfaction with the operation and organization of the program, its content, and its providers are additional elements to consider in the improvement of the program.

Differential Value

The differential value of a program needs to be appraised. This evaluation refers to all the previous evaluation questions and addresses the issues of equity and disparity. The intervention program should be reviewed to discover whether there were differences in the effectiveness or the process of the program among different ethnic or racial groups or according to the participants' educational background or other characteristics. It should also be determined whether the equipment and material and human resources were equally available to members of the community.

Dissemination of Results

The evaluation results need to be shared among those involved in the process; that is, service providers and community members. For team members, information on the effectiveness of the program, in its entirety or in parts, and the success of all or some of the activities provides insights regarding the sustainability of the program, the need for modifications, or possible program cancellation. For the community, the evaluation results provide knowledge on changes in their own health status, strengthen the links with the providers, and may offer incentives for continued participation.

It is also necessary to provide evaluation results to funding agencies and different levels within the organization that performed the intervention. Sharing the results with the wider population through publications, especially in the academic field, may provide the opportunity for reproduction or adaptation of the intervention in other communities.

RESOURCES IN COMMUNITY HEALTH INTERVENTIONS

The planning of resources for community health interventions includes both human and material resources. All of the resources are translated into a time allocation and budget.

Human Resources

Human resources should be planned in accordance with all the activities that will be carried out by the program, from those that are specifically related to the health assessment and intervention activities to administrative tasks. For these activities, specialized personnel might be required, like epidemiologists, statisticians, educators, health promoters, doctors, nurses, and other healthcare professionals. Administrative personnel are needed for coordination tasks, budget management, and other managerial tasks. A professional should be designated to coordinate and overview the whole process. The time of the available human resources needs to be allocated for the new activities, and their capacity should be built up so the program can run smoothly.

Community members can also be part of the needs assessment process, such as in participatory research endeavors[73] when they are agreed upon by the healthcare professionals and community members. Issues of confidentiality should be carefully considered, especially in close-knit communities.

Throughout the process of the intervention, accountability in the form of a continuous and transparent reporting system should exist for updates of events, methodological follow-up, and general information for the relevant stakeholders. Accountability is used in decision making regarding program components, continuation, modification, or discontinuation.

Material Resources

Material resources include the materials, instruments, and equipment needed for the health assessment and the intervention. They include questionnaires, office supplies, machines, audiovisual aids, and various means of communication.

TIME LINE AND BUDGET IN COMMUNITY HEALTH INTERVENTIONS

The proposal for an intervention and its implementation requires allocating adequate time for each stage, as well as budget planning. The budget preparation needs to consider the human resources, materials and equipment, and all other requirements of the institution through which the intervention will be delivered.

As demonstrated in Table 2-5, the time line is usually presented in a Gantt chart that features the schedule of activities to be performed during the program. In the first row, the time (frequently in months) is depicted; the first column lists the scheduled activities, which could overlap. The details included in the Gantt chart will depend on the program requirements.

SUMMARY

Community health interventions are systematic and organized processes that address health problems affecting a community. The interventions can be carried out in different settings, from family homes to clinical settings, schools, or workplaces. Community involvement throughout the intervention could include observing, complying with the program, or fully partnering with the healthcare team, depending on the organization of the community and its willingness to participate.

TABLE 2-5 Gantt Chart

	1	2	3	4	5	6	7	8	9–24	25	26	27	28–30
Health assessment	█	█											
Prioritization			█	█									
Selective assessment					█	█	█						
Planning of intervention						█	█	█					
Implementation of intervention									█	█			
Evaluation										█	█	█	
Report and dissemination													█

The intervention requires baseline knowledge of the situation, which can be gathered through qualitative or quantitative methods or both. The planned intervention can address changes of behavior or changes in the environment for prevention and health promotion, early diagnosis, or treatment and rehabilitation. It can also include health policies and the enactment of laws.

Clear objectives and descriptions of the activities to be performed are the basis for the evaluation of outcomes, processes, and the structure of the program. The evaluation can be based on a before-and-after design or use a control community in which the intervention is not performed for comparison of results.

Box 2-2 A road map for the design of interventions

Health assessment	Gather existing health information
	Prioritize health problems and plan a selective assessment on the priority condition
	Design the health assessment—target population, objectives, definition of variables
	Select data collection methods and plan of analysis
Intervention planning and implementation	Review the literature to discover what has already been done and look for evidence of program effectiveness
	Select the type of intervention
	Define the target population
	Define objectives and activities
Evaluation	Analyze the program effectiveness, performance of activities, use of resources, efficiency, satisfaction, and differential value
	Disseminate evaluation results
Resources	Plan for human and material resources
	Build capacity
Time line and budget	Determine the sequence in which activities will be performed
	Analyze the cost of the different components of the program

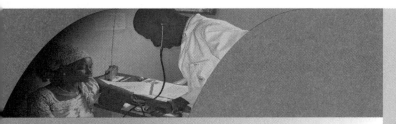

Discussion Questions

- How do you select a setting for an intervention?
- How involved should community members be in the process of community interventions?
- How would you decide whether a comprehensive or selective health assessment should be carried out?
- What are the benefits of using a model to guide interventions?
- What are the benefits of learning about evidence-based interventions?

Review Questions

- What settings are used for interventions?
- What steps should be followed for a health assessment?
- What steps should be followed in designing an intervention?
- Which types of evaluations are used for assessing outcomes?
- How are resources for community interventions planned?

REFERENCES

1. American Academy of Pediatrics. Childrens' health topics: immunizations/vaccines. http://www.aap.org/healthtopics/Immunizations.cfm. Accessed May 30, 2009.

2. Centers for Disease Control and Prevention. Achievements in public health, 1900–1999 impact of vaccines universally recommended for children—United States, 1990–1998. *MMWR Weekly.* 1999;48:243–248. http://www.cdc.gov/mmwr/preview/mmwrhtml/00056803.htm. Accessed May 30, 2009.

3. UNICEF. The state of the world's children 2009. http://www.unicef.org/sowc09/report/report.php and http://www.unicef.org/sowc09/docs/SOWC09_Table_3.pdf. Accessed March 2009.

4. Centers for Disease Control and Prevention. National, state, and local area vaccination coverage among children aged 19–35 months—United States, 2007. *MMWR.* 2008;5;57:961–966.

5. Choi YH, Gay N, Fraser G, Ramsay M. The potential for measles transmission in England. *BMC Public Health.* 2008;8:338.

6. US Department of Health and Human Services. US Preventive Services Task Force. http://www.ahrq.gov/clinic/uspstfix.htm. Accessed January 2009.

7. Canadian Task Force on Preventive Health Care. Evidence-based clinical prevention. http://www.ctfphc.org/. Accessed January 2009.

8. Cochrane Library. What are systematic reviews and protocols? http://www3.interscience.wiley.com/cgi-bin/mrwhome/106568753/WhatAreSystematicReviews.html. Accessed January 2009.

9. World Health Organization. Health promotion glossary. WHO/HPR/HEP/98.1. http://www.who.int/hpr/NPH/docs/hp_glossary_en.pdf. Accessed December 2008.

10. Merriam-Webster Online. http://www.merriam-webster.com/. Accessed January 2009.

11. Christensen P. The health-promoting family: a conceptual framework for future research. *Soc Sci & Med.* 2004;59:377–388.

12. Kreuter MW, Alcaraz KI, Pfeiffer D, Christopher K. Using dissemination research to identify optimal community settings for tailored breast cancer information kiosks. *J Public Health Manag Pract.* 2008;14:160–169.

13. Spinks A, Turner C, Nixon J, McClure RJ. The "WHO Safe Communities" model for the prevention of injury in whole populations. *Cochrane Database Syst Rev.* 2005;(2):CD004445. doi:10.1002/14651858.CD004445.pub3.

14. Cashman SB, Stenger J. Healthy communities: a natural ally for community-oriented primary care [letter]. *Am J Public Health.* 2003;93:1379–1380.

15. Whittaker R, Maddison R, McRobbie H, et al. A multimedia mobile phone-based youth smoking cessation intervention: findings from content development and piloting studies. *J Med Internet Res.* 2008;10:e49.

16. Community-Campus Partnerships for Health. Community-based participatory research. http://depts.washington.edu/ccph/commbas.html. Accessed December 2008.

17. Israel BA, Schulz AJ, Parker EA, Becker AB. Review of community-based research: assessing partnership approaches to improve health. *Annu Rev Public Health.* 1998;19:173–202.

18. Nguyen TT, McPhee SJ, Bui-Tong N, et al. Community-based participatory research increases cervical cancer screening among Vietnamese-Americans. *J Health Care Poor Underserved.* 2006;17:31–54.

19. Cashman SB, Adeky S, Allen AJ III, et al. The power and the promise: working with communities to analyze data, interpret findings and get outcomes. *Am J Public Health.* 2008;98:1407–1417.

20. Christopher S, Watts V, McCormick AKHG, Young S. Building and maintaining trust in community-based participatory research partnership. *Am J Public Health.* 2008;98:1398–1406.

21. Geographic Information Systems (GIS) at CDC. http://www.cdc.gov/gis/. Accessed February 2010.

22. Kazda MJ, Beel E, Villegas D, Martinez JG, Patel N, Migala W. Methodological complexities and the use of GIS in conducting a community needs assessment of a large US municipality. *J Community Health.* 2009;34:210–215.

23. Abramson JH. WINPEPI (PEPI-for-Windows): computer programs for epidemiologists. *Epidemiol Perspect Innov.* 2004;1:6. http://www.brixtonhealth.com/pepi4windows.html. Accessed July 2009.

24. Blumberg SJ, Luke JV. Reevaluating the need for concern regarding noncoverage bias in landline surveys. *Am J Public Health.* 2009;99:1806–1810.

25. O'Toole J, Sinclair M, Leder K. Maximizing response rates in household telephone surveys. *BMC Med Res Methodol.* 2008;8:71.

26. Lefever JB, Howard KS, Lanzi RG, et al; Centers for the Prevention of Child Neglect. Cell phones and the measurement of child neglect: the validity of the parent–child activities interview. *Child Maltreat.* 2008;13:320–333.

27. Raymond HF, Rebchook G, Curotto A, et al. Comparing Internet-based and venue-based methods to sample MSM in the San Francisco Bay Area [published online and ahead of print January 22, 2009]. *AIDS Behav.*

28. Rankin KM, Rauscher GH, McCarthy B, et al. Comparing the reliability of response to telephone-administered versus self-administered Web-based surveys in a case-control study of adult malignant brain cancer. *Cancer Epidemiol Biomarkers Prev.* 2008;17:2639–2646.

29. Robertson AS, Rivara FP, Ebel BE, Lymp JF, Christakis DA. Validation of parent self reported home safety practices. *Inj Prev.* 2005;11:209–212.

30. Korn T, Katz-Leurer M, Meyer S, Gofin R. How children with special needs travel with their parents: observed versus reported use of vehicle restraints. *Pediatrics.* 2007;119:e637–e642.

31. Rose G. Sick individuals and sick populations. *Int J Epidemiol.* 2001;30:427–432.

32. Becker M, ed. The Health Belief Model and personal health behavior. *Health Educ Monogr.* 1974;2:324–473.

33. Bandura A. Self-efficacy: toward a unifying theory of behavioral change. *Psychol Rev.* 1977;84:191–215.

34. Bandura A. *Social Foundations of Thought and Action: A Social Cognitive Theory.* Englewood Cliffs, NJ: Prentice-Hall; 1986.

35. Fishbein M, Ajzen I. *Belief, Attitude, Intention, and Behavior: An Introduction to Theory and Research.* Reading, MA: Addison-Wesley; 1975.

36. Ajzen I, Fishbein M. *Understanding Attitudes and Predicting Social Behavior.* Englewood Cliffs, NJ: Prentice-Hall; 1980.

37. Prochaska JO, Velicer WF. The transtheoretical model of health behavior change. *Am J Health Promot.* 1997;12:38–48.

38. Wright JA, Velicer WF, Prochaska JO. Testing the predictive power of the transtheoretical model of behavior change applied to dietary fat intake. *Health Edu Res.* 2009;24:224–236.

39. Sun X, Prochaska JO, Laforge RG. Transtheoretical principles and processes for quitting smoking: a 24-month comparison of a representative sample of quitters, relapsers and non-quitters. *Addict Behav.* 2007;32:2707–2726.

40. Kotler P, Zaltman G. Social marketing: an approach to planned social change. *J Mark.* 1971;35:3–12.

41. DeBuono B, González AR, Rosenbaum S. Reducing the risk of preventable injury and disease. In: DeBuono B, González AR, Rosenbaum S, eds. *Moments in Leadership: Case Studies in Public Health Policy and Practice.* New York, NY: Pfizer Global Pharmaceuticals; 2007. 105-109.

42. Health Act 2006. http://www.opsi.gov.uk/acts/acts2006/pdf/ukpga_20060028_en.pdf. Accessed February 2009.

43. Thrasher JF, Boado M, Sebrie EM, Bianco E. Smoke-free policies and social acceptability of smoking in Uruguay and Mexico: findings from the international control policy evaluation project. *Nicotine Tob Res.* 2009;11;591–599.

44. Shafir S, Parks J, Gentilello L. Cost benefits of reduction in motor vehicle injuries with a nationwide speed limit of 65 miles per hour (mph). *J Trauma.* 2008;65:1122–1125.

45. Wagenaar AC, Wiviott MB. Effects of mandating seatbelt use: a series of surveys on compliance in Michigan. *Public Health Rep.* 1986;101:505–513.

46. Winston FK, Kallan MJ, Elliott MR, Xie D, Durbin DR. Effect of booster seat laws on appropriate restraint use by children 4 to 7 years old involved in crashes. *Arch Pediatr Adolesc Med.* 2007;161:270–275.

47. Homer J, French M. Motorcycle helmet laws in the United States from 1990 to 2005: politics and public health. *Am J Public Health*. 2009;99:415–423.

48. Mayrose J. The effects of a mandatory motorcycle helmet law on helmet use and injury patterns among motorcycle fatalities. *J Safety Res*. 2008;39:429–432.

49. Liu BC, Ivers R, Norton R, Boufous S, Blows S, Lo SK. Helmets for preventing injury in motorcycle riders. *Cochrane Database Syst Rev*. 2008: Issue 1. Art. No. CD004333. DOI: 10.1002/14651858.CD004333.pub3

50. Yeung CA. A systematic review of the efficacy and safety of fluoridation. *Evid Based Dent*. 2008;9:39–43.

51. Mertz KJ, Weiss HB. Changes in motorcycle-related head injury deaths, hospitalizations, and hospital charges following repeal of Pennsylvania's mandatory motorcycle helmet law. *Am J Public Health*. 2008;98:1464–1467.

52. National Health Service South Central. Public board paper HA09/020 meeting—26 February 2009. Water fluoridation—the scientific evidence. http://www.southcentral.nhs.uk/document_store/12351421641_ha09-020 (i)_water_fluoridation_-_the_scientific_evidence.pdf. Accessed March 2009.

53. Rabb-Waytowich D. Water fluoridation in Canada: past and present. *J Can Dental Assoc*. 2009;75:451–454.

54. Walton WW. An evaluation of the Poison Prevention Packaging Act. *Pediatrics*. 1982;69:363–370.

55. Spiegel CN, Lindaman FC. Children can't fly: a program to prevent childhood morbidity and mortality from window falls. *Am J Public Health*. 1977;6:1143–1147.

56. Health and Safety Commission; ACSNI Study Group on Human Factors. *Third Report: Organizing for Safety*. London, England: HMSO; 1993:23.

57. Brownson RC, Housemann RA, Brown DR, et al. Promoting physical activity in rural communities: walking trail access, use, and effects. *Am J Prev Med*. 2000;18:2235–2241.

58. Centers for Disease Control and Prevention. Guide to community preventive services: promoting physical activity. www.thecommunityguide.org/pa. Accessed January 2009.

59. Wang G, Macera CA, Scudder-Soucie B, Schmid T, Pratt M, Buchner D. A cost–benefit analysis of physical activity using bike/pedestrian trails. *Health Promot Pract*. 2006;6:174–179.

60. Wilson JMG, Jungner G. *Principles and Practice of Screening Disease*. Geneva, Switzerland: World Health Organization; 1968. http://wholibdoc.who.int/php/WHO_PHP_34.pdf. Accessed December 2008.

61. Papadakis S, Moroz I. Population-level interventions for coronary heart disease prevention: what have we learned since the North Karelia Project? *Curr Opin Cardiol*. 2008;23:452–461.

62. Krug EG, Dahlberg L, Mercy JA, Zwi AB, Lozano R. *World Report on Violence and Health*. Geneva, Switzerland: World Health Organization; 2002.

63. Peden M, Oyegbite K, Ozanne-Smith J, et al.; World Health Organization, UNICEF, eds. *World Report on Child Injury Prevention*. Geneva, Switzerland; 2008.

64. Calhoun AD, Clark-Jones F. Developmental psychopathology, the public health approach to violence, and the cycle of violence. *Ped Clin N Am*. 1998;45:281–291.

65. Gofin R. Preparedness and response to terrorism. A framework for public health action. *Eur J Public Health*. 2005;15:100–104.

66. Christakis DA, Zimmerman FJ, Rivara FP, Ebel B. Improving pediatric prevention via the Internet: a randomized, controlled trial. *Pediatrics*. 2006;118:1157–1166.

67. Van Voorhees BW, Fogel J, Reinecke MA, et al. Randomized clinical trial of an Internet-based depression prevention program for adolescents (Project CATCH-IT) in primary care: 12-week outcomes. *J Dev Behav Pediatr*. 2009;30:23–37.

68. Brendryen H, Drozd F, Kraft P. A digital smoking cessation program delivered through Internet and cell phone without nicotine replacement (happy ending): randomized controlled trial. *J Med Internet Res*. 2008;10:e51.

69. Healthy People 2010. Health communication. http://www.healthypeople.gov/document/html/volume1/11healthcom.htm#_Toc490471359. Accessed January 2009.

70. Kickbusch I. *Healthy Societies: Addressing 21st Century Health Challenges*. Health Literacy: addressing the double inequity. Adelaide: Government of South Australia; 2009: 44–47.

71. Abramson JH, Abramson ZH. *Research Methods in Community Medicine*. 6th ed. West Sussex, England: John Wiley & Sons; 2008.

72. National Institutes of Health. Women's health initiative. http://www.nhlbi.nih.gov/whi/. Accessed February 2009.

73. Glover Blackwell A. Active living research and the movement for healthy communities. *Am J Prev Med*. 2009;36(2S):S50–S52.

APPENDIX 2-1

Selected Sources of Information on Health Status in the United States

CDC WONDER from the Centers for Disease Control and Prevention (CDC) allows users to search data sets of vital statistics and other health data for information about cancer, birth, mortality, and more by region and nation. It includes the Healthy People 2010 objectives and data.	http://wonder.cdc.gov www.cdc.gov
The Youth Risk Behavior Surveillance System (YRBSS), produced by the CDC with input from states, tracks health behaviors at the state level over time	http://www.cdc.gov/HealthyYouth/yrbs/index.htm Also searchable through CDC WONDER
The US Census Bureau Web site has multiple access points to national and local data.	http://www.census.gov
The US Bureau of Labor Statistics provides access to their time series data and table of economic indicators.	http://www.bls.gov
The National Center for Health Statistics provides data sets on national health and social indicators, including Healthy People 2010, youth and adolescent health and behavior, and much more.	http://cdc.gov/nchswww/
The District of Columbia Department of Health presents epidemiological reports on health at its various Web sites.	http://dchealth.dc.gov
The National Neighborhood Indicators Partnership from the Urban Institute incorporates geographic tools and neighborhood data.	http://www.urban.org/nnip/about.html http://www.urban.org/nnip/partners.html
The American Anthropological Association's Statement on Race describes the organization's conclusion that inequalities based on race are not based on biological factors.	http://www.aaanet.org/stmts/racepp.htm
The *Community Guide's* Model for Linking the Social Environment to Health by Laurie M. Anderson, PhD, et al., and the Task Force on Community Preventive Services examines social environments, communities' social resource needs, and community interventions.	http://academicdepartments.musc.edu/nursing/departments/researchoffice/documents/Anderson%202003.pdf Anderson LM, Scrimshaw SC, Fullilove MT, Fielding JE; Task Force on Community Preventive Services. The *Community Guide's* model for linking the social environment to health. *Am J Prev Med.* 2003;24:3S.
The History of Race in Science Web site, sponsored by the University of Toronto, MIT, and others, captures bibliographies, syllabi, links, and conferences that critically evaluate the role of race and racism in health, science, and related fields.	http://web.mit.edu/racescience/links/index.html

Unequal Treatment: Confronting Racial and Ethnic Disparities in Health Care characterizes the racial disparities that exist in health care, including differences in pain medication, cardiac procedures, and other aspects of health care.

http://www.nap.edu/catalog/10260.html
Smedley BD, Stith AY, Nelson AR, eds.; Committee on Understanding and Eliminating Racial and Ethnic Disparities in Health Care. *Unequal Treatment: Confronting Racial and Ethnic Disparities in Health Care.* Washington, DC: National Academies Press; 2003.

The National Center on Minority Health and Health Disparities is NIH's center for the reduction and elimination of health disparities.

http://ncmhd.nih.gov

The Office of Minority Health provides links to federal agencies and nongovernmental organizations that are involved in minority health care.

http://www.omhrc.gov

The Kaiser Family Foundation reports on disparities in health care and health status in their State Health Reports.

http://www.kff.org/minorityhealth/disparities.cfm

PolicyLink's 2002 report *Reducing Health Disparities Through a Focus on Communities* is based on research from around the United States.

http://www.policylink.org/atf/cf/%7B97c6d565-bb43-406d-a6d5-eca3bbf35af0%7D/REDUCINGHEALTHDISPARITIES_FINAL.PDF

Applied Research Center, *Closing the Gap: Solutions to Race-Based Health Disparities*

http://www.arc.org/content/view/250/481

THRIVE—Guide to health disparities reduction. From the Prevention Institute, this provides communities with factors to evaluate when addressing community health and racial health disparities.

Foundations for the Future: A Backgrounder on the Social Determinants of Health and Health Inequities is a publication from the Canadian Women's Health Network on the key social determinants of health.

http://www.cwhn.ca/en/node/40540

The WHO's Commission on the Social Determinants of Health publishes reports on the relationship between social factors and public health.

http://www.who.int/social_determinants/en
(follow the Publications link)

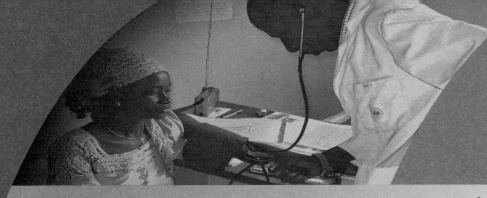

CHAPTER 3

Community-Oriented Primary Care (COPC): History and Principles

KEY TERMS

community-oriented
    primary care
community participation
COPC
healthcare team
identification of health needs
    at the community level

integration
natural history of diseases
primary care
prioritization
public health

INTRODUCTION

Community-Oriented Primary Care (COPC) is a primary care delivery approach that originated from Sidney L. Kark and Emily Kark's work in Pholela, South Africa, in the 1940s and 1950s and has further been developed in Jerusalem since the 1960s.[1] Notably, the term *Community-Oriented Primary Care* was coined by Sidney Kark in 1981,[2] although COPC principles and practice were the backbone of the work done in South Africa. The approach is characterized by the integration of clinical care and public health.

Prior to the Karks' work in South Africa, there were experiences of extending primary care to include a population approach. One of those experiences was introduced by John Grant during 1921 in a Chinese medical school. This was done through a *health station*, which was deemed to need facilities as good as a hospital's.[3] Years later, in 1939, William Pickles began using epidemiology, the basic science of population health, as part of his UK primary care practice.[4] These experiences continued afterward in other places around the world. A notable example is that of Tudor Hart, a pioneer of general practice in the United Kingdom, who introduced a community orientation in his general practice in Wales during the 1960s.[5]

Despite individual experiences with integrating a population approach into primary care, worldwide recognition did not come until the World Health Organization's (WHO) International Conference on Primary Health Care in 1978 at Alma-Ata.[6] At that conference it was declared that primary health care is an essential component in the delivery of healthcare services at the community level and is the key to delivery of "Health for All." Notably, several authors established a link between that conference and the Karks' pioneering work in South Africa[7-11] to such an extent that their work was credited, among others, with its origin.

In this chapter the various definitions of COPC will be analyzed, and its origins and development will be presented. The conceptual and methodological frameworks and service characteristics, as well as the values involved in COPC, will be examined. Additionally, factors and opportunities that facilitate the application and development of COPC in different healthcare systems will be assessed as well as its worldwide application.

DEFINITIONS OF COPC

As summarized in Box 3-1, several definitions of COPC have been proposed by the Karks and other authors or organizations.

The common elements in these definitions are individual and community care (community medicine); the integration of primary care and public health (promotion and prevention); and the provision of care to defined, entire populations, healthy or sick, based on identification of needs. It is important to note that community participation and intersectoral collaboration are not common to all definitions, although nowadays they are considered integral to the practice of COPC.

THE ORIGIN OF COPC IN SOUTH AFRICA

Sidney L. Kark expressed his broad view of the social, cultural, economic, and political determinants of health as a medical student. His publications *The Economic Factor in the Health of the Bantu in South Africa*[18] and *Problems of National Health*[19] are an expression of these views. As student activists, Sidney and his wife, Emily Kark, founded the Society for the Study of Medical Conditions Among the Bantu in 1935.

On the basis of their exemplary work and activities as medical students at the University of the Witwatersrand Medical School, the government's chief medical officer recruited the Karks in 1940 to create the Pholela Health Unit in the rural area known today as KwaZulu-Natal.[20] Services offered at the Pholela Health Unit were more extensive than what was offered at a typical clinic. This unit embraced a new concept of healthcare service—the *community health center*—integrating individual-based care with community health activities.

The first steps of the care offered in Pholela were the framework of what Kark referred to as Social Medicine.[21,22] The main features included the following:

- consideration of the community as a whole
- recognition that behavioral, cultural, and social characteristics are crucial components of health assessment and care planning
- provision of health care by a healthcare team
- use of epidemiology as a tool for assessing health determinants
- evaluation of care and the application of teaching and research as integral parts of healthcare services

Box 3-1 Definitions of COPC*

Kark SL, 1981[2]	"There is a strong case for enlarging the traditional horizons of the primary care practitioner from the strictly *clinical* to the *epidemiological and community aspects of care*; it is this which I refer to as community-oriented primary health care."
Kark SL, Kark E, 1983[12]	"A way of practicing medicine and nursing, or of providing primary care, which is focused on *care of the individual who is well or sick, or at risk for illness or disease*, while also focusing on promoting the health of the *community as a whole* or any of its subgroups."
Institute of Medicine (IOM) United States[13]	"The provision of primary care services to a *defined community*, coupled with systematic efforts to identify and address the major health problems of that community through *effective modifications in both the primary care services* and other appropriate *community health programs*."
King Edward's Hospital Fund for London and the Department of Social Medicine of Hebrew University-Hadassah School of Public Health and Community Medicine[14]	"A continuous process by which primary health care is provided to a *defined community* on the basis of its *assessed health needs* by the planned *integration of public health with primary care practice*."
A Dictionary of Epidemiology[15]	"In this form of practice the primary health care practitioner or team is *responsible for health care both at the individual and at the community or population level*."
Rhyne RL, Bogue R, Kukulka A, Fulmer H[16]	"A process by which a *defined population's health problems are systematically identified and addressed*."
Foz G, Gofin J, Montaner I[17]	"The practice of *primary care* with *population responsibility*, oriented to the *health improvement* of a defined community served by the health service, with the progressive *participation of the community and in coordination with all services involved* with the health of the community or its determinants."

*Emphasis is added in all definitions.

Health care in Pholela was based on a healthcare team composed primarily of doctors and nurses. They were responsible for health assessments at the individual, family, and community levels. A family diagnosis was done, which required both epidemiological and clinical skills. This diagnosis formed part of the overall community diagnosis upon which health promotion and preventive and curative services were provided. The family and community diagnosis by the healthcare team and the integration of services have a present significance because they are being proposed for the integration of clinical care and public health.[23]

Another innovative feature of the Karks' practice was their inclusion of information on the habitat and environment as an integral part of the community diagnosis. For example, there was a meteorological unit of the health center that collected information on rainfall, temperature, and humidity.

The Health Status and the Intervention Programs

One of the first problems that the Karks set out to address in their time at Pholela was malnutrition. This was done through promotion and treatment activities by both the health center's team and the population.[24] The activities involved growing vegetables that supplied the family's needs and the creation of a daily market run by the local producers. Competitions of home vegetable gardens were organized by community members and the health center team. Additionally, in an effort to improve crop production, methods to make compost using refuse were taught. The gardens were also used for other local activities, such as cooking lessons and health education. In addition, the health center promoted milk consumption by making it available to the community at affordable prices and encouraging local people to sell milk at the roadside. An evaluation of these activities showed an increase in the number of summer gardens from 65% to 89% in 10 years and an increase in winter gardens from 54% to 69% in 2 years. Compost was applied by nearly half the families in a 10-year period.

As a consequence of all these activities, the nutritional status of mothers and children improved. Children's growth patterns were positively affected, and signs of vitamin and micronutrient deficiencies were greatly reduced. Infant mortality decreased from 275/1000 to 82/1000 live births during the period from 1942 to 1957. Although no comparison group was available to demonstrate that the changes were due to the health center's activities, a time trend analysis that compared the initially defined area that received care at the health center with areas later incorporated showed the positive effect of the interventions that were implemented.

The success of the healthcare model created in Pholela prompted the recommendation by the National Health Services Commission (Gluckman Report) to develop a nationwide network of community health centers.[25] The Pholela unit itself became part of the Institute of Family and Community Health in Durban, South Africa.[1] Sidney L. Kark was named as director of this institute in 1946, and afterward he became the chair of the Department of Social, Preventive, and Family Medicine of Natal University Medical School in Durban. The South African government planned to develop more than 200 health centers similar to Pholela. By 1949, 44 community health centers were already founded, but unfortunately political changes in South Africa—which introduced the apartheid policy—interrupted the development of new health centers and ultimately forced all of them to close. The Karks, together with many of their team members, were compelled to leave the country because these closures were representative of the apartheid regime's efforts to negate their ideas and achievements.[26] Nonetheless, the seeds of the COPC approach were planted by the Karks and their team, and afterward COPC was developed and practiced in Jerusalem and elsewhere.

Among the many publications from Karks' experience is *The Social Pathology of Syphilis in Africans.*[27] This seminal work analyzed the historic background of the disease, which was unknown among the African population. In the late 19th century, the economic impact of the discovery of diamonds in Kimberley and gold in the Witwatersrand forced Africans to migrate to work, leaving behind their families. The migrants lived in poverty and unhealthy environments, and they returned to their homes only after long absences. The study stressed not only individual behavior, but also the social context and "the pattern of society that does not allow for the healthy development of the individual."

In 1958, Sidney L. Kark and his family moved to the United States, where he became the founding chairman of the Department of Epidemiology in the School of Public Health at the University of North Carolina at Chapel Hill. One year later, the Karks left North Carolina for Jerusalem.

THE DEVELOPMENT OF COPC IN JERUSALEM

Upon their arrival in Jerusalem, and together with a multidisciplinary team of their colleagues from South Africa, the Karks continued their work in social and community medicine.

Project in Social Medicine at the Medical School

In 1959, the WHO Israel Project in Social Medicine was created as part of the Department of Social Medicine of the Hebrew University and Hadassah Medical School.[1] Sidney L. Kark was the visiting WHO professor of Social Medicine, and the project included former members of the Institute of Family and Community Health in Durban, as well as Israeli professionals. The former South African members of the institute were skilled in epidemiology, family and community practice, and health education. Some of the original South African professionals in the Social Medicine project moved to the United States and the United Kingdom after a few years.

Two of the primary goals of the project were the creation of academic units at the Hebrew University, including epidemiology, biostatistics, family and community health, maternal and child health, health education, community nursing, and culture and health, as well as the creation of a community health center.

The Community Health Center

Established in 1953, the Hadassah Community Health Center was located in the outskirts of Jerusalem, where a few housing projects had been built during the previous 2 years for new immigrants (from North African, Middle Eastern, and central and eastern European countries) and for veteran Israeli civil servants. The Community Health Center became the field training area for residents in family practice, residents in public health, medical and nursing students, social workers, and public health students from Hebrew University. Research studies (carried out by team members and MPH, PhD, and medical students) were mostly service oriented and were one of the foundations of the community-oriented practice and teaching center. Additionally, epidemiological studies and studies in social epidemiology were carried out at the health center.

Services and Healthcare Team at the Health Center

The health center consisted of a family practice (FP) and a mother and child health (MCH) clinic. Both clinics provided care to a geographically defined area within the neighborhood. Homebound care was provided to the entire area.

The FP clinic offered integrated curative and preventive care through the life course for a defined population of approximately 2700 individuals. The clinic was financed by a contractual agreement between the Hadassah Medical Organization and the Trade Union Sick Fund (the largest sick fund—health maintenance organization—in the country during that time, to which the vast majority of the area population was affiliated). The population was registered in records designed by the center. These records included sociodemographic information, family trees, medical history, and ongoing consultations. Each family member had his or her own record, and family members could be identified through a special number that linked all of them. These records could also be used for a health surveillance purpose and linked with data from the intervention programs. The paper records were transferred to electronic records in the following years.

The core healthcare team at the health center included family doctors, pediatricians, nurses (with public health training), and a health educator. Epidemiologists, statisticians, sociologists, and a social psychiatrist were part of the supportive team. All of them were proficient or, if needed, trained in the community approach to health care.

For the purpose of care, the area was divided into clusters of homes to which teams of one family physician and two nurses were assigned. Studies by the healthcare team and students provided an ongoing picture of the physical (housing, close environment) and social characteristics of the defined area and population. The teams were responsible for the ongoing provision of routine care, as well as the community programs. The teams worked in the clinic, performed outreach activities, and were also involved in the community health programs. This allowed for the teams to have a good knowledge of the neighborhood and population and assured continuity of care. Nurses were responsible for demographic surveillance, which was facilitated by visiting each home at least once a year. These outreach activities also allowed the identification of determinants of health (individual and familial), available resources, and barriers to attend the health center.

The MCH clinic provided care for a larger geographic area within the neighborhood, including approximately 25,000 people and 400 births per year. Preventive antenatal care and preventive care for infants and children through age 6 years and for school children was provided by a combination of the MCH clinic and the School Health Services. The main providers were nurses, who were in charge of growth and development, surveillance, immunizations, screening activities, and providing counseling to parents. Pediatricians and generalists were also team members, and obstetricians attended to high-risk pregnant women. Curative care to the MCH population was provided by the sick fund. For details on the service and COPC programs, refer to Case Studies 13 and 14.

The COPC Practice at the Community Health Center

The community orientation of the health services developed by the healthcare team, included several new activities. Among others, the identification of community health needs implemented through a community health study, the promotion of community participation, and the integration of primary care and public health in the care of individuals and the community.

The Identification of Health Needs One of the sources of information for community health problems in the 1960s was an ongoing collection of health information from clinical records. Although the recording system was established with a community orientation in the FP, it became evident that not all the information was available, either because some residents, mainly the young adults, did not frequent the clinic or because the information was not always recorded.

The nurses facilitated outreach activities to identify residents who were not attending the center and assess their reasons for nonattendance. The team assisted in decreasing barriers of access. Special efforts were done to improve recording, and a survey was carried out to complete the identification of needs and provide a community diagnosis of the health status of the population.

The Community Health Study As part of this community diagnosis process, the Kiryat Hayovel Community Health Study was carried out between 1969 and 1971 in the defined geographic area of the Hadassah Community Health Center and the adjacent area, covering all adults and a sample of 50% of the children. One of the purposes of the study was to obtain baseline information for the planning of community programs and future evaluation of health interventions. A quasi-experimental design was determined. As a control group, the study incorporated the adjacent population in the neighborhood that received regular care from another clinic. The objectives of the study were to determine the prevalence of cardiovascular and other chronic health conditions, their risk factors, and their determinants.[28,29] Successive rounds of examinations were carried out from 1975 to 1976 and again from 1985 to 1987, which were used for the study of trends and evaluation purposes. The follow-up evaluation of the population regarding survival continued during the 1990s.

The Integration of Primary Care and Public Health The health center services integrated curative, preventive, and promotional activities addressing all stages of the natural history of disease. The integration of individual care with public health was completely realized in the FP area, where COPC was applied (see Case Study 14 regarding the control of cardiovascular risk factors in Jerusalem).

The MCH service provided mainly preventive care and also developed COPC programs (see Case Study 13). Curative care, as mentioned, was provided by the sick funds in which children and mothers were enrolled. Both the preventive and curative care at the Community Health Center were connected by a referral system.

Epidemiology in Practice All members of the health center, as well as the Department of Social Medicine, participated in weekly meetings called Epidemiology in Practice. In the meetings, the changing health needs of the community and the community program activities were discussed. These forums were instrumental for quality assurance and were integral in developing new community programs according to changing community needs, modification of existing programs, and assessment of effectiveness. A periodic analysis of acute morbidity, which identified developing epidemic trends by using Pickles charts,[30] was presented in the sessions, and mortality trends were reviewed. Studies performed by faculty and students pertaining to the community health status or evaluation of programs were also presented. The Epidemiology in Practice meetings resembled grand rounds; the patient was the community and constituted an in-service training to all members of the health center and the Department of Social Medicine.

Community Participation Since its inception, the Community Health Center was utilized by the population for varied community activities. One section of the center also functioned as a synagogue, and a large hall was used for weddings and other celebrations. One of these celebrations was the 25th an-niversary of the health center, which was organized by the community, giving expression to the cultural diversity of the different ethnic groups in the area. A library also functioned in the premises, and the center was the meeting place for a diabetics club and an elderly club.

In the early stages of the community health center, relationships were established between the team and the community. The involvement of community members in activities of the health center declined over time in parallel to an increase in the standard of living, characterized by better housing and environmental conditions and improved levels of education and social status. In the late 1970s, and as community participation dwindled, the health center took the initiative to renew the community members' involvement. Residents, community services representatives, and healthcare team members participated in a series of meetings. It was decided that there was a need for coordination of the welfare, education, and healthcare services of the community. Working groups were formed, which functioned for several years and included additional activities prioritized by the healthcare team and members of the community. During this period, a multifunctional community center with cultural, sports, and educational activities was built adjacent to the health center. This prompted collaboration between the two centers and the transference of some of the activities performed at the health center.

With the passing of time, community participation had to be encouraged again. A new director of the health center in the early 1980s invited selected community members to form an advisory committee for the health center. At its monthly meetings, this committee suggested changes for improving services and running the health programs, which were discussed and later implemented. When economic conditions threatened the health center's operation and its closure was inevitable, the committee organized demonstrations that were effective in postponing any interruption of the activities.

Master of Public Health Programs

In 1960, the Department of Social Medicine established a Master of Public Health (MPH) program for Israeli healthcare professionals, which was the first and only such program in the country until the late 1990s. Further, in 1970 the Department of Social Medicine created the International MPH Program. On the basis of the work done by the department and the community health center, in 1980 the School of Public Health and Community Medicine of Hadassah and Hebrew University was created.[31] This was the first school of public health in the country. Currently in Israel there are two other schools of public health and two other MPH programs. The Hebrew University Hadassah School of Public Health and Community Medicine has approximately 1200 MPH graduates from Israel and 85 other countries, mainly from Africa, Latin America, and Southeast Asia, with some students from Australia, the United States, and western Europe. Starting in 1990, students also attended from eastern and central European countries.

One of the main features of the MPH program in Jerusalem is a workshop core course, which was named Family and Community Health in the 1960s. Later, the course was renamed Community Medicine in and Through Primary Care, and since 1981 it has been called Community Oriented Primary Care—COPC. This workshop teaches the basic principles and practice of COPC. In evaluations carried out by the workshop's team and completed by MPH graduates in the 1980s and 1990s (75% response rate), more than half of the graduates reportedly apply COPC principles in their functions, whether in practice, teaching, administration, or research.[32]

With a similar structure and organization as in the MPH program, the workshop was also included in the Family Medicine Residency Program in Jerusalem in the 1980s. An evaluation implemented a few years after the first workshops had a 75% response rate, and family physicians reported usefulness and application of the COPC approach in their practice.[33]

Sustainability and the End of an Era

The close link among the Community Health Center, the academic Department of Social Medicine, and the School of Public Health and Community Medicine achieved sustainability of the practice, teaching, and research of COPC throughout the years. Most of the COPC programs in Jerusalem were evaluated on short- and long-term criteria and different methods, which demonstrated the feasibility and effectiveness of this approach when it is implemented in family practice and MCH settings in primary care (see Case Studies 13 and 14).

The Hadassah Community Health Center was closed in 1999 when the Hadassah Medical Organization considered the center no longer viable. Thus, 50 years after the center was founded, and after 30 years of practicing COPC, the health center was transferred to another organization, and COPC was no longer practiced at the center. The lessons learned from the 30 years in which the feasibility, effectiveness, and sustainability of the approach were demonstrated continue to have their effects throughout teaching and the development of the COPC approach in selected practices in Israel and other countries. In 1999, 60 years after the development, practice, teaching, and research of the Social Medicine dimension, the Karks published their last book, *Promoting Community Health: From Pholela to Jerusalem.*[1] Some years later, in 2003, the Department of Social Medicine was also closed "despite notwithstanding its worldwide recognition."[34]

Even with the shutting down of centers of excellence in academic and practical endeavors, the practice of COPC continues elsewhere. In Israel, some or part of the programs were adapted by the sick funds[35] and the MCH clinics, and occasionally they were adopted as national policies. The international dissemination of COPC continues in different parts of the globe and is adapted to varied health systems, health problems, and populations. Some of these examples are presented in the case studies in this book. Many others can be found in the academic literature. Some of this work is carried out by members of Kark's Jerusalem team and the graduates of the MPH program of the School of Public Health and Community Medicine. Many others are applying COPC principles given the implicit values of the approach and its relevance to their populations.

THE CONCEPTUAL FRAMEWORK OF COPC

The conceptual elements of COPC develop from social medicine and community medicine approaches. It addresses the health status of a population and its socio-cultural-economic determinants by implementing and evaluating community interventions. It considers the health of individuals in the context of their families and communities, addressing not only personal needs but community health needs as well. This is realized through the integration of primary care with public health (see Chapter 7).

This conceptual framework is translated into practice following a six-step process (see Chapter 4). Its methodological framework entails the use of epidemiology as the basic science for the assessment of health needs and determinants and the identification of risk groups. Concomitantly, social and behavioral sciences are used for an in-depth analysis and understanding of the individual and community dimensions of health and health care.

The definition of *community* is essential in COPC because in this approach the healthcare team takes responsibility for the health care of all members of the community, whether geographically or otherwise defined. The principles of taking responsibility for the community's identified health needs and the intervention in the natural history of a prioritized health problem in which the community has an active, participative role are the essence of the COPC process. This is realized in a healthcare service that is characterized as being accessible, providing pro-active and comprehensive care, and implementing interventions based on health needs carried out by a multidisciplinary team that performs outreach activities, with intersectorial cooperation.

The *adoption* of the principles of COPC has to be accompanied by the *adaptation* of the methodology to the local realities and healthcare system. See Figure 3-1.

FIGURE 3-1 The Community-Oriented Primary Care (COPC) Approach

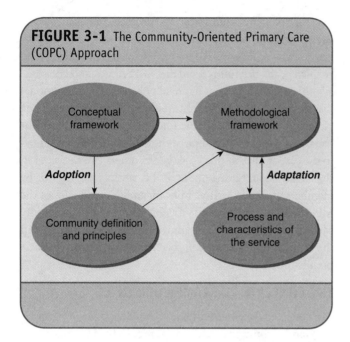

THE FIVE COPC PRINCIPLES

The five COPC principles are (1) responsibility for the health and health care of a defined population; (2) health care based on identified health needs at the population level; (3) prioritization; (4) interventions covering all stages of the health–illness continuum of a selected condition; and (5) community participation (see Table 3-1).

Responsibility for the Health and Health Care of a Defined Population

By taking responsibility for the health and health care of a defined population, COPC goes further than considering health at the individual level and care based on the demand. This principle requires having a defined population that includes not only health clinic users or sick individuals, but also healthy individuals for which preventive and promotional activities can be developed. The defined population determines the denominator for the measurement of health status (morbidity

TABLE 3-1 The COPC Principles

Responsibility for the health of a defined population	• Considers the defined community as the target and as a partner • Includes healthy and sick individuals, not only clinic users • Determines the denominator for calculations of rates and for health surveillance
Care is based on the identified health needs and determinants at the population level	• Promotes the fulfillment of responsibility that care is not based only on demand • Considers the determinants of health • Allows for an objective prioritization process of health needs and opportunities to organize the service accordingly
Prioritization	• Allows a rational use of resources • Allows the priority health condition(s) to be decided by the healthcare team and community members • Applies an objective and transparent process that follows predetermined criteria
Program of intervention covers all the stages of the health–illness continuum	• Addresses the health condition at all stages from its asymptomatic stage to symptom manifestation and its outcomes (identifies the determinants and risk factors at each stage) • Provides care through health promotion, prevention, and curative treatment • Promotes continuity of care
Community participation	• Works *with* the community, not only *in* the community • Involves community members and community organizations • Requires the willingness of the community to exercise its right to participate in its own care

and mortality rates, case-fatality rates, etc.), health indexes (infant mortality, low birth weight, birth rate, adolescent pregnancy rate, etc.), and the use of healthcare services (proportion of the population using the service, referral rates, compliance with advice, etc.). It allows for surveillance of these measurements over time and identifies at-risk populations.

Health Care Based on Identified Health Needs at the Population Level

The community's health needs reach beyond clinical cases because they might convey only the tip of the iceberg. For example, some individuals in need of health care may not consult the clinic for different reasons, such as lack of access due to language, financial barriers, or lack of legal residence documentation. Hence, health needs have to be identified through information provided by all the community members, beyond individual consultations. It includes not only physical health, but also mental and emotional health and behaviors and their sociocultural, environmental, and biological determinants.

For example, the prevalence of children with asthma may be higher than is revealed by clinic records because not all patients who experience the condition seek care. Depression might not be identified in a clinical contact, or patients may not consult for it. Furthermore, blood pressure, weight, and height are not often measured in clinics because of lack of time or human resources. Additionally, other problems may exist that the healthcare professionals do not consider. Those problems may not be specifically examined and would not be known among members of the community who do not attend the clinic. Those conditions could include poor vision, anemia in infancy, lack of breastfeeding, poor dental health, urinary incontinence, or mental health problems.

One of the reasons for persistent disparities in the health of a population is the magnitude of undiagnosed cases of specific conditions that are prevalent in the population and the lack of knowledge or understanding of the determinants of health. This may affect the success of interventions.

Prioritization

The identification of the most prevalent health problems in the community allows for a prioritization process and the organization of healthcare services accordingly, in terms of structure, expertise, and allocation of resources. The various community health problems that are faced by a healthcare service and a community at any given point in time compete for the limited human and economic resources both inside and outside the healthcare sector. Diabetes, hypertension, and obesity may coexist in a community alongside asthma, HIV, teenage pregnancy, depression, and other conditions. This requires a process of prioritization by the healthcare service and the community that offers opportunities for starting on common ground and engaging the community in its own care. (See Chapter 4 for a discussion of prioritization methodology.)

Intervention Covering All Stages of the Health–Illness Continuum of a Selected Condition

By providing care to a whole population, including ill and healthy people, the healthcare service takes the responsibility for disease prevention, health promotion, treatment, and rehabilitation. This is relevant for all conditions. For example, with hypertension, the initiative of the service for an early diagnosis is important because half of the people suffering from the condition are not diagnosed. Moreover, half of those who are diagnosed remain untreated, and half of those who are treated do not have their blood pressure under control.[36] This requires the healthcare service providers to take a proactive role in all the stages of the condition. Considering that this is one of the well-known risk factors for cardiovascular diseases, health care requires a comprehensive approach, including prevention, promotion, treatment, and rehabilitation. Additionally, the identification of other risk factors, such as hypercholesterolemia, obesity, diabetes, sedentary life habits, and smoking, also require comprehensive interventions, which need multisectoral coordination to assure an appropriate environment that supports healthy living habits.

Community Participation

Community participation entails working *with* the community, not only *in* the community. In each community, the nature of its members' participation in their health care will depend on, among other things, the level of community organization, the cultural and social characteristics of the community members, the degree of social cohesion, and both the community's and the healthcare providers' expectations (see Chapter 6).

Dialogue, mutual respect, and cooperation between the healthcare team and the community is an important component in achieving continuity and sustainable changes in healthcare delivery and the success of health intervention programs. The healthcare team should proactively promote and facilitate community participation in all the steps of the approach as a principle that characterizes COPC.

Some of the challenges in community participation are the vested interests of some groups that advocate for their special concerns and not the common good. The eroding sense of community, especially in places where diverse backgrounds, organizations, and sectors exist, may affect mutual trust and preclude problem solving.

The application of the five COPC principles are evident in different programs in various countries,[21,37–42] and some of them are described in the cases studies in this book. The COPC principles are recognized by the Canadian Health Services Research Foundation as one of the few collaboration approaches between primary care and public health that uses a theoretical framework.[43] This view is shared by New Zealand primary care organizations[44] and the Pan American Health Organization (PAHO).[45]

Do all five principles need to be present for a service to be defined as a COPC practice? A definite answer does not exist. Although applying the five principles in a primary care practice would definitely provide a positive answer, a practice that is applying some of the principles may be in the process of developing COPC services. The development may not be realized in a short time because the pace of implementation needs to be adapted to the local realities regarding material and human resources. A practice that provides good, quality care in treating or rehabilitating patients or that engages in preventive services, promotional activities, or epidemiological studies may benefit a defined population. Yet it may not necessarily constitute a COPC practice if these activities are done with an individual focus, without considering the community context. Community participation itself could be an excellent example of inclusion, but it may not necessarily constitute a COPC practice if all the other principles are lacking. Although COPC shouldn't pretend to be prescriptive, the focus in the total defined community, care based on the identified health needs, and community participation must be considered.

CHARACTERISTICS OF A COPC SERVICE

The characteristics of a COPC service depends on the specific healthcare system where it is developed and its organization and resources, as expressed in Table 3-2.

COPC AND COMMUNITY DEVELOPMENT

Is community development inherent to the conceptual framework of COPC? Community development goes beyond active community involvement in the improvement of the various dimensions of social life and health care. The community is not an object; it is an actor of community development. Geiger stated that "although community development and social change are not explicit goals of COPC, they are implicit in COPC's emphasis on community organization and local participation with health professionals in the assessment of health problems."[46]

Community development is related to empowerment, the highest level of community participation (see Chapter 6), when aspects other than health are part of the process. When community members have the option and the ability to take an active role in decisions related to their health care and social life, they may experience their own personal, familial, and com-

TABLE 3-2 Characteristics of a COPC Service

Accessibility	Be aware of and reduce barriers to accessibility—geographic, economic (insurance), religious, cultural, communication.
Comprehensive care	Identify and care for physical, mental, and social dimensions of individuals, families, and communities.
Multidisciplinary team	The varied health needs require the input of different disciplines, based on available resources.
Outreach	Work outside of clinic walls Identify microenvironment (housing) determinants of health and identify available resources at family and neighborhood levels.
Proactive approach	Identify healthcare needs at the community level and subsequently initiate care.
Intersectorial cooperation	Addressing the health problems of a community may need the coordination and cooperation of other sectors, such as education, social services, NGO's, etc.

munity development. It is important to emphasize that community development initiated and promoted from external organizations or experts may have a different impact than when it is initiated and promoted by community members or local organizations.

In Kark's pioneering work in Pholela, community development, as mentioned earlier, was expressed through intervention programs. For example, vegetable gardens were grown for family use and for selling products, in which community members, children, patients, and staff were involved.[21] In parallel, residents of the area were trained and became the majority of the healthcare team.

During the 1960s in the United States, the federal Office of Economic Opportunity initiated a "war on poverty." The agency promoted a war on deprivation and inequality by different social movements. COPC-based healthcare centers were included in this program, and the Tufts School of Medicine, working in Bolivar County in the Mississippi Delta, had the opportunity to experiment with community development by combining the actions of different local institutions. The COPC healthcare programs, in addition to the curative and preventive roles, became an instrument of community development. In these communities, malnutrition was one of the main health problems. The healthcare team handled prescriptions for food (milk, fruits, meat, vegetables), and in addition to a cooperative to grow vegetables, they created a new occupation called *nutritional sharecropping*.[47] In that way, the health center was able to succeed in nutritional improvement and in creating new opportunities for employment that supported economic growth for the community.

Although this process of community development entails coordination with other relevant community services (education, culture, welfare), the COPC team must consider its role as promoter, leader, or partner. For that purpose, the team needs to have knowledge and understanding of the degree of social cohesion in the community and take into account the position and capabilities of the healthcare service.

THE DISCIPLINES OF COPC

Epidemiology plays an essential role in COPC. It complements the clinical assessment of a health condition by providing its population dimension (see Chapter 8). The epidemiology of primary care[48,49] or local research,[50] which is community oriented and service oriented, serves two purposes: (1) identifying community needs by analyzing existing data or carrying out surveys in the defined population to establish baseline information; and (2) evaluating performance and outcomes. It is the epidemiological reasoning that helps practitioners to realize that the causes of consultations

at the clinical level are not necessarily representative of the problems at community level. "The inverse care law"[51] expresses that people with the least need of healthcare services use those services more frequently.

Social and behavioral sciences are needed for an understanding of the determinants of health. The influence of cultural practices and the social, economic, and political contexts of communities and their governing bodies all impact the individuals' and the community's health. The use of qualitative methods, in addition to quantitative measures, creates a comprehensive picture of the community, which allows for a better understanding of community needs and practices. A process of triangulation—integrating the knowledge from different sources and by different methods—strengthens the interpretation of the available information. The use of epidemiological methods and social and behavioral sciences alone in a primary care setting do not assure a COPC approach unless it is integrated into the identification of needs that are followed by programs to address those needs.

COPC AND FAMILY MEDICINE

Family medicine can be considered the basic specialty in COPC. Its wide focus on the individual's or family's medical and psychosocial dimension is parallel to some of the elements of COPC, but it does not always fulfill the community dimension. Experience shows that there are two different trends among family physicians and general practitioners: (1) physicians whose focus and interest are on the quality of clinical care and the importance of communication skills in the physician–patient relationship, and (2) physicians who, in addition to the previously mentioned attributes, extend their expertise to a community orientation.

The second approach was studied in a sample of 500 young primary care physicians in the United States; the study measured the physicians' interaction with the community.[52] Their activities were categorized in four distinctive groups: (1) identifying and intervening in community health problems, (2) responding to the cultural features of the community, (3) coordinating the use of community resources, and (4) contributing beyond care to individual patients. The study results demonstrated a limited community dimension, showing no interaction of the COPC features.[53]

As an indicator of a welcome turning point in its organizational policy, the World Organization of Family Doctors (Wonca) recommended the development of a community-orientated approach in the Durban Declaration.[54] It emphasized the need for a combination of approaches, including primary health care, public health, and clinical and community development. This new policy was reinforced in a 2002 Wonca guidebook[55] that considers COPC to be a component of family doctors' strategies for implementing primary health care, based on previous COPC published experiences.

A notable example of the extension of family medicine to incorporate a community orientation in their profession and practice was developed in Catalonia, Spain (see Case Study 12) with the formation of a COPC Working Group within the Catalan Society of Family and Community Medicine. COPC capacity-building programs influenced the creation and development of a network of 43 community-oriented practices.[38] The 20 years of experience in Catalonia shows that both family medicine and COPC benefit from the extension of the scope of care to the community. Family medicine enriches its quality of care by being aware of the community determinants of health. COPC benefits by continuously adapting its methods to the local reality of the healthcare system. Through the team approach of family medicine in Catalonia, other professional members of the primary care team became aware and interested in the content and practice of COPC. See Figure 3-2.

COPC AND NURSING

Nursing care has a special role in COPC. By training and vocation, nurses' perspective of care is broad and is a natural fit for their role in the COPC functions of promotion, prevention, treatment, and rehabilitation. Their activities could be at the individual, family, or community levels. Their involvement requires the necessary skills for the identification and care of the socio-cultural-economic determinants of health. Training in public health with an emphasis on sociobehavioral sciences, health education, counseling, and outreach activities provides nurses with skills and knowledge for the practice of community health care. This provides a better understanding and closer relationship with individuals and families. Nurses have a major role in the promotion and facilitation of community participation activities.[56,57]

COPC AS AN INTEGRATION OF PRIMARY CARE AND PUBLIC HEALTH FUNCTIONS

The functions of COPC are an encounter between primary care and public health. As demonstrated in Table 3-3, the approach is integrative in purpose (protect and maintain health at the individual and community level), in content (carry out activities of health promotion, prevention, and treatment), and in process (carry out primary care and public health functions by the same team or service).

According to these functions, COPC could also be an interface between top–down planning (vertical programs) and bottom–up activities (generated by the local team and the community). (See Case Study 16.)

COPC EFFECTIVENESS

The application of COPC throughout the years in different countries and healthcare systems showed the effectiveness of the approach. In 1988, an exhaustive review of the effectiveness of COPC since the early experiences in South Africa showed the reduction of infant mortality, improvement in children's growth and development, a reduction in the incidence and prevalence of infectious diseases, increased coverage of immunizations, control of risk factors for chronic conditions, and changes in population health behaviors.[58]

A special issue of the *American Journal of Public Health* in 2002 analyzed the application of COPC in five countries. The experience in Dallas, Texas, regarding programs in several clinics showed an improvement in the access to healthcare services, a reduction in children's and adults'

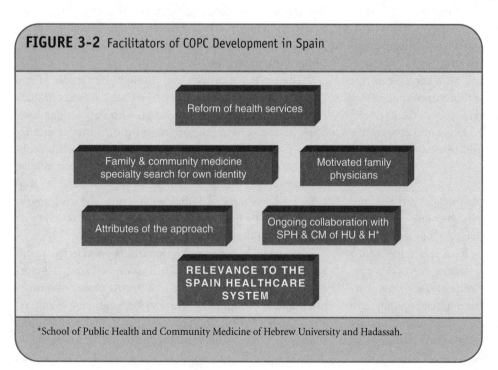

FIGURE 3-2 Facilitators of COPC Development in Spain

Reform of health services

Family & community medicine specialty search for own identity

Motivated family physicians

Attributes of the approach

Ongoing collaboration with SPH & CM of HU & H*

RELEVANCE TO THE SPAIN HEALTHCARE SYSTEM

*School of Public Health and Community Medicine of Hebrew University and Hadassah.

TABLE 3-3 COPC: An Integration of Primary Care and Public Health Functions

Primary care functions	Public health functions
Performs demographic and health surveillance	Provides healthcare services to a defined total population
Screens and treats in clinical care	Uses epidemiology and behavioral and social sciences
Counsels at individual, family, and community levels	Identifies and promotes community participation
Team identifies healthcare needs	Promotes intersectorial coordination
Team addresses the prioritized health conditions	

length of hospitalization, and lower neonatal mortality rates.[37] Additionally, there was an increase in community participation, including decision making about health priorities. In a different social and health system, COPC services in Jerusalem[32] improved children's development, increased breastfeeding, improved oral health, and reduced the prevalence of anemia in children and pregnant women. For the adult population, there was a decreased prevalence of smoking habits and improvement of hypertension control. Experiences in Pholela and Mississippi[21,46] displayed an increase in community participation and community organization, improvement of the economic and social conditions, and the reduction of poverty. In the United Kingdom, COPC improved the working organization of primary care practice teams, enabled teams to acquire skills to make community diagnoses, and modestly reduced community members' behavioral risk factors.[59]

In addition, a literature review in 2008 based on 170 peer-reviewed articles analyzed the completeness in the application of the COPC model and its effectiveness, with the recommendation for more research in both aspects.

CAPACITY BUILDING IN COPC

Clinical care and community medicine are the bases of COPC. Although clinical knowledge and skills are acquired in medical schools, students are rarely exposed to community medicine or even learning in community settings. Only a few hours of the total curriculum is dedicated to epidemiology, public health, and social sciences. Family medicine and pediatrics are the specialties whose field of action is primary care, but mostly they are dedicated to individuals.

A 1961 article titled *The Ecology of Medical Care*,[61] based on studies from the United States and Britain and reproduced in 2001 in the United States,[62] is a case in point to demonstrate the vision that a medical student may have of the health problems afflicting the population. The studies consistently

showed that when subjects were asked about illnesses experienced in an average month, about 750/1000 responded positively. Subsequently, the subjects were asked whether they consulted a physician, and 250 responded affirmatively; 10 of them were referred to a hospital, 1 of which was hospitalized in a university teaching hospital (see Figure 3-3).

From that reality, the vision that a medical student may have of community health problems is really limited (see Figure 3-4). An improvement of that vision could be provided by primary care clinics, which have the potential to see a patient in the family context, although not always in the community context (see Figure 3-5).

To have a complete picture of community health problems and to identify populations at risk or those who do not consult services because of different types of barriers, the population

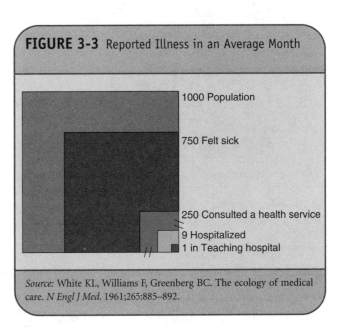

FIGURE 3-3 Reported Illness in an Average Month

1000 Population

750 Felt sick

250 Consulted a health service

9 Hospitalized

1 in Teaching hospital

Source: White KL, Williams F, Greenberg BC. The ecology of medical care. *N Engl J Med.* 1961;265:885–892.

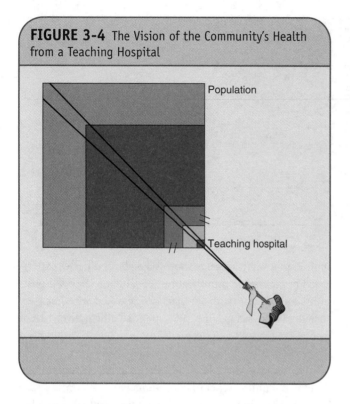

FIGURE 3-4 The Vision of the Community's Health from a Teaching Hospital

approach provided by COPC is needed. This vision also includes healthy people for which preventive care and health promotion are needed. This constitutes the training needed for the COPC approach (see Figure 3-6).

Although other professions, such as nursing, may have more comprehensive training in community health, a need for integration of the disciplines still exists. Capacity building in COPC can best be realized by interprofessional training where the different disciplines involved in community health care share the same learning space, which should be community based. To achieve the vision established in Figure 3-6, there are two requirements: (1) having primary care settings that practice COPC and (2) training professionals on COPC.

The different domains that are related to COPC and the teaching–learning process require that this approach not be taught in a lecture-based course. One option, whenever it is possible according to the type and number of participants (students of health sciences, healthcare professionals, and people with other positions in the healthcare system), the time available, and academic requirements, is to carry out an intensive educational program. It could be a program based on interactive

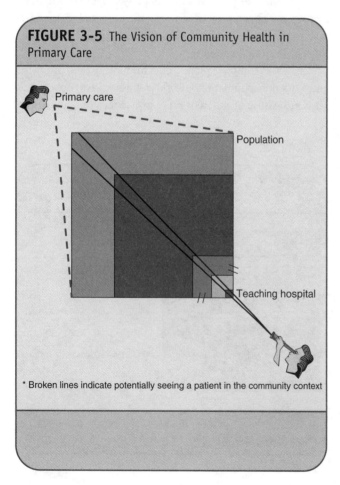

FIGURE 3-5 The Vision of Community Health in Primary Care

* Broken lines indicate potentially seeing a patient in the community context

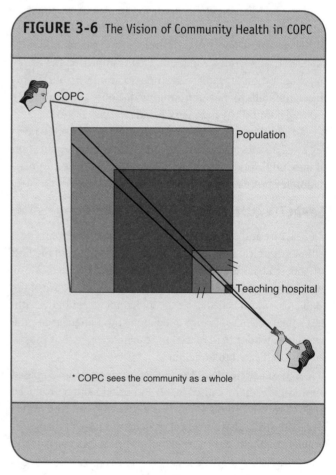

FIGURE 3-6 The Vision of Community Health in COPC

* COPC sees the community as a whole

work, such a workshop with relatively small groups of participants that focus on knowledge, experience, and competencies or skills to be used in a proposal for a COPC program based on real data.

Example of a COPC Workshop

The format of this example is based on the experience of the COPC Workshop, a core course for public health students in the Jerusalem MPH program.[63] The workshop was later adapted to an intensive and concentrated method, a 5-day, 40-hour program[38] carried out in different countries and with different professionals. The adaptation also took into account the target audience such as with family physicians and general practitioners in residency programs; district administrators in health management programs; and in-services for physicians and nurses in diverse health institutions.

Objectives

- Learn the principles and methods of community-oriented primary care (COPC).
- Apply the COPC approach in the participant's healthcare services.

Content

- integration of curative, promotive, and preventive care
- health needs assessment
- stages of COPC development
- development of population-based health programs
- evaluation of effectiveness
- approaches to community participation
- intersectoral cooperation
- multidisciplinary team and outreach
- uses of epidemiology in primary care

Participants

- healthcare workers related to primary care
- professionals with responsibilities in planning and management of healthcare service delivery
- public health students
- nursing students
- students of other health sciences

Methods

The format of the workshop combines short introductory lectures and the work of small groups that are, whenever possible, made up of people from different professions to resemble a healthcare team. The groups of six or seven participants will have the assignment of planning a proposal for the development of COPC in their own services. For this purpose, the participants are required to prepare and bring data from their own practices. The work in groups will constitute 60–70% of the total time of the workshop. A tutor is assigned to work in each group throughout the workshop. Relevant literature are distributed to the participants in advance of the workshop.

Workshop Planning, Preparation, and Evaluation

The planning and preparation of a workshop requires the involvement of teachers and healthcare professionals who are working in the same healthcare system as the participants. Whenever possible, it is relevant to carry out a workshop on the premises of a COPC practice setting where the practice's healthcare team leads the teaching. Otherwise, because of the assignment to prepare a feasible proposal for a COPC program in the actual practice, it is appropriate to use real data from the participants' practices and populations to reproduce a real-life situation in a classroom environment.

Evaluations of workshops by MPH graduates and family physicians in Israel[33] and Spain[38] have shown that the workshops were useful in the respondent's current work. Several of the case studies presented in this book (Benin, Chad, Colombia, Moldova, Spain, and Uruguay) are outcome expressions of COPC academic training and its adaptability to the reality of different countries, systems, and contexts.

GLOBAL DISSEMINATION OF COPC

COPC is being practiced across the globe in different settings and healthcare systems. Some examples are a professional society in Catalonia, Spain; a training center for healthcare professionals in the United Kingdom; the Ministry of Public Health in Uruguay; and a university in Washington, DC. In addition to these developments, COPC has been applied in various countries.[64–70] The settings determine the focus of the programs, whether teaching, practice, or a combination of both. As mentioned, COPC programs dissemination have been influenced by the teaching and practice of the Jerusalem team[32] and the graduates of the School of Public Health, as illustrated by the some of the case studies in this book.

Notably, there are models based on the same elements of COPC but denominated differently, such as the census-based, impact–oriented (CBIO) approach[71] in Bolivia, Haiti, and Bangladesh. Additionally, there are applications of COPC, though not under this name, at the national level in Cuba[72,73] and Costa Rica,[74] at the regional level in Brazil,[75,76] and in Canada.[77] At the international healthcare organization level, there are also developments related to COPC, notably the Pan American Health Organization (PAHO), Wonca, and The Network: Towards Unity for Health.

With the purpose to reexamine the 25-year application of the primary-healthcare model after the Alma-Ata conference,

PAHO decided to analyze the experience in the American Region of the WHO. Intensive and extensive studies of different experiences in the region were carried out, resulting in the recommendation of a new strategy for a primary-healthcare-based system. The recommendation expressed in the Declaration of Montevideo considers primary-healthcare approaches like COPC. One of the results of these recommendations was a PAHO report on a primary-healthcare-oriented medical training proposal, where COPC is also considered.[78] The WHO's *World Health Report 2008* emphasized the role of a renewed primary-healthcare approach, which is close to the concepts and practices of COPC.[79]

Additionally, the PAHO, through its Health of the Indigenous People of the Americas Program, organized a COPC experts meeting in Ecuador in 2008. The experts analyzed the application of this approach in indigenous populations. The meeting's recommendation suggested testing the application of COPC in two sites in the region. As previously described, the World Organization of Family Doctors (Wonca) considers COPC to be an approach to new roles of family physicians in the community. Also, The Network: Towards Unity For Health,[80] an NGO officially related to the WHO, represents about 150 academic institutions of health sciences worldwide, mainly medical schools, whose teaching curricula are community oriented. As part of The Network, the Integrating Medicine and Public Health Task Force works and promotes the integration of medicine and public health through the COPC approach, among others.

Factors Contributing to the Application of COPC

An analysis of this accumulated experience identifies factors that contribute to the application of COPC in different healthcare systems (see Figure 3-7). Although all of these factors are expressed as a framework, not all of these elements played the same role in each application. The essential factor is the attributes and relevance of the COPC approach to the local healthcare system. It constitutes the promoter and catalytic factor that requires the presence (in minor or major degree) of all the other factors to facilitate the application. Special mention should be given to motivation, a needed factor in any process of change and

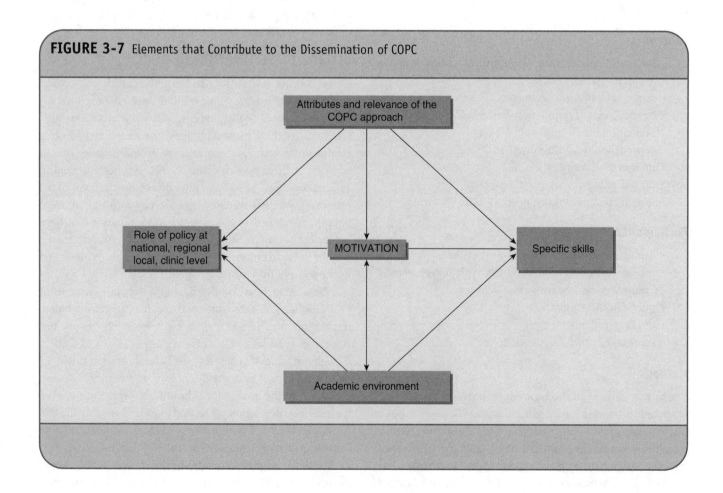

FIGURE 3-7 Elements that Contribute to the Dissemination of COPC

development. Healthcare structure and organization are mentioned frequently as the obstacle to a larger application of COPC.[81]

COPC IN THE UNITED STATES

There is a history of more than 50 years in the teaching and application of the COPC approach in the United States.

Teaching

Residency Programs

The teaching of COPC in the United States primarily occurs in residency programs of family medicine, family practice, preventive medicine, and community medicine. COPC is also incorporated into rural healthcare programs and fellowship programs, with very few programs for medical students.[82] In the United States, where a major concentration of interest exists in the education and practice of COPC, there is a gap between the teaching and practice of COPC. An example of this gap was evidenced in the literature review of 300 articles on community health. Among them, 170 referred explicitly to COPC[60] in family medicine or nursing, mainly from the United States, England, and Israel. Although 60% of the articles were related to general theory and education, only 25% were categorized as project reports and research.

In relation to the recommendation by the Association of Family Practice Residency Directors (AFPRD) to include COPC as a required component of curricula, a survey about community medicine training, administered to 244 randomly selected family practice residency programs, found that less than half of the programs included COPC in their curricula.[83] Further examples of the gap between teaching and practice was provided by another survey carried out among 400 practicing physicians and 470 residency directors. It was found that almost 40% of the programs teach COPC, but only 7% of physicians reported the practice of COPC.[84] Despite the gap between teaching and practice, the considerable interest in COPC in the United States is expressed in the aforementioned literature review.[60] Other authors analyze the meaning, relevance, and recommendations for new methodological tools to facilitate the application of COPC.[85–89]

Area Health Education Center

The Area Health Education Center (AHEC), a national program geared toward health sciences students, has also developed COPC programs. In the District of Columbia, AHEC's mission is to improve the health status of the disadvantaged residents of the district.[90] Activities are taking place through clinical placements of health sciences students throughout the district. COPC was naturally included as part of the curriculum. The COPC module covers a description of the principles, characteristics, and steps for COPC implementation, essay questions for students and scholars, and selected sources of information on demographics and health status in the United States.

Health Resources and Services Administration

Another development was made by the Health Resources and Services Administration (HRSA) of the US Department of Health and Human Services through its Center for Quality. HRSA adopted COPC principles into its Health Disparities Collaborative program, which has been operating for more than a decade. COPC was also considered for practice and training programs at community healthcare centers (CHCs) throughout the country. This national quality improvement effort linking primary care and public health was described in a document prepared by the George Washington University COPC team. In this document COPC competencies were formulated to align COPC training curricula with two other models that were already implemented: the Communities of Practice Model and the Chronic Care Model. This has resulted in the creation of the Expanded Care Model framework, which is now being used in the Health Disparities Collaborative program. It is a patient-centered, expanded-care team approach to the delivery of care within a comprehensive healthcare service. The George Washington University document includes teaching material to be used in training health sciences professionals at CHCs and is reported to have been used extensively for HRSA internal dialogues. It is also used as reference for HRSA's report to the US Congress on the national work in progress on quality improvement. COPC principles are specifically referenced in upcoming publications about these quality improvement collaboratives.[91]

George Washington University

In 1992, the Program of Public Health at George Washington University (GWU) engaged in exploratory discussions about the community medicine dimension in its teaching. This was followed by COPC training programs for primary care practitioners working in Washington, DC. In 1996, these activities were the seminal background that developed into the first MPH COPC program in the country at the GWU School of Public Health and Health Services in the Department of Prevention and Community Health.[92] A 1-year COPC International Certificate Distance Learning Program was launched in 1998 as a joint program by GWU and Hebrew University in Jerusalem.

Development of the George Washington University COPC Activities
A process was initiated in 2004 for the COPC team

to extend GWU's academic activities beyond the teaching program. As a result, the COPC team has been involved in several activities outside the university field. At the invitation of PAHO, the team prepared a document on the community-oriented dimension of family and community health for the WHO's American Region. The document was distributed to the countries in the region and became one of the bases of a renewed Family and Community Health program in the American Region, which was recently approved by PAHO.

The COPC team was also involved in several activities with the leadership of city hospitals interested in enlarging their community orientation role. The activities included suggestions on COPC programs and on the process of coalition building. Participants included managers, physicians, and nurses from primary care settings in the area.

Additionally, in 2008 the US Department of Health and Human Services, along with five of its federal agencies, decided to develop healthcare programs for elderly Hispanics in the United States. Eight sites with the largest populations of elderly Hispanics were included in the program. Technical assistance on community orientation in the planned intervention was provided by the GWU COPC team, based on the elements of the COPC approach (see Case Study 9).

Practice

Early practices in the 1950s

By the 1950s in the United States, there were community practices based on similar principles of the Karks' work. One of them was at the Navajo Nation's Many Farms community in Arizona. The practice was initiated by Dr. Deuschle and his team in conjunction with the Indian Health Services, and it demonstrated an impact on quality of care. The project later developed into an academic department of community medicine in Kentucky.[93]

In 1957, Jack Geiger, then a young physician and today a recognized public health personality, visited Pholela to learn about the innovations in the delivery of primary care developed by the Karks. Shortly after, Geiger[46,94] played a key role in the development of neighborhood health centers that today include a network of about 1200 community health centers around the United States, providing care to about 20 million people.[95]

Practices of COPC

There are numerous COPC practices in the United States, including family practice in Arkansas[56]; Ramsey Family and Community Medicine in Minneapolis, Minnesota[42]; Mound Bayou, Mississippi Indian health services[46]; adolescent school-based services in Dartmouth, New Hampshire, and in Southwest New Mexico,[96] for children and adults in Rochester, New York,[39] and Dallas, Texas[37]; the Rural Health initiative in Rockford, Illinois[97]; underserved communities in St. Louis, Missouri[98]; the MetroHealth Clement Center in Cleveland, Ohio[85]; and Rush Medical College in Chicago, Illinois.[99]

Recommendation for further implementation of COPC

The previously mentioned International Conference on COPC, which was organized by the IOM in 1982, was instrumental in the analysis of numerous COPC experiences in the country. The organization recommended that the COPC approach be implemented throughout the United States, including program expansion outside of deprived areas.[100] There are also renewed recommendations for COPC to be applied in the United States,[101] and discussions are taking place about the feasibility and applicability of the COPC approach in the American healthcare system.[81] There are numerous other health approaches that refer and include community activities, although they are not focused on a total community and primary care services.[102–106]

THE FUTURE OF COPC

What could be the future of COPC? What could be the possible determinants of increasing the application of COPC? Although the practices and case studies included in this book reflect a worldwide practice of the COPC approach, challenges and barriers exist. Among them are the increasing costs of healthcare services with the subsequent cost-containment policies; the fee-for-service reimbursement system; the threat of an increasing shortage of human resources in primary care; the lack of health sciences professionals training in community orientation; and the lack of primary care settings in which to learn and practice community orientation.

However, there are also developments in health care that could have a positive influence for an increased application of the COPC approach, such as the following:

- Studies of different healthcare systems in developed and developing countries show that a strong primary care infrastructure determines better population health, lower costs, and increased satisfaction.[107–108]
- Hospitals are interested in extending their care to the community level.
- There is a need to have appropriate approaches for the care of aged populations with the concomitant increasing prevalence of chronic conditions.
- The PAHO, WHO, and Wonca have made recommendations for a renewed primary care approach (similar to COPC) in developing and underdeveloped countries.

- There are current healthcare services reforms with an emphasis on primary care, such as in Brazil's Family Health Program,[75] New Zealand's primary healthcare organization,[44] and Catalonia's new law on public health and primary care.[109]

In addition to these developments, the increasing interest in and knowledge about the role of social determinants of health in community health, the initiatives to reduce inequalities and inequities, and the social justice attributes of COPC offer an appropriate methodology for the development of the approach.

SUMMARY

COPC is a primary care delivery approach that was pioneered by Sidney L. Kark and Emily Kark in Pholela, South Africa in the 1940s and 1950s; it has been further developed in Jerusalem since the 1960s. COPC is based on providing primary care to well and sick individuals and also focusing on promoting the health of the community as a whole or any of its subgroups. It addresses the healthcare needs of the community through the integration of primary care and public health. The application and effectiveness of COPC have been demonstrated in different settings and healthcare systems globally.

There are five principles of COPC: (1) responsibility for the health and health care of a defined population; (2) care based on the identified health needs at the population level; (3) prioritization; (4) interventions covering all stages of the health–illness continuum of a selected condition; and (5) community participation. The characteristics of services where COPC is applied include (1) accessibility; (2) comprehensive care; (3) a multidisciplinary team; (4) outreach activities; and (5) a proactive approach; (6) and intersectorial cooperation. The adoption of the principles for a given practice needs to be paired with the adaptation of the methodology to the realities of the specific community and service.

Some of the constraints for the development of COPC are a fragmented healthcare system, a limited workforce, and a fee-for-service reimbursement system. The opportunities for the development of COPC are reforms in healthcare services, national and international initiatives to integrate primary care and public health, increased community interest and involvement in health and health care, information technology, and policies that emphasize and support the essential role of primary care in the healthcare system.

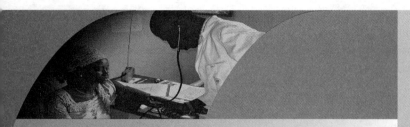

Discussion Questions

- How relevant are the principles of COPC to the current organization of the healthcare system in your country?

- How pertinent is it to adapt the methodology of COPC to the current primary care services in your country?

- Are all principles needed to fulfill the COPC approach?

- To what extent is the training of physicians and nurses appropriate for the practice of COPC?

- How could COPC increase its role in the practice of public health?

Review Questions

- What is COPC?

- What are the elements of Social Medicine as practiced in Pholela?

- What are the principles of COPC?

- What characteristics should a COPC service have?

- What are the disciplines used by COPC?

- What are some of the factors that facilitate the application of COPC?

REFERENCES

1. Kark SL, Kark E. Promoting community health: from Pholela to Jerusalem. Johannesburg, South Africa: Witwatersrand University Press; 1999.

2. Kark SL. The practice of community-oriented primary health care. New York, NY: Appleton-Century-Crofts; 1981.

3. Seipp C, ed. *Health Care for the Community: Selected Papers of John B. Grant.* Baltimore, MD: Johns Hopkins University Press; 1963.

4. Pickles WM. *Epidemiology in Country Practice.* Bristol, England: John Wright; 1939.

5. Hart JT. *A New Kind of Doctor.* London, England: Merlin Press; 1988.

6. World Health Organization, United Nations Children's Fund. *Primary Health Care: Report of the International Conference on Primary Health Care, Alma Ata, USSR, 6–12 September, 1978.* Geneva, Switzerland: World Health Organization; 1978. Health for All Series No. 1.

7. Susser M. Pioneering community oriented primary care. *Bull World Health Org.* 1999;77:436–438.

8. Crampton P, Dowell A, Woodward A. Third sector primary care for vulnerable populations. *Soc Sci & Med.* 2001;53:1491–1502.

9. Litsios S. The Christian medical commission and development of the World Health Organization's primary health care approach. *Am J Public Health.* 2004;94:1884–1893.

10. Gofin J, Gofin R. Community oriented primary care and primary health care. *Am J Public Health.* 2005;95:757.

11. Schaay N, Sanders D. *International Perspective on Primary Health Care over the Past 30 Years.* Cape Town, South Africa: School of Public Health, University of the Western Cape; date unknown. http://www.hst.org.za/uploads/files/chap1_08.pdf. Accessed November 2009.

12. Kark SL, Kark E. An alternative strategy in community health care: community oriented primary health care. *Isr J Med Sci.* 1983;19:756–759.

13. Nutting P, Connor EM. Community *Oriented Primary Care: A Practical Assessment*, Vol II, p.3 Institute of Medicine, National Academy Press, Washington DC, 1984. www.nap.edu/openbook.php?record_id=672&page=R1. Accessed January 2010.

14. King Edward's Hospital Fund for London, Department of Social Medicine of the Hebrew University-Hadassah School of Public Health and Community Medicine. *Community-Oriented Primary Care: A Resource for Developers.* London, England: King's Fund; 1994.

15. Porta M, ed. *A Dictionary of Epidemiology.* 5th ed. New York, NY: Oxford University Press; 2008.

16. Rhyne RL, Bogue R, Kukulka A, Fulmer H, eds. *Community Oriented Primary Care: Health Care for the 21st Century.* Washington, DC: American Public Health Association; 1998.

17. Foz G, Gofin J, Montaner I. Atención primaria orientada a la comunidad: una visión actual. In: Martín Zurro A, Cano Pérez JF, eds. *Atención primaria—conceptos, organización y práctica clínica.* 6th ed. Madrid, Spain: Elsevier; 2008: 345–366.

18. Kark SL. The economic factor in the health of the Bantu in South Africa. *Leech.* 1934;5:18–22.

19. Kark SL. Problems of national health. *Leech.* 1935;6:12–19.

20. Susser M. A South African odyssey in community health: a memoir of the impact of the teachings of Sidney Kark. *Am J Public Health.* 1993;83:1039–1042.

21. Kark SL, Steuart GW, eds. *A Practice of Social Medicine.* Edinburgh, Scotland: Livingstone; 1962.

22. Gofin J. On "a practice of social medicine" by Sidney and Emily Kark. *Soc Med.* 2006;1:107–115. www.socialmedicine.info. Accessed January 28, 2010.

23. Gofin J. Integrating medicine and public health. http://www.the-networktufh.org/publications_resources/positioncontent.asp?id=8&t=Position+Papers. Accessed November 2009.

24. Slome C. Community health in rural Pholela. In: Kark SL, Steuart GW, eds. *A Practice of Social Medicine.* Edinburgh, Scotland: Livingstone; 1962: 269–291.

25. Phillips HT. The 1945 Gluckman report and the establishment of South Africa's health centers. *Am J Public Health.* 1993;83:1037.

26. Tollman S. Community oriented primary care: origins, evolution, applications. *Soc Sci & Med.* 1991;32:633–642.

27. Kark SL. The social pathology of syphilis in Africa. *Int J Epidemiol.* 2003;32:181–186. Original publication: Kark SL. The social pathology of syphilis in Africa. *S Afr Med J.* 1949:23:77–84.

28. Kark SL, Gofin J, Abramson JH, et al. Prevalence of selected health characteristics in men—a community health survey in Jerusalem. *Isr J Med Sci.* 1979;15:732–741.

29. Gofin J, Kark E, Mainemer N, et al. Prevalence of selected health characteristics of women and comparison with men. A community health survey in Jerusalem. *Isr J Med Sci.* 1981;17:145–159.

30. Kark SL. *Epidemiology and Community Medicine.* New York, NY: Appleton-Century-Crofts; 1974.

31. The Braun School of Public Health and Community Medicine – Hadassah and Hebrew University of Jerusalem. http://publichealth.huji.ac.il/eng/about.asp. Accessed November 2009.

32. Epstein L, Gofin J, Gofin R, Neumark Y. The Jerusalem experience: three decades of service, research, and training in community-oriented primary care. *Am J Public Health.* 2002;92:1717–1721.

33. Gofin J, Gofin R, Knishkowy B. Evaluation of a workshop on community oriented primary care (COPC) for family medicine residents in Jerusalem. *Fam Med.* 1995;27:28–34.

34. Kark JD, Abramson JH. Sidney Kark's contributions to epidemiology and community medicine. *Int J Epid.* 2003;32:882–884.

35. Silberberg DS, Baltuch L, Hermoni Y, Viskoper R, Paran E. The role of the doctor–nurse team in control of hypertension in family practice in Israel. *Isr J Med Sci.* 1983;19:752–755.

36. Herman J. Second thoughts: the law of halves. *J Clin Epidemiol.* 1996;49:595–598.

37. Pickens S, Boumbulian P, Anderson RJ, et al. Community-oriented primary care in action: a Dallas story. *Am J Public Health.* 2002;92:1728–1732.

38. Gofin J, Foz G. Training and application of community-oriented primary care (COPC) through family medicine in Catalonia, Spain. *Fam Med.* 2008;40:196–202.

39. Bayer WH, Fiscella K. Patients and community together: a family medicine community-oriented primary care project in an urban private practice. *Arch Fam Med.* 1999;8:546–549.

40. Carter D, Green D. Health promotion: applying COPC to incontinence. *Nurs Times.* 1994;90:44–45.

41. Abramson JH, Gofin J, Hopp C, Schein MH, Naveh P. The CHAD program for the control of cardiovascular risk factors in a Jerusalem community: a 24-year retrospect. *Isr J Med Sci.* 1994;30:108–119.

42. Baker NJ, Harper PG, Reif CJ. Use of clinical indicators to evaluate COPC projects. *J Am Board Fam Pract.* 2002;15:355–360.

43. Martin-Misener R, Valaitis R; Canadian Health Services Research Foundation. *A Scoping Literature Review of Collaboration Between Primary Care and Public Health: A Report.* Ottawa, Ontario, Canada: Canadian Health Services Research Foundation; 2008.

44. Crampton P. The exceptional potential in each primary health organisation: a public health perspective. Opinion piece on the relationship between public health and primary care for the National Health Committee. http://www.phac.health.govt.nz/moh.nsf/pagescm/769/$File/PHandPrimaryCare.doc. Published February 23, 2004. Accessed January 2010.

45. Pan American Health Organization, Serie: The Renewal of Primary Health Care in the Americas, No.2: Medical Education for Primary Health Care. Health Systems and Services Area and Human Resources for Health Development Project, Washington DC, 2009.

46. Geiger JH. Community-oriented primary care: a path to community development. *Am J Public Health.* 2002;92:1713–1716.

47. DeBuono B, González AR, Rosenbaum S, eds. National case study: Jack Geiger and the community health center movement. In: DeBuono B,

González AR, Rosenbaum S, eds. *Moments in Leadership: Case Studies in Public Health Policy and Practice*. New York, NY: Pfizer Global Pharmaceuticals; 2007: 14–26.

48. Abramson JH. Application of epidemiology in community-oriented primary care. *Public Health Rep*. 1984;12:348–353.

49. Mullan F. Primary care epidemiology: new uses of old tools. *Fam Med*. 1986;18:221–225.

50. Goodman A. President Obama's health plan and community-based prevention. *Am J Public Health*. 2009;99:1736–1738.

51. Hart JT. The inverse care law. *Lancet*. 1971;1:405–412.

52. Pathman DC, Steiner BD, Williams E, Riggins T. The four community dimensions of primary care practice. *J Fam Pract*. 1998;46:293–303.

53. Garr DR, Rhyne RL. Primary care and the community [editorial]. *J Fam Pract*. 1998;46:291–292.

54. Wonca Working Party on Rural Practice. Health for all rural people: the Durban Declaration. http://www.globalfamilydoctor.com/aboutWonca/working_groups/rural_training/durban_declaration.htm. Published September 2004. Accessed September 2009.

55. Boelen C, Haq C, Hunt V, Rivo M, Shahady E. Improving health systems: the contribution of family medicine: a guidebook. Singapore: Wonca Best Printing Company; 2002.

56. Hartwig MS, Landis BJ. The Arkansas AHEC model of community oriented primary care. *Holistic Nurs Pract*. 1999;13:28–37.

57. Orpaz R, Korenblit M. Family nursing in community-oriented primary health care. *Int Nurs Rev*. 1994;41:155–159.

58. Abramson JH. Community-oriented primary care: strategy, approaches, and practice—a health care program. *Pub Health Rev*. 1988;16: 35–98.

59. Gillam S, Schamroth A. The community-oriented primary care experience in the United Kingdom. *Am J Public Health*. 2002;92:1721–1725.

60. Gavagan T. A systematic review of COPC: evidence for effectiveness. *J Health Care for Poor and Underserved*. 2008;19:963–980.

61. White KL, Williams F, Greenberg BG. The ecology of medical care. *N Engl J Med*. 1961;265:885–892.

62. Green LA, Fryer GE Jr, Yawn BP, Lanier D, Dovey SM. The ecology of medical care revisited. *N Engl J Med*. 2001;344:2021–2025.

63. Gofin J. Planning the teaching of community health (COPC) in an MPH program. *Pub Health Rev*. 2002;30:293–301.

64. Art B, Deroo L, De Maeseneer J. Towards unity for health utilising community-oriented primary care in education and practice. *Educ Health*. 2007;20(2). http://www.educationforhealth.net. Accessed September 2009.

65. Aday LA, Youssef A, Sheng-wen L, Weihua C, Chen Z. Estimating the risks and prevalence of hypertension in a suburban area of Beijing. *J Community Health*. 1994;19:331–341.

66. Ryne RL, Hertzman PA. Pursing community-oriented primary care in a Russian closed nuclear city: the Sarov-Los Alamos community health partnership. *Am J Public Health*. 2002;92:1740–1742.

67. Tollman SM, Pick WM. Roots, shoots, but too little fruit: assessing the contribution of COPC in South Africa. *Am J Public Health*. 2002;92: 1725–1728.

68. Kazakh Ministry of Health, Ministry of Labor and Social Welfare, and AIHA set to launch national expansion of community-oriented primary healthcare projects [press release]. Washington, DC and Astana, Kazakhstan: American International Health Alliance; December 3, 2004.

69. Nirola DR, Tshering J, Brodie J, Huntington MK. The impact of community-oriented primary care in Trongsa Dzongkhag, Kingdom of Bhutan. *Indian J Community Med*. 2006;31:18–23.

70. Muhammad Gadit AA. Manora Island project: a model primary care project in Pakistan. *J Med Biol Sci*. 2007;1:1–20. http://www.scientificjournals.org/journals2007/articles/1111.pdf. Accessed November 2009.

71. Perry H, Robinson N, Chavez D, et al. Attaining health for all through community partnerships: priniciples of the census-based, impact-oriented (CBIO) approach to primary health care developed in Boliva, South America. *Soc Sci & Med*. 1999;48:1053–1067.

72. Dresang LT, Brebrick L, Murray D, Shallue A, Sullivan-Vedder L. Family medicine in Cuba: community-oriented primary care and complementary and alternative medicine. *J Am Board Fam Pract*. 2005;18:297–303.

73. Huish R. Going where no doctor has gone before: the role of Cuba's Latin American School of Medicine in meeting the needs of some of the world's most vulnerable populations. *Public Health*. 2008;122:552–557.

74. Bertondano I de. The Costa Rican health system: low cost, high value. *Bull World Health Org*. 2003;81:626–627.

75. Escorel S, Giovanella L, Magalhães de Mendocnça MH, De Castro Maia Senna MC. The Family Health Program and the construction of a new model for primary care in Brazil. *Rev Panam Salud Pública*. 2007;21:164–176.

76. Guanais F, Macinko J. Primary care and avoidable hospitalizations: evidence from Brazil. *J Ambul Care Manage*. 2009;32:115–122.

77. Stevenson Rowan M, Hogg W, Huston P. Integrating public health and primary care. *Healthc Policy*. 2007;3:161–181.

78. Pan American Health Organization, 46th Directing Council, Regional Declaration on the new orientations for primary health care (Declaration of Montevideo), Washington, DC, September 2005. www.paho.org/English/GOV/CD/CD46-decl-e.pdf. Accessed February 2010.

79. World Health Organization. *The World Health Report 2008: Primary Health Care (Now More Than Ever)*. Geneva, Switzerland: World Health Organization; 2008.

80. The Network: Towards Unity for Health. What is The Network: Towards Unity for Health? http://www.the-networktufh.org/home/index.asp. Accessed November 2009.

81. Williams RL. Motherhood, apple pie, and COPC. *Ann Fam Med*. 2004;2:100–102. Followed by publication of electronic letters: Farley T, Conundrum, April 2, 2004; Kaufman A, Commentary of Dr. Williams' editorial, April 3, 2004; Like RC, Whiter. COPC and family medicine practice-based research, April 11, 2004; Smith DR, When all else fails, April 22, 2004; Strelnick AH, Community-oriented public health & primary care: learning to share mom's apple pie, May 12, 2004; Gofin J, Gofin R, The relevance of community oriented primary care (COPC)—a comment on the editorial of *Annals of Family Medicine*, June 7, 2004; Cashman SB, Community-oriented primary care: more pies than just apple, August 12, 2004.

82. Glasser M, Hunsaker M, Sweet K, MacDowell M, Meurer M. A comprehensive medical education program response to rural primary care needs. *J Assoc of Am Med Coll*. 2008;83:952–961.

83. Plescia M, Konen JC, Lincourt A. The state of community medicine training in family practice residency programs. *Fam Med*. 2002;34:177–182.

84. Longlett SK, Phillips DM, Wesley RM. Prevalence of community-oriented primary care knowledge, training, and practice. *Fam Med*. 2002; 34:183–189.

85. Williams RL, Crabtree BF, O'Brien C, et al. Practical tools for qualitative community-oriented primary care community assessment. *Fam Med*. 1999;31:488–494.

86. Mettee TM, Martin KB, Williams RL. Tools for community-oriented primary care: a process for linking practice and community data. *J Am Board Fam Pract*. 1998;11:28–33.

87. Williams RL, Flocke SA, Zyzanski SJ, et al. A practical tool for community-oriented primary care community diagnosis using a personal computer. *Fam Med*. 1995;27:39–43.

88. Williams RL, Snider R, Ryan MJ. A key informant "tree" as a tool for community oriented primary care—the Cleveland COPC group. *Fam Pract Res J*. 1994;14:273–280.

89. Gillanders WR, Buss TF, Gemmel D. Assessing the denominator problem in community-oriented primary care. *Fam Med*. 1991;23:275–278.

90. Program Office of the District of Columbia—Area Health Education Center. Mission. http://dcahec.gwumc.edu/html/mission.html. Accessed November 2009.

91. Calvo A, Rainsford Calvo L, Bezold C. Comprehensive Health Homes: using the Expanded Care Model of the HRSA Health Disparities Collaboratives. http://www.altfutures.com/draproject/pdfs/A_Comprehensive_Health_Home_-Using_the_Expanded_Care_Model_of_The_Collaboratives_--_11-21-08_Draft.pdf. Accessed April 2010.

92. Mullan F, Epstein L. Community-oriented primary care: new relevance in a changing world. *Am J Public Health.* 2002;92:1748–1755.

93. Deuschle KW. Community-oriented primary care: lessons learned in three decades. *J Community Health.* 1982;8:13–22.

94. Geiger HJ. The meaning of community oriented primary care in an American context. In: Connor E, Mullan F, eds. *Community Oriented Primary Care. New Directions for Health Services.* Washington, DC: National Academies Press; 1983:60–103.

95. Bureau of Primary Health Care, HRSA, DHHS. 2008 Uniform Data System. Washington, DC; 2009. http://www.ncsddc.org/upload/wysiwyg/2009%20Annual%20Meeting%20Materials/McNamara%20-%20National%20Association%20of%20Community%20Health%20Centers.pdf. Accessed January 2010.

96. Summers LC, Williams J. School-based health center viability: application of the COPC model. *Issues Compr Pediatr Nurs.* 2003;26:231–251.

97. Glasser M, Hunsaker M, Sweet K, MacDowell M, Meurer M. A comprehensive medical education program response to rural primary care needs. *Acad Med.* 2008 Oct;83:952-61.

98. Saint Louis University School of Medicine. SLU AHEC Program. http://medschool.slu.edu/comfam/index.php?page=slu-ahec-program. Accessed November 2009.

99. Bardack M, Thomspon SH. Model prenatal program of Rush Medical College at St. Basil's Free Peoples Clinic, Chicago. *Public Health Rep.* 1993; 108(2):161–165.

100. Nutting PA, Connor EM; Division of Health Care Services, Institute of Medicine. *Community Oriented Primary Care: A Practical Assessment.* Vol 2. Washington, DC: National Academies Press; 1984.

101. Wright RA. Community-oriented primary care: the cornerstone of health care reform. *JAMA.* 1993;269(19):2544–2547.

102. Sanders J, Baisch MJ. *Community based participatory action: Impact on a neighborhood level.* Community Health Improvement Process, Project MUSE, Scholarly Journals online, 2008, John Hopkins University Press http://muse.jhu.edu/journals/progress_in_community_health_partnerships_research_education_and_action/v002/2.1sanders02.pdf. Accessed February 2010.

103. Noris T, Pittman M. The healthy communities movement and the coalition for healthier cities and communities. *Public Health Rep.* 2000;115: 118–124.

104. Centers for Disease Control and Prevention. CDC's Healthy Communities Program. http://www.cdc.gov/HealthyCommunitiesProgram/. Accessed September 2009.

105. Parker E, Margolis LH, Eng E, Henriquez-Roldán C. Assessing the capacity of health departments to engage in community-based participatory public health. *Am J Public Health.* 2003;93:472–476.

106. Citrin T. Enhancing public health research and learning through community–academic partnerships: the Michigan experience. *Public Health Rep.* 2001;116:74–78.

107. Macinko J, Starfield B, Shi L. The contribution of primary care systems to health outcomes within Organization for Economic Cooperation and Development (OECD) countries, 1970–1998. *Health Serv Res.* 2003;38: 831–865.

108. Macinko J, Starfield B, Erinosho T. The impact of primary healthcare on population health in low- and middle-income countries. *J Ambul Care Manage.* 2009;32:150–171.

109. España (Cataluña). Ley 18/2009, 22 de octubre, de salud pública. Diari Oficial de la Generalitat de Catalunya, 30 de octubre de 2009, núm. 5495, 8107–8116.

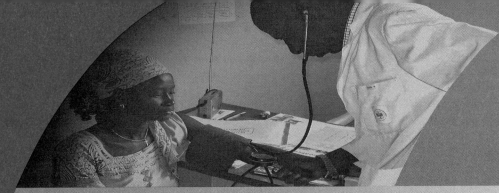

CHAPTER 4

The Methodology of the Community-Oriented Primary Care (COPC) Process

INTRODUCTION

Community-oriented primary care (COPC) is an approach that goes beyond addressing the healthcare demands of a defined community. It addresses the health needs of all its members—those who attend the health service and those who do not, those who are healthy or at risk (addressed through prevention and promotion activities), and those who are sick (addressed through treatment and rehabilitation). COPC also addresses the determinants of health and disease.

The practice of COPC requires a certain harmony in the conceptualization of health and its determinants by primary care professionals and the community, which is not always present. Professionals may consider mainly the medical aspects of a community's health status, but the community may emphasize the cultural and social context of its ailments. Although these may be extreme examples of the community's reality, a bridge between the two is essential to implement the COPC approach, which blends clinical individual care with public health principles and practice. Specifically, it deals with individual care, but it also has a population focus.

In this chapter we will review the process and implementation of the COPC approach. The principles that were explored in Chapter 3 are followed by the practical steps in this chapter.

INDIVIDUAL CARE AND COMMUNITY CARE

There is a parallel between the individuals' and the community's care, and similar steps are followed to examine their states of health and to provide treatment and follow-up (see Table 4-1). Both the background and the health problem must be understood. For an individual patient, this is done through an anamnesis. For a community, the process includes the characterization of the community and a detailed assessment of a

TABLE 4-1 Individual and Community Care

	Individual care	Community care
Getting to know the individual and the community	Anamnesis, family history, physical examination, and tests	Characterization of the community by its sociodemographic characteristics, culture, environment, and resources
Diagnosis	Assessment of main complaint, results of physical exam and tests to rule out other diagnoses	Community diagnosis through health indicators, rates and distributions, assessment of health needs and determinants of health, prioritization of pressing problems, and detailed assessment of the health problem
Treatment or intervention	Medicines, procedures, counseling on behavior change	Intervention for the whole community through an organized set of activities, including prevention, promotion, treatment, and rehabilitation
Evaluation	Assessment of compliance with intervention and of health status after treatment	Assessment of program effectiveness through evaluation of changes in health status of the community, performance of program activities, and resources used
Reassessment	Follow-up for assessment of health status, recurrence, and need for change in treatment	Decision on modifications, continuation, or discontinuation of the program; start a new prioritization process

prioritized problem. Care is provided to an individual according to the disease or condition. Care to a community is administered through an organized set of activities, and this constitutes an intervention program. An evaluation of care and follow-up is also conducted for both, as well as reexamination after the treatment of an individual or after a community intervention program. The latter step provides an assessment of the situation and is the basis for making decisions about the need to continue with the treatment or community intervention, and starting a new prioritization process.

The necessary skills in the COPC approach are clinical (for individual care) and are complemented by epidemiology, biostatistics, qualitative methods (for community assessments), and behavioral and anthropological sciences, which are vital for both individual and community care. The strength of the COPC approach is that it takes care of the individual in the context of the community, and it addresses and assesses changes in health status and behaviors not only at the individual level, but also at the community level.

STARTING A COPC PROGRAM

The decision to start a COPC program may be initiated by a healthcare organization at the central level, or it might be proposed by a healthcare professional or a healthcare team at the clinic or health center level if they have independence in decision making. If approval is needed at a higher level, or if the central level needs to approve the adoption and adaptation of COPC, this initial step may need to involve different players and decision makers. The community seldom initiates the process, although community members might be interested in participating or partnering with the program. Although this initiative may be advantageous for program development and facilitates the process, community participation should be sought by the healthcare team and built into the process.

A strategic plan should be delineated in which those involved in the process will be familiarized with the COPC approach and will be motivated to follow it. Knowledge about the entire COPC process is required. Although this might be obvious, sometimes not all members of a practice are knowledgeable on the principles and the methodology of COPC.

An initial study period might be required. This needs to be combined with consideration of the effectiveness of the approach and the interest of the practice members or the organization to adopt or further develop the principles of social justice in health care. An analysis of the flexibility and capabilities of the clinic to accommodate new activities and distribute its time differently is required. Also necessary is an analysis of whether financial incentives would be required. The support of the organization and members of the local team, as well as members of the community, is invaluable in the development

of a COPC practice. When the decision to follow the COPC approach is made, the process delineated in the following sections requires a decision about the involvement of different members of the practice, team building activities, and the definition of roles for each member. Capacity-building activities are needed, not only on the principles and steps of COPC, but also on the specific program or programs to be developed in the practice.[1–3]

THE SETTING IN COPC

The primary care setting is essential to COPC and distinguishes it from the settings of other community programs. COPC places primary care at the core of community programs. It might include a single primary care practice in a certain neighborhood or area, or it could be a group of practices that are under the same health maintenance organization (HMO).

The links between primary care practices and other healthcare services, such as specialty clinics or hospitals, have the potential for providing continuity of care for individual patients and the community. The person, not the disease, is at the center of attention in the community context. Community care in COPC is not only where care takes place; it is also the care that considers individuals and their micro- and macroenvironments as well as their interrelation with the collective state of health. The coordination and cooperation with other levels of care and health-related services or sectors and professionals is an essential component in the delivery of COPC.

THE COMMUNITY IN COPC

The need to define the community is based on one of the principles of COPC—*to know whom the primary care service is responsible for* and whom the COPC programs will be developed for. This is important not only for the healthcare professionals (knowing who and how many people to reach and how to engage the community in its care), but also for the members of the community (knowing who is taking care of their health). Both the professionals and the community must clearly understand the definition of community to ensure a smooth-running practice. The definition assists in the assessment of demographic and health data and in identifying available resources.

The task of defining the community could be handled by the clinic professionals themselves, according to their degree of organizational independence or by the organization they belong to. This can be accomplished in consultation with the community, and in some instances a community may decide which clinic they prefer to belong to. In the latter case, negotiations for the conditions of enrollment might be needed. Some problems may arise when insurance is a precondition for enrollment in a service or documentation is required in a community that is largely undocumented.

For any of the definitions that are adopted in accordance with the local reality, it is crucial to include *all* the potential members of the community (in accordance with the principles of COPC). Therefore, the definition should be inclusive of those who are usually underserved for any reason, whether the barriers to healthcare services are financial, legal, or some other type. Thus, an exhaustive examination needs to be done of the community members that the service will potentially be responsible for. The exclusion of community members has a direct impact on their health status, whether it is the lack of immunizations for uninsured children or the diagnosis of cancer at a late stage. In general, health disparities in the population may be widened by lack of care.

Geographic Definition

The classical geographic definition of a community for a primary care practice, limited by specific boundaries or encompassing certain statistical areas, might not always be applicable in COPC. In rural areas, this might be an appropriate definition. However, defining a community geographically might be challenging, with the diffusion of services provided by HMOs, national or governmental sources, nongovernmental organizations (NGOs), the closeness to an urban area, or the freedom to choose among healthcare providers. In urban settings, the multiplicity of providers within the same area might be the prevailing situation. In these cases alternatives for defining the community need to be considered to determine who the health service is responsible for.

People Registered in a Primary Care Clinic

A list of people who receive care in a primary care practice is one of the alternatives for a definition of community. A decision must be made regarding the meaning of being enrolled in a clinic, whether by choice or by inclusion of those who visited the clinic once and were consequently registered. Consideration should be given to whether that criterion qualifies an individual to be a member of that community. Geographic information systems (GISs)[4] can be used to determine the geographic spread of the patient population (those who went to the clinic in the last year, for example). The patients' addresses can be retrofitted[5] and displayed on a map. This can provide a good grasp of the penetration of the clinic in the community (defined as the percentage of persons in that area who were registered in the clinic, or the percentage of persons residing in specific census tracts, wards, or zip code areas).

Initial Defined Area

Another alternative to defining the community is an initial selection of an area close to the service, the initial defined area (IDA). This may assist in identifying a total population to begin with, and it can be enlarged progressively, as feasible, by the health service and existing resources.[6]

The concept of distance between the health service and community is important not only for the geographic accessibility of the service, but also for a possible closer contact between the health service and community members to facilitate outreach activities and community involvement. To ease this process, especially in the case of large populations attending a primary care service, the area can be subdivided and the members allocated to different teams.

Within a certain population receiving care in a primary care practice, there might be different subgroups identified according to their social or support networks. They may deserve special attention with regard to their health needs or to stimulate their participation in the process of individual or community care.

Other Types of Communities

Other definitions of communities can be used, such as children in a school, workers in a factory, inmates in a prison, or persons in a refugee camp.

THE COPC PROCESS

The COPC process is customarily presented through a cycle with six steps. They are depicted in Figure 4-1. Although these six steps exemplify a sequence, the different steps may overlap. This is a spiral process that builds on each one of the steps se-

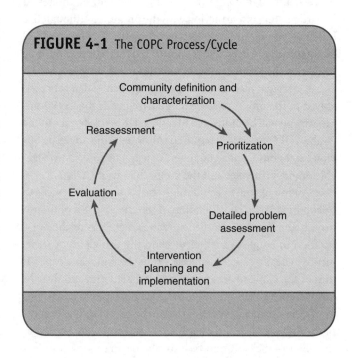

FIGURE 4-1 The COPC Process/Cycle

quentially and advances while completing the previous step. The process allows for flexibility and interaction in the development of the approach. This can be an iterative approach; a previous step may need reconsideration, and on occasion the intervention can be implemented as the detailed assessment is being performed.

CHARACTERIZATION OF THE COMMUNITY

After the community is defined, it is necessary to get to know it and to delineate its profile. The characterization of the community entails knowing about its physical and sociodemographic characteristics, its resources and assets, and its health status.

The characterization of the community initiates the process of community diagnosis. Similar to an individual clinical diagnosis, the community diagnosis provides comprehensive information about the community, its health and health-related problems and their determinants, and the available resources and assets for addressing these problems. This will be the basis for determining the health priorities of the particular community and the subsequent process of programming and implementing the COPC program.

Physical Characteristics of the Community

The physical characteristics of the community include a description of its location and environmental characteristics, as well as its communications availability and use. Rural areas situated in close proximity to a river that can overflow, crowded urban areas, locations near industrial complexes whose waste materials can pollute the environment, and housing characteristics (type of construction and materials used, such as asbestos and lead paint) all have implications for the safety and health of the community members. The communication facilities, the condition of the roads, and the availability of transportation have implications for the use of the health service and for the ability of the health service to conduct outreach activities. Available green spaces and spaces for recreation are invaluable for leisure activities for individuals and families, as well as for community activities. The general outlook of a community regarding cleanliness and beautification may be an indication of the community's available resources and the community members' attitude toward their immediate environment.

Sociodemographic Characteristics of the Community

The sociodemographic characteristics of the community include its demographic and sociocultural characteristics, its cultural health-related practices, and its organization and governing bodies.

The age and sex distribution, best represented in a population pyramid as depicted in Figures 4-2A, B, and C (please note that the figures are for countries, not specific communities),[7] may evidence a high proportion of children or elderly, or some age–sex brackets may be missing in a migrant population. This initial analysis of the population provides an indication of the types of problems that might be prevalent in the community. The number of people in each age–sex bracket will be used for the calculation of specific rates, for example, in a baseline study of health status or the study of changes over time. The constitution of family units and other sociodemographic characteristics, such as education, marital status, or race or ethnicity, provide additional information that will be useful for identifying and addressing inequalities in health status and the use of services before and after an intervention.

Specific health behaviors might be practiced by a group, and certain conditions in specific ethnic groups may alert the program managers of the need for performing screening tests (e.g., thalassemia among a population of Greek origin, Tay-Sachs among a Jewish population, or sickle cell anemia among a population with African ancestry). An individual or group religion, as well as the degree of religiosity, may also have implications for health behavior and use of services. Occupations may put community members at risk for specific health problems, for example, if the community is centered around a specific industry. During economic crises, the rates of unemployment may be markers of distress in a certain community. This may suggest the need for assessing mental health status or deleterious practices, such as alcohol abuse or family violence.

Length of permanence in the community is another characteristic that may be important to know. Communities with constant turnover may have poor social cohesion and organization, which are characteristics with health impacts, and they may be more difficult to engage. Migration affects the health status of the immigrants as well as those who are left behind, especially when the family unit is disrupted, such as when the breadwinner or parents of small children migrate to another country.[8–10]

Knowledge of the community's cultural characteristics and sociocultural practices with regard to health, and understanding the community and its involvement in its health care is invaluable in program design. Familiarity with the organization of the community, the identification of community organizations (formal and informal groups), and knowledge about social cohesion and networks all provide the basis for an understanding between the healthcare providers and the community members.

FIGURE 4-2 Population pyramids

A.

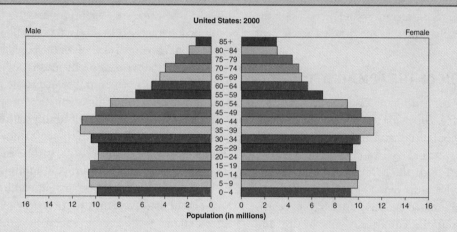

United States: 2000

B.

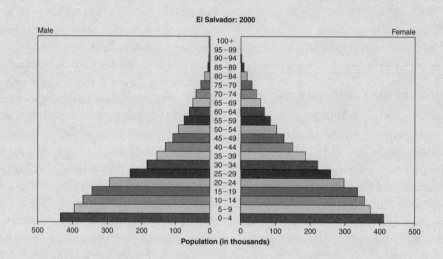

El Salvador: 2000

C.

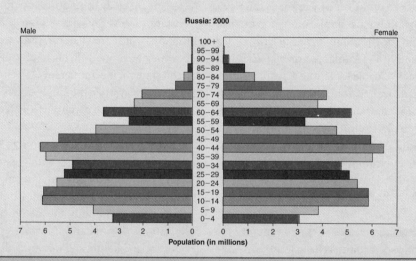

Russia: 2000

Source: Data from U.S. Census Bureau. International Database

Resources and Assets of the Community

An assessment of the services and assets available to the community—in terms of health and health-related issues, as well as their organization and linkages among them—is needed to appraise their availability for the health care and well-being of the population. This information will be important for intervention programming. Identifying different providers in the community may assist in coordinating activities, as will identifying overlapping healthcare services and gaps in the provision of care. Barriers to accessing care and referral systems need to be understood because they could hinder or facilitate the care provided to members of the community or the performance of interventions.

In certain communities it is important to know the nonofficial healthcare resources, such as traditional healers, espiritistas, and curanderos, which may be the source of care for community members. Nonofficial sources of care may be sought as an alternative to health clinics, but they also might be used as the sole providers when a family does not have resources to attend the clinic or when conventional medicine is deemed to be ineffective. Establishing relations with this sector and incorporating them in the care of target populations may be valuable. Services external to the health sector—such as social and welfare services or educational, cultural, and sports centers and spaces for youngsters—provide knowledge about additional venues or settings for health activities. Additionally, religious leaders may have a direct bearing in the collective health behavior of some communities.

Overall, knowledge of the available resources provides the basis for establishing collaboration among different institutions and building networks that are necessary when developing the COPC approach. Mapping the resources (and the different population groups) can assist the healthcare team in locating the community members and their assets.

Health Status of the Community

The assessment of the community's health status, in terms of vital statistics and health indexes, is the basis for determining the health needs and demands of the community. This information includes birth and fertility rates and mortality rates. Those rates contribute to the understanding of population growth. Mortality rates are also measured by specific causes and by age and sex. This latter information, as the tip of the iceberg of the community's health problems, will provide information on the most severe problems and their scope. The maternal mortality ratio (MMR), infant mortality (IM), and under-five mortality (U-5M) rates are indicators not only of the health status of a population but also of the quality of the healthcare services in the community. Cause-specific morbidity information helps identify the demands of community members who attended primary care clinic or hospitals.

In addition, anthropometric measurements, such as weight and height distribution or blood pressure and cholesterol levels, are useful for the understanding of growth patterns and risk factors. Information on health behaviors, such as substance abuse, physical activity, and eating habits, may help in understanding the community's state of health and providing direction for intervention programs.

Detailed community characterization features are provided in Box 4-1. The list is not exhaustive, and the various items might not be applicable to all communities; conversely, specific characteristics may not have been included in the list but can be incorporated as needed.

A comparison of the information gathered for the specific community should be compared with data from a larger area (for example, a district or state) for the estimation of the relative extent of the community health problems and the identification of health inequalities (gender, ethnicity, socioeconomic status, geographic distribution, etc.).

Sources of Information for Community Characterization

The characterization of a community is based on available information from different sources, according to the type of information needed. The quality of the information should be evaluated for completeness, accuracy, and reliability.

Vital statistics, for example, can be obtained from statistical bureaus or local authorities. The data may not always coincide with the defined community, or it may be available only for a larger area than the community. In this case the data can be used as a proxy measure for the community. IM rates might vary greatly in cases where the community under care is a relatively small one. The increase or decrease in one or two infant deaths might produce large variations in the rate; a period of 5 years, for example, could be a reasonable alternative for the presentation of the IM rate. The MMR, even in places where the rate is relatively high, still constitutes rare events because they are counted per 100,000 live births. A better indication of maternal health can often be obtained from morbidity data or pregnancy-related events or procedures (e.g., hemorrhage, preeclampsia, and cesarean sections). Morbidity data from the community's primary care clinic will provide information on the specific community, and hospital data may provide it for a larger area.

Additional sources of information, especially for child and adolescent health, might be provided by school records. Surveys on the community done by academic institutions, research institutes, or NGOs can also provide valuable information on the community. Interviews with key community members, as well as focus groups with community leaders and

Box 4-1 Characterization of a community

Physical Features

Geographic location (statistical areas, census tracts, wards, or zip code areas), natural borders
Size
Climate
Soil
Natural resources
Communications (landline and cell phones, Internet availability and penetration, TV)
Transportation
Housing characteristics, commodities
Recreation areas
Shopping facilities
Other features
Environmental characteristics:
Pollution
Maintenance of roads
Presence of wild animals, rodents, insects
Cleanliness

Community Resources, Services, Assets

Personal healthcare services:
Primary, secondary, and tertiary care
Emergency care
Referral system
Accessibility, availability, and barriers, such as location, hours, and financing (percentage of insured costs, out-of-pocket expenses)
Consultation rates, hospitalization rates
Number of doctors, nurses, healthcare workers/population; training
Nonpersonal healthcare services:
Waste and excreta disposal
Water supply
Other services
Educational services:
Schools
Day care, kindergarten
Institutions of higher education
Enrollment and dropout percentages by gender
Recreational services:
Youth clubs
Community centers
Cultural institutions
Sports institutions or spaces
Welfare services:
Disadvantaged populations
People with disabilities
Percentage receiving services or compensation
Other services

Sociodemographic Features

Age and gender distribution
Occupation or unemployment
Social class distribution
Educational status
Marital status
Ethnic or racial groups
Religiosity
Family structure (nuclear, extended)
Number of members in the family
Crowding index
Mobility and migration
Social characteristics:
Family formation
Gender preference
Community organization and participation
Social networks, social capital
Crime and security
Cultural practices related to health (consanguineous marriages, weaning practices, consultation of traditional practitioners)
Languages spoken
History of the community
Other characteristics

Health Status of the Community

Vital statistics:
Mortality rates (general and cause specific)
Infant mortality (neonatal and postneonatal)
Under-five mortality rate
Maternal mortality
Birth rate, fertility rate
Health indexes:
Morbidity (causes of consultations to clinics, hospitalizations)
Somatic characteristics (weight, height, blood pressure, cholesterol)
Psychological characteristics (IQ, personality type, depression)
Behavior (smoking, drugs, alcohol, violence, physical activity, breastfeeding, use of seat belts, use of services)
Other indexes

members of specific groups (mothers, adolescents, etc.), are additional sources of information. Healthcare professionals may also share their knowledge and perspective on the community's health problems.

Assembling this information will provide knowledge and insights on the perceived health problems and their determinants, as well as the community's beliefs and associated customs, use of services, and barriers encountered in health care. The process of gathering this information is also a means of communication between healthcare professionals and the community, which can establish the grounds for cooperation and a common vision to improve the health of the community through sustainable interventions.

The information gathered, especially information on the health status of the community, answers the COPC principle of *addressing the health needs of the community* as the basis for developing and implementing programs.

The analysis of information from different sources—which includes not only conditions or diseases that generate demand for healthcare services, but other health issues as well—offers the opportunity to have a more comprehensive picture of what the health problems and their determinants might be. This will be the basis for making decisions on the priority(ies) to address the major health problems of the community.

PRIORITIZATION

An organized, systematized, and efficient response is called for to address the health needs of the community. This implies the need to prioritize, a process that aims to select a specific health condition, problem, set of related problems, or health behaviors that are deemed to take precedence among others. The focus and systematic development of an intervention program for the prioritized condition(s) will be done in parallel with the health service's usual care for all other health demands.

The goals of the prioritization process are to have a rational investment of human resources and financing, and produce a collaborative effort to achieve a reduction in the burden of disease at the individual, family, and community levels. The ultimate goal is to contribute to the reduction of inequalities in health status and inequities in the use of healthcare services. Prioritization should not be confused with rationing, which is restriction in the provision and use of services.

To carry out the prioritization process, a life course approach can be taken in which the whole age spectrum is considered. However, first consideration should be given to the age distribution of the community. If the community has a large proportion of children, they might be selected as the focus of attention, as well as pregnant women or women of reproductive age. A similar decision can be made for an aging population. Alternatively, a prioritization process can be fol-

lowed within specific specialties within a clinic (pediatrics, geriatrics, mental health).

Prioritization is initiated by listing the health problems that were identified when the community was characterized. These health problems may include conditions that are vague or poorly defined. They can also include organizational problems of the service. It is advisable to narrow the list to the most significant five or six problems to make prioritization a manageable process. During prioritization, it is also advisable to consider the organizational problems separately from the health problems. Solving organizational problems is necessary for the improvement of the quality of the service, but it is not guaranteed that it will improve the health situation of the community. Moreover, organizational aspects need to be addressed in the context of the intervention.

One obstacle often encountered in the prioritization process is the limited amount of available information (in terms of quantity or quality) about the specific community and its health problems. It may be necessary to rely on proxy measures, such as health indicators of a nearby comparable community or the larger area to which the community belongs.

The prioritization process is an additional opportunity for involvement of the community, for which there is a growing interest among the public.[11] However, this may vary according to the degree of community organization. Interests and value judgment may be inevitable when different people, professionals, and organizations are involved. The organization of the process should take into account reducing subjectivity to a minimum and be both systematic and transparent.

Practical Steps in the Prioritization Process

In preparation for the prioritization process, some practical steps are suggested (see Table 4-2).

Prioritization Criteria and Scoring

The process of prioritization is done according to specific criteria and scoring. Four criteria and scoring from 1-lowest to 3-highest (see Box 4-2) in a scoring grid (see Box 4-3) are suggested here.[13] This helps to systematize the process and diminish subjectivity. The criteria suggested can be applied in its entirety, or some of its components can be selected or modified.

The health problem that receives the highest overall score is then selected for intervention. It is advised to compare the health problems within each column to ensure consistency. The type of scoring and how it will be allocated to each criterion needs to be decided in advance. One approach is that each participant proposes a score and the mean of the scores is calculated for each criterion. Another approach could be assigning the scores by consensus. Different discussion techniques

TABLE 4-2 Prioritization Process

Deciding who will be involved in the process and the work methodology	This entails determining who among the healthcare professionals, community members (also considering marginalized people), and organizations will be part of the process. The working approach and ethics should be set up in a way that will maximize the abilities and competencies of the participants.
Defining responsibilities of the stakeholders and goals of the process	This needs to be done at the outset of the process to start on common ground and agreed-upon premises. It also contributes to the transparency of the process.
Deciding on a time table for the process	Establishing time limits increases the likelihood of conducting an efficient process.
Organizing the available information	This entails making data sources available to the team, searching for literature on the effectiveness of programs, consulting with experts, or gathering additional information about the health problems under consideration in the defined community.
Selecting the methods and criteria for prioritization	This step establishes the overall methodology of the process. The most widely used criteria are those related to the burden of disease, availability of effective interventions, and costs. Other criteria, such as interest of providers and decision makers, are also used.[12]

can be carried out for that purpose. A Delphi process,[a] general discussions, or nominal group technique[b] can be used with the presence of those involved, live or virtual. A competent and trained group leader (internal or external to the practice) is helpful for this process.[14] There might be a need for a revision or appeal of the selected condition when the scores are close. A joint decision by team members is necessary in this case.

DETAILED ASSESSMENT

The detailed assessment completes the *community diagnosis*, which started with the characterization of the community and the process of prioritization. The goal of the detailed assessment is to measure the size and distribution of the health problem, according to relevant sociodemographic variables, and its determinants at each stage of its natural history. These determinants are the ones that can be modified through an intervention.

The detailed assessment of the prioritized condition serves several purposes: (1) The identification of at-risk populations, based on age, gender, ethnicity or race, educational status, place of residence, or other relevant characteristics, may help in the

decision as to whether the program should address the total population or selected populations; (2) the assessment provides the basis for planning the intervention in accordance with the local findings; (3) a baseline can be established for comparison during program evaluation to assess changes after the program implementation.

Because the detailed assessment may entail active data collection, and given the significance of the detailed assessment regarding program implementation and future evaluation, some questions need to be addressed. First of all, during the process of community characterization, data on the selected condition were available in a certain form. Careful consideration should be given as to whether the information available is sufficient for the assessment purposes:

• Does the information cover the specific community? In some instances the data partially address the community, and it will not be possible to distinguish information from those who are not under the responsibility of the service. Information that covers a larger area might include a completely different population than that of the specific community.

• Does the information have the same case definition for the health condition under study? Did the information include the determinants of interest and relevance in the targeted community?

---

[a]This method is used to reach consensus. Participants contribute ideas or answer questions that are discussed and refined in successive iterative rounds. Face-to-face contact and even identity disclosure is not necessary.
[b]Participants get together in groups to generate ideas in writing, share them with the group, and then discuss them with the group. This is followed by a preliminary vote, a discussion, and a final vote.

Box 4-2 Criteria for prioritization and their scoring

Criteria	Components	Justification	Scoring
Relative importance	*Magnitude*	Measured according to prevalence and incidence rates. A decision has to be taken regarding scoring, given to different types of measurements. The information available on these criteria may not be comparable among the different conditions, or may not refer specifically to the community. Ascribing the scores to these different types of measurements may then require an agreement between the participants. Assigning the scores comparing one condition to the other may assist in this process.	low = 1 to 3 = high
	Seriousness	Measured according to case fatality or disability measures such as disability adjusted life years–DALYs, performance of activities of daily living, proportion of bed or homebound as a consequence of the condition. This may also require, comparisons between the different measurements and agreement between the participants.	low = 1 to 3 = high
	Economic impact	This criteria is mainly based on the health condition impact on work earnings, whether directly (when the program is for adults) or indirectly when minors are involved and it affects a caretaker (parent or other)	Minor (absenteeism from work) = 1 Intermediate (loss of salary) = 2 Major (affects the community) = 3
Feasibility of intervention	*Resources*	This criteria is based on the existing human and financial resources and facilities available, and whether there is need for additional resources	If resources are not available = 1 If new resources are required = 2 If financial, human resources, and facilities are available = 3
	Conformity with health policies	Health policies, whether at national, regional or local level, or from the health maintenance organization need to be considered, as they may facilitate or hinder the development of an intervention program	No supportive policy = 1 There are existing policies but they are not implemented = 2 There is a health policy that has been implemented = 3
	Cultural acceptability	The cultural make up of a community and their health believes might be a decisive factor regarding the acceptance of an intervention program.	In conflict with cultural norms in the community = 1 Acceptable only to subgroups of the community = 2 Consistent with existing cultural frameworks and norms = 3
	Interest of healthcare personnel	The cooperation of the existing healthcare personnel is needed for an efficient running of the program.	No expression of interest = 1 Some interest = 2 Teams are ready to act = 3
Predictive effectiveness of the intervention	*Evidence of effectiveness according to literature*	Published material on the effectiveness of interventions programs, mainly in peer reviewed journals are needed to assist in the decision to develop the intervention program.	No evidence or poor evidence = 1 Some evidence = 2 Good evidence = 3
	Local factors related to effectiveness	In order to be able to implement the program, the availability of resources, especially personnel, and the possibility of training needs to be assessed	No trained personnel or no possibility of training = 1 Some trained personnel or some possibility of training = 2 Personnel are trained or there is the possibility of training = 3.
Community concern and interest		The cooperation of the community is essential in planning and carrying out a program. Their concern and interest need to be assessed	No expression of interest or perception of barriers = 1 Expression of interest = 2 Community requests action = 3

The justification of each program costs should be considered within the whole process.

Box 4-3 COPC priority-setting matrix

Health problems	Relative importance			Feasibility of intervention				Predicted effectiveness of intervention		Community concern and interest	Total score
	Magnitude	Seriousness	Economic impact	Resources	Conformity with health policies	Cultural acceptability	Interest of healthcare personnel	Evidence of effectiveness	Local factors related to effectiveness		

- Is the time frame of data collection sufficiently recent? Data that was collected too far in advance may be irrelevant if demographic or other changes occurred in the community.
- Is the quality of the information adequate? A thorough methodological assessment regarding reliability and completeness will provide the answer.

In the prioritization process it may become evident that there are health problems or conditions that are difficult to dissociate from one another, such as diarrheal diseases and malnutrition, which might also have common socioeconomic, cultural, and environmental determinants. The coprevalence and the interaction of different conditions, behaviors, somatic characteristics, and psychological characteristics, as well as their shared determinants, was denominated *community syndrome* by Sidney L. Kark, similar to the symptoms and signs that form a clinical syndrome.[6] See Figure 4-3 for an example diagram of a community syndrome.

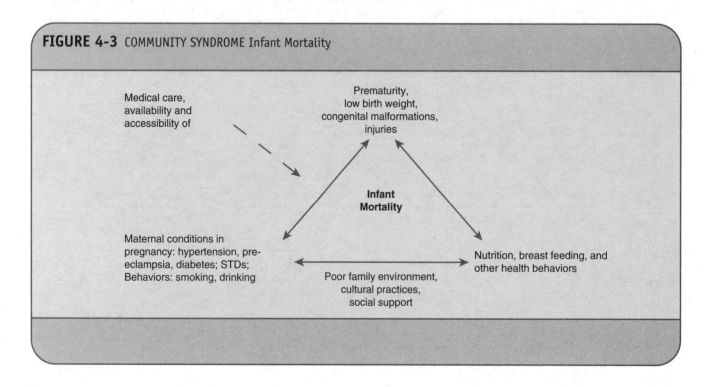

FIGURE 4-3 COMMUNITY SYNDROME Infant Mortality

Planning and Implementation of the Detailed Assessment

The planning and implementing of the detailed assessment should be, as much as possible, integrated into the practice to minimize interference with the clinic activities. Integrating the different healthcare team members in the process is important to develop a sense of ownership and commitment from early on in the process. For the same reasons, community participation should also be considered, in accordance with their capabilities and the training that the clinic members can offer. The institutional resources allocated to the task should consider the existing resources. Some of the personnel's time can be diverted to these activities, or additional funding through grants or other sources can be sought for specific tasks.

Decision on the Population for the Detailed Assessment

The COPC principle of *addressing the health needs of* all *members of the community* is considered here—not only those who are sick or those who attend the clinic, but also people who are healthy or at risk for the condition. The population can include all members of the community or any of its subgroups (such as age groups, racial and ethnic groups, or those who live in the initially defined area). Even if selecting a subgroup of the community is justifiable, all of its members should be included.

Additionally, it needs to be decided if the detailed assessment will be carried out for a sample that is representative of the whole population or whether it will include all of the target population. These decisions will depend not only on the community's size, but also on the health problem selected. For example, the primary care practice might need to have information on each one of its members, such as blood pressure in a program for the control of hypertension. The available human and financial resources also need to be considered.

Another consideration is whether the program is intended as a program trial (see Chapter 2) in which case the design calls for a control community (one that will not receive the program but from which data will be collected at baseline and during the evaluation) that will be compared with the trial group to assess if the intervention itself caused favorable outcomes.

Formulation of Objectives for the Detailed Assessment

The detailed assessment objectives are designed to answer a variety of questions regarding the prioritized health condition. For example, what is the prevalence of the selected condition? How it is distributed in the community in terms of sociodemographic and other relevant characteristics? Additional questions should address the different determinants of the specific health condition or those that will need to be modified by the intervention.

The detailed assessment could also include the appraisal of knowledge, attitudes, beliefs, and practices (KABP) if they are the target of the intervention or if they are a required step in achieving an expected outcome. This has to be carefully weighted in the planning of the detailed assessment (and in the intervention) because the link between knowledge and practices has been questioned (for example, the prevalence of smoking behavior among healthcare professionals). Environmental conditions, cultural factors, use of services, and compliance with treatment and advice also need to be considered when defining the objectives.

Addressing the Natural History of the Health Condition In a given community the different stages of the *natural history of the disease*, or the health–illness continuum, are represented (see Figure 4-4 and Figure 4-5). Members of the community might be exposed (+) or not exposed (−) to a certain risk to contract a disease. Among those who are exposed, some of them will develop the disease or the particular behavior (+), and others will not (−). Among those who experience the disease, some will continue to a chronic state or be disabled by the condition, others will recover, and others may have a premature death. Similarly, the consequences of a poor health behavior can be outlined (see Figure 4-6).

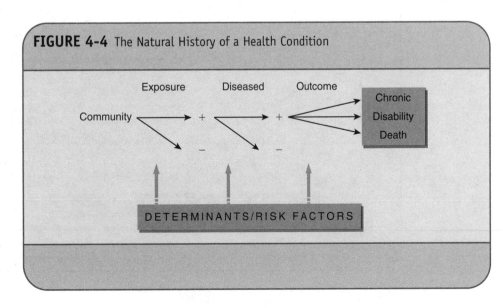

FIGURE 4-4 The Natural History of a Health Condition

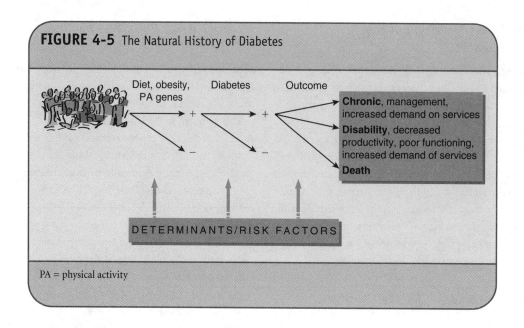

FIGURE 4-5 The Natural History of Diabetes

PA = physical activity

At all these stages there are determinants that may protect the individual or the community, or that jointly with the risk factors may accelerate the development of the condition. The determinants can be of a social and cultural nature, or they can be biological or environmental. The health service and the access or barriers to it should also be considered at all stages of the natural history of the condition.

Healthcare professionals and community members should decide which determinants they consider relevant. For that purpose, theoretical knowledge, learned from the literature, and individual experience should be utilized. This knowledge will guide not only the detailed assessment, but also the planning of the intervention.

Methods of Data Collection and Analysis

Data collection methods will depend on the prioritized condition and the resources available to the health service. Data collection can be done with quantitative or qualitative methods.

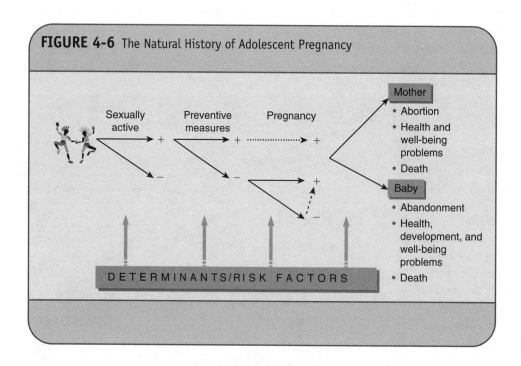

FIGURE 4-6 The Natural History of Adolescent Pregnancy

Quantitative Methods Information from the service itself, through its *clinic records*, will be useful if all members of the community have access to the service and attended the service during the planned information collection period. Clinical records will provide diagnoses, in the form of codes from the International Classification of Diseases (ICD),[15] International Classification of Primary Care,[16] and *Diagnostic and Statistical Manual of Mental Disorders*,[17] results of laboratory tests (such as lipid profile or hemoglobin), measurements (blood pressure, weight, and height), or the number of visits to the clinic. Behaviors such as substance abuse and physical activity may also be included in the records. The reliability and validity of the records, whether in relation to the diagnosis, laboratory tests, or measurements, must be determined if they are going to be used for a community diagnosis.

Birth records, in hard copy or electronic form, can be another valuable source of information for the study of pregnancy outcomes. These records may contain some information on sociodemographic characteristics, which is valuable for the study of the outcomes among different population groups and the identification of high-risk populations. Information on other characteristics, such as psychosocial characteristics, may not be available from these records.

Hospital records will provide additional information on general morbidity, injuries, treatment, prognosis, and length of stay. This information can be linked to clinic records to tackle the issue of severity of the condition.

Depending on the condition selected, *registers* might also be available, such as in the case of mental health conditions or congenital anomalies when addressing pregnancy outcomes. The registries might have been designed in and for the specific clinic, or they might be available for a district or larger area. In the latter case, if addresses are provided and there is a waiver for the release of those records, they may constitute a useful source.

Because the planning of the intervention will also be based on addressing the different determinants of the health condition, the information available from records may not always be suitable or available, and there may be a need for alternative sources. It may be necessary to conduct *surveys* (self-administered—in hard copies, through the Internet or other electronic means—face to face or phone) to collect the relevant information. The surveys can be organized as a screening procedure (for example, depression, postpartum depression, or hypertension) with the confirmation of a diagnosis in successive steps.

The detailed assessment may take a *descriptive* form by the measurement of the nature and extent of the selected health condition according to sociodemographic variables (age, sex, education, occupation). It can be expressed as a mortality rate (for example, the rate of cardiovascular conditions) and morbidity rate expressed by prevalence and incidence rates. This type of assessment provides information on the distribution of the condition across the relevant variables. It also gives an indication of how the condition varies among different groups and can signal inequalities in health status.

An *analytical* approach to the study of the health condition will add to the previous analysis, aiming to identify associations between conditions and behaviors, coprevalence, and relevant determinants, as well as the identification of community syndromes.

Qualitative Methods These methods are used to get a more thorough understanding of the health problem and its determinants by observing the community and asking individuals about their perspectives, attitudes, and behaviors surrounding the condition. *Focus groups* and *in-depth interviews* with community members provide information on behaviors and cultural practices that may not be as easily elicited and understandable through the quantitative methods.[14] This information can also guide data collection through quantitative methods.

INTERVENTION

COPC interventions follow a systematic and organized set of activities that are carried out in a predetermined sequence. The planning may begin while the detailed assessment of the conditions is taking place. For example, in a program for the control of hypertension, when a person is screened to have high blood pressure, he or she needs to be referred for diagnostic purposes. Similarly, in a mental health program, when a community member reports indicators of depression, a referral is warranted. Occasionally, health education activities are initiated during the detailed assessment, or inquiring about certain conditions may elicit a response from the community members who may then seek advice or care, thus jump-starting the intervention.

An assessment of the literature to determine the best practices for interventions on the selected health condition should be done well in advance to guide and prepare the program activities. The use of specific models and theories should be considered (see Chapter 2). For this purpose, *evidence of effectiveness* for different types of interventions, activities, and the means of delivering them will be searched for in the literature.

The *feasibility* of applying any of these interventions will depend on the cultural and social acceptability of the targeted community or subgroup, the social and political context, and the resources available (budget and facilities) to the healthcare practice and the community members.

Planning and Implementation of the Intervention

The first step in planning the intervention is to learn what has already been done in relation to the selected condition by the healthcare services and other agencies and by the community. These might be sporadic or well-organized activities, and it is important to learn from their successes and failures.

For example, if the selected condition is diabetes, some of the questions to be asked are as follows:

- Is the existing intervention evidence based?
- Which age group is the program targeting?
- Were case-finding activities carried out?
- What were the specific criteria to define diabetes?
- Are treatment and referral guidelines available?
- What is the level of compliance with advice and treatment?
- What outreach activities are in place?
- What training has the healthcare team received with regard to the care of diabetes and its complications?
- What has been the involvement of the community to date?

In another case, if the targeted intervention is teenage pregnancy, questions may include the following:

- What is the target group? Does it include boys and girls?
- What are the methods used for contraception? Are contraceptives available to teenagers?
- What activities have been carried out for the prevention of pregnancy and leaning about sexuality, for follow-up with the pregnant teenagers, and for dealing with risk during pregnancy? Is it evidence based?
- Are services used in a timely manner when the pregnancy is diagnosed? Are schools involved, and do they have any activities or services for pregnant teens or teenage mothers?
- What are the attitudes of the community regarding teen pregnancy? What is the extent of family and community support regarding teenage pregnancy?

Defining the Target Population for the Intervention

In the detailed assessment, the target population was already defined, and the intervention might be carried out on the same population. It might also be that although a certain intervention was planned for a specific age group, for example, those who are 25 years old and older, it will be initially implemented for a subgroup, such as those who are 35 years old and older or those who live in a certain location. This decision would depend on the resources available; also, beginning with a small-scale program may be reasonable before including the total defined population. Whether an initial subpopulation or the total community will be included, it is important to stress that *all members within the selected community* are included in the program.

Formulating the Objectives for the Intervention

The objectives of the intervention indicate what we want to achieve in terms of decreasing morbidity and mortality, modifying behaviors or the environment, and modifying the determinants of the health condition. They are distinguished from the objectives of the detailed assessment, which provided a snapshot of the selected health condition and its determinants.

The intervention objectives need to be phrased in measurable terms and include a time dimension. A time dimension should address what the intervention intends to achieve in what amount of time. For example, in an injury prevention program, the objective might be to decrease the incidence of injuries by 50% among adolescents in a 5-year period. Both the intended objective and the time in which it is to be achieved will be based on what pertinent literature has shown to be possible in other communities. Most importantly, the objectives should be feasible and adapted to the local context. Additional objectives, or intermediate objectives, can be formulated to achieve the primary objectives of the program. For example, in a program to decrease the incidence of motor vehicle injury mortality, the objectives could include increasing the use of seat belts, decrease driving under the influence of alcohol, or increasing knowledge regarding injury prevention.

In accordance with the COPC principle of *addressing the natural history of the condition*, as previously discussed, the objectives should include promotion, prevention, early diagnosis, treatment, and rehabilitation (Figure 4-7). This is possible where there is a comprehensive and integrated service offering this continuum of care. In some cases, such as in maternal and child healthcare services, most of the program objectives will focus on prevention and promotion, whereas the curative and rehabilitative services would need to be continued by other services in coordination with the clinic (see Case Study 13).

The importance of developing realistic and well-defined objectives cannot be overemphasized. They are the foundation for planning and implementing the program, assessing the resources needed, and defining the targets to be measured during the evaluation.

Formulating Activities for the Intervention

The intervention activities are geared toward meeting each of the proposed program objectives. Multiple activities can be implemented for each objective, addressing prevention and promotion, treatment, or rehabilitation, according to the prob-

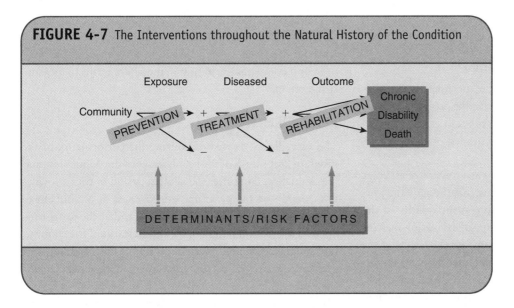

FIGURE 4-7 The Interventions throughout the Natural History of the Condition

tracking the health status of the population and for monitoring the program activities.

SURVEILLANCE AND MONITORING

Surveillance activities are implemented to continuously identify and assess changes in the health status of the population. Surveillance is a natural continuation of the community diagnosis and can be based on an analysis of records or surveys. The analysis of hospitalizations or clinical records will help the service to monitor the health status of the community.

lem. Educational activities carried out face to face in individual clinic contacts or in groups can address issues of prevention and promotion, as well as appropriate treatment of a certain condition. Communication technologies, such as text messaging and e-mails, are increasingly used in primary care for varied problems, such as drinking[18,19] and depression,[20] with promising results.

When planning the intervention activities, the team should develop *culturally sensitive* and appropriate activities in which the language and content of the intervention respect the community makeup or different groups within a heterogeneous community. Environmental changes can also be appropriate activities, such as in an injury prevention program. Although this may not be considered an activity at the primary care level, healthcare professionals and community members may be effective coalition builders and advocates for these changes. The intervention may need to be coordinated with the organization of a referral system, and it may need to liaise with other organizations or levels of care, such as specialty clinics or hospitals.

If resources are available, surveys can be carried out to analyze specific aspects of the intervention and its effects on the population. Qualitative and quantitative methods can be used for that purpose.

Surveillance may also include a follow-up of the demographic characteristics of the population, such as births (which are essential in programs dealing with pregnancies), deaths (when their reduction is a program goal), and migration. The follow-up of the planned activities and their degree of performance is usually called *monitoring*. It follows up on the process of the program according to the preestablished set of activities and alerts program managers of the need for changes.[21]

Surveillance and monitoring are ongoing processes that provide a continuous look at the program. They facilitate identifying problems in the performance of activities that need to be reassessed during the course of the program and alerts program managers of changes in the health situation that need to be considered. This process is naturally followed by the final assessments that are done in the evaluation.

Designing Records

For keeping track of the program activities, a record system is needed. It could be a system that is already in use at the clinic or a specially designed system. For example, for a hypertension control program, the usual recording of blood pressure and medications will be used. The same holds for early identification, diagnosis, treatment, and follow-up of diabetes. If additional records are designed, they should be incorporated into the clinical file (whether electronic or hard copy). This would also facilitate the integration of the program in the routines of the clinic. Well-organized records are invaluable for

EVALUATION

Evaluation provides information about the intervention program's achievements. It provides the healthcare team and the community with empirical evidence regarding the program's degree of effectiveness. An evaluation also provides information on what worked and what did not, and it analyzes the extent of resource utilization and whether the resources were used efficiently; consequently, it indicates the need for continuation or modification of the program.

The evaluation might be performed by an external or an internal team. An external team is required to assure objectivity in the evaluation. An internal team may be used if an interim evaluation is planned.

The Methodology of the Evaluation

Program trials (see Chapter 2) are experiments or quasi-experiments that seek to appraise whether the program outcome is due to the specific intervention and not to extraneous factors.[22–24] They are used when the effectiveness of innovative interventions need to be proven.

A *program review* is carried out when there is an assumption, as shown in similar interventions, that the activities produced a beneficial outcome and to test the quality of the program. The performance of this type of evaluation may include *before and after* surveys that compare the results of the detailed assessment with those obtained after the program implementation.[25] In services that are progressively expanded, the use of *after* data from a given population can be compared with the *before* data from the new added population, assuming that both populations are similar. These data in turn can be compared with its own *after* data. *Time series* (outcomes over a period of time) can also be used for evaluation.[26,27]

What Is Being Evaluated?

In a COPC program, several issues need to be addressed.[14] *Outcomes* refers to the program *effectiveness*, whether the program worked or the extent to which the stated program objectives were achieved (e.g., decrease in hypertension prevalence, decrease in injury incidence). It answers the question, does it work? Effectiveness is differentiated from *efficacy*, which assesses the degree of beneficial results expected from a particular intervention carried out under ideal conditions. It answers the question, can it work? Program effectiveness should also address whether the outcomes were achieved for all groups within a community (e.g., those with high and low education levels, immigrants and veteran residents, varied ethnic and racial groups).

A *process* evaluation relates to the performance of the program activities. It is measured against the established plan (e.g., measurement of hemoglobin levels according to protocol, coverage of the population in the immunization program), the utilization of offered services, and the degree of compliance with advice (taking hypertension medicines, doing physical exercise).

The *program structure* includes the physical setting, the facilities and equipment, the availability and accessibility of the services, and the barriers of use (geographic, physical, economic, cultural, etc.). The process of accountability (to whom to report) should also be considered. The population's and the healthcare team's satisfaction with the process and the outcomes of the program should also be evaluated.

Efficiency measures the cost incurred in achieving the results. It compares the input (manpower, time, equipment, etc.) with the effectiveness of the program to assess cost-effectiveness, or it compares the output in monetary terms to measure cost–benefit.

REASSESSMENT

The surveillance carried out during the performance of the program keeps track of the health status of the population, and the evaluation done after the allotted period of time provides information on the program's effectiveness or attainment of objectives. It closes the COPC process and at the same time opens it for reexamination of the health status of the community and the decision to continue or modify the program. Most intervention programs constantly integrate new participants (new people in the community, those reaching the age of admission, women who become pregnant, newborns, recent enrollees). The reassessment also addresses the changing needs of the community, whether due to the intervention or further sociodemographic, environmental, or other changes in the population, and it starts a renewed appraisal of priorities.

THE HEALTHCARE TEAM IN COPC

The healthcare team should attend to the needs of individuals and families and also to the community as a whole. It should address not only sick people, but also promote the health of the community members and prevent the development of diseases. These latter tasks need to be done without medicalization of the process.

The composition of the team will vary in accordance to the place, the community's health problems, the program to be developed, and the existing resources or those that can be obtained. Physicians and nurses comprise the core team in a COPC practice. Other members of the team can be professionals that are in daily contact with community members, such as health educators or health promoters. Social workers, nutritionists, psychologists, and environmentalists can form part of the team, depending on the program needs. Team members can all be part of the same institution, or the team can be built through intersectoral cooperation or links with other institutions or organizations that serve the same community. Epidemiologists and statisticians are members of the team who will assist and support the core team in the community orientation. These members of the team may be available within the clinic or the institution that develops the COPC approach, or they can be part of the public healthcare services or academic institutions recruited to work with the clinic.

Traditional doctors, such as espiritistas, curanderos, or shamans, may be incorporated into the healthcare team in places where they are part of the informal healthcare system, and they can be approached by community members as their first contact or for consultations. The incorporation of traditional practitioners requires an agreement about their functions and an understanding of their practices and influence on the community members. A community organizer may be needed to bridge the practice activities with the community.

The roles of all the team members need to be clearly defined to assure a smooth functioning of the clinic and the health programs and so all members know what is expected from them.

SUSTAINABILITY

A healthy condition seldom disappears; therefore continued action is needed, or in other words, a program must be sustainable. This means that a managerial process should be in place to assure that the services and activities have enough materials and human resources to function over the long term.[28] Alternatively, as proposed by the Stanford Five-City Project,[29] sustainability is achieved when the community has access to the knowledge, skills, and resources needed to conduct effective health promotion programs.

Sustainability is facilitated when the activities are integrated into the routine of the service. The program, as opposed to a project (which might have narrower aims and is meant to operate for a limited period of time), is intended to be part of the service. Sustainability might be more viable when there is community involvement and participation because the sense of ownership and need might be shared with the health service. Both can address the barriers that may appear with the needed continuation of the program. Presenting the evidence of positive changes in health status and its determinants and the cost-effectiveness of the intervention is also important because this justifies the investment in the COPC approach. It might also support extending the program to other clinics.

The support of the institution leadership is an invaluable resource for sustainability. The leadership's commitment to the delivery of the COPC approach provides not only economic support, but also support for its principles and adaptation to the clinical setting. In case of competing services or institutional priorities, this support can be decisive for the sustainability of COPC.

RESOURCES AND BUDGET PLANNING

The integration of the program in the routines of the clinic might necessitate reallocating human resources or time to different activities. Occasionally, additional human resources may be required. They can also be procured from other agencies (social workers) or universities (epidemiologists, statisticians) that could

cooperate with the program. Community members can also be team members (community health workers, health promoters).

To introduce the healthcare team to the culture of the COPC approach, capacity building is needed to acquire new knowledge and skills and for the development of a team spirit and positive attitudes toward the new approach. Clear definitions of the roles of each member of the healthcare team should be established, and a fair distribution of tasks and responsibilities should be delineated. Accountability processes within the health service and the community should be established. The budget will be organized in accordance with the human and material resources needed for implementing the program.

INTERSECTORAL COOPERATION

The burden of disease experienced by a community, and the complexity of its determinants, needs the cooperation of professionals, organizations, and institutions outside the healthcare field. This intersectoral cooperation does not always develop naturally. However, health services are well positioned to initiate partnerships with other sectors because of the sensitivity and importance of the service. This intersectoral cooperation needs to be organized to maximize resources, avoid duplication, and strengthen the local capacity for problem solving.

Consideration has been given to issues of *sharing* (responsibilities, values, decision making, or data), *partnership* (with open and honest communications, mutual trust, respect, and common goals), *interdependency* (to reach synergy in addressing common goals), *power* (the empowerment of each participant whose respective powers are recognized by all involved), and *team work* (multidisciplinary teams with different professions, interdisciplinary teams with a common goal and decision-making process, and transdisciplinary teams that open professional territories) to achieve an effective practice.[30] Intersectoral cooperation entails the professional and personal aspects of those involved and accepting potential trade-offs for achieving a common goal. It also needs an interprofessional learning program.[31]

OPPORTUNITIES AND CONSTRAINTS IN THE APPLICATION OF THE COPC APPROACH

There are organizational setups that facilitate the implementation of the COPC approach. In a system where there is universal insurance, barriers to accessing healthcare services are notoriously diminished. Additionally, when a service is geographically allocated, the development of COPC is facilitated. Even within this setup, there might be a free choice of providers, which may necessarily require a readjustment of the definition of the target community. National, local, or services policies might be additional facilitators in the development of COPC. The motivation of the healthcare team members also contributes to the successful introduction of a program.

Toward the end of the first decade of the 21st century, there was momentum for the renewal of primary health care (PHC), initiated by the Pan American Health Organization (PAHO)[32] and driven by the World Health Organization (WHO) in the World Health Report 2008,[33] with the vision of PHC as "a set of values and principles for guiding the development of health systems." The report addresses the reforms that are needed to improve health through universal coverage, people-centered healthcare systems, public policies to promote and protect the health of communities, and making health authorities more reliable. All of these reforms can provide fertile ground where COPC can be developed.

In the United States, the high cost of health care that left 45.7 million people uninsured in 2007 (15.3% of the population, of which 18% were children),[34] the fragmentation of services, and the diminishing workforce of primary care professionals might make it difficult to develop COPC. However, organizations such as Federally Qualified Health Centers[35] can further their activities using COPC. Recent recognition by the government that this should be a priority ought to provide further support.

The reforms of healthcare systems that are occurring around the world, and the expected reform in the United States, offer opportunities and challenges for the development of COPC. The reforms also work to promote just and equitable services to diminish inequities and inequalities in the health of the community.

The WHO World Health Assembly of May 2009[36] further exhorted member states "to put people at the centre of health care by adopting, as appropriate, delivery models focused on the local and district levels that provide comprehensive primary health care services, including health promotion, disease prevention, curative care and palliative care, that are integrated and coordinated according to needs, while ensuring effective referral system[s]." It also calls for universal access to primary care by providing equitable, efficient, and sustainable financial systems, promoting active participation of people in their own care, training of appropriate resources, and strengthening health information and surveillance of the systems to facilitate evidence-based policies and program evaluation.

SUMMARY

Community-oriented primary care (COPC) is an approach of service delivery in primary care that attends to the perceived and assessed health needs of a defined community. COPC incorporates all the members of that community or the community's subgroups, and it addresses the priority health problems through an intervention covering the natural history of the condition. Thus, the intervention programs include preventive care, health promotion activities, treatment, and rehabilitation. The community is an active participant or partner in this endeavor, and cooperation with other sectors is sought as needed. The approach is applied through a series of steps, starting with the definition and characterization of the community, a prioritization process to decide on a pressing health condition, a detailed assessment of that condition, and the planning and implementation of the intervention. The surveillance, monitoring, and evaluation of the program leads to the reassessment of the condition and the continuation, modification, or discontinuation of the program. The incorporation of the program into the routine activities of a service facilitates its sustainability.

Box 4-4 A road map for the development of COPC programs

<table>
<tr>
<td rowspan="10" style="writing-mode: vertical">C O M M U N I T Y   D I A G N O S I S</td>
<td>Definition of the community</td>
<td>According to the service, it could be the following:
Geographically-defined area
Initial defined area (IDA) close to the service
Registered or insured people in a clinic
School, factory, refugee camp
Any definition should be all inclusive</td>
</tr>
<tr>
<td>Characterization of the community</td>
<td>Physical characteristics
Socio-cultural-demographic characteristics
Resources and assets (healthcare and other services, NGOs)
Health status of the community</td>
</tr>
<tr>
<td>Prioritization</td>
<td>Decision on who will be involved and their responsibilities
Decision on method and criteria
List of health conditions
Perform prioritization</td>
</tr>
<tr>
<td>Detailed assessment of the selected condition and its determinants</td>
<td>Analyze literature
Formulate objectives (What do we want to know about the condition and its determinants?) and define the population (Among whom?)
Gather available information
Collect new information</td>
</tr>
<tr>
<td>Intervention</td>
<td>Formulate objectives and define the target population (What do we want to achieve and in what period of time? Among whom?)
Formulate activities
Design records</td>
</tr>
<tr>
<td>Surveillance and monitoring</td>
<td>Ongoing assessment of health status and performance of activities</td>
</tr>
<tr>
<td>Evaluation</td>
<td>Assessment of effectiveness
Outcomes, process, structure
Differential value
Satisfaction
Efficiency</td>
</tr>
<tr>
<td>Resources and budget planning</td>
<td>Human resources, time allocation, and budget needed</td>
</tr>
<tr>
<td>Reassessment</td>
<td>Revision of the program and its achievements. Is there a need for change? Initiate a new prioritization process?</td>
</tr>
</table>

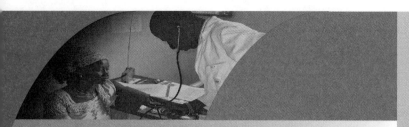

Discussion Questions

- How feasible is it to develop a COPC practice in a fragmented healthcare system?

- Do all COPC principles need to be applied in practice?

- Can different steps of the COPC process be applied separately?

- How feasible is it to involve the community in the COPC process?

- Why is intersectoral cooperation needed in COPC?

Review Questions

- What are the steps of the COPC process?

- Which criteria are useful for prioritization?

- How can the use of available data be assessed for the purpose of a detailed assessment?

- Which approaches can be used for the COPC intervention to address the health–illness continuum?

- Which types of evaluation are used in COPC and for what purpose?

REFERENCES

1. Gofin J, Gofin R, Knishkowy B. Evaluation of a community-oriented primary care workshop for family practice residents in Jerusalem. *Fam Med.* 1995;27:28–34.

2. Gofin J. Planning the teaching of community health (COPC) in an MPH program. *Public Health Rev.* 2002;30:293–301.

3. Gofin J, Foz G. Training and application of community-oriented primary care (COPC) through family medicine in Catalonia, Spain. *Fam Med.* 2008;40:196–202.

4. Geographic Information Systems (GIS) at CDC. http://www.cdc.gov/gis/ Accessed January 2010.

5. Mullan F. Geographic retrofitting: a method of community definition in community-oriented primary care practices. *Fam Med.* 2004;36:440–446.

6. Kark SL. *The Practice of Community-Oriented Primary Health Care.* New York, NY: Appleton Century Crofts; 1981.

7. US Census Bureau. International data base. http://www.census.gov/ipc/www/idb/. Accessed February 2009.

8. Lassetter JH, Callister LC. The impact of migration on the health of voluntary migrants in Western societies. *J Transcult Nurs.* 2009;20:93–104.

9. Maffla C. Health in the age of migration: migration and health in the EU. *Community Pract.* 2008;81:32–35.

10. Burazeri G, Goda A, Tavanxhi N, Sulo G, Stefa J, Kark JD. The health effects of emigration on those who remain at home. *Int J Epidemiol.* 2007;36:1265–1272.

11. Wiseman U, Mooney G, Berry G, Tang KC. Involving the general public in priority setting: experiences from Australia. *Soc Sci & Med.* 2003;56:1001–1012.

12. Oxman AD, Schunemann HJ, Fretheim A. Improving the use of research evidence in guideline development: 2. priority setting. *BioMed Central.* Health Research Policy Systems 2006;4:14. doi:10.1186/1478-4505-4-14.

13. Gofin J, Gofin R. Community-oriented primary care: a public health model in primary care. *Rev Panam Salud Pública.* 2007;21:177–184.

14. Abramson JH, Abramson ZH. *Research Methods in Community Medicine.* 6th ed. West Sussex, England: John Wiley & Sons; 2008.

15. World Health Organization. International classification of diseases. http://www.who.int/classifications/icd/en/. Accessed February 2009.

16. World Health Organization. International classification of primary care, second edition (ICPC-2). http://www.who.int/classifications/icd/adaptations/icpc2/en/index.html. Accessed February 2009.

17. American Psychiatric Association. DSM-IV-TR: The current manual. http://www.dsmivtr.org/. Accessed February 2009.

18. Kypri K, Langley JD, Saunders JB, Cashell-Smith ML, Herbison P. Randomized control trial of a web-based alcohol screening and brief intervention in primary care. *Arch Int Med.* 2008;168:530–536.

19. Linke S, Harrison R, Wallace P. A web-based intervention used in general practice for people with excessive alcohol consumption. *J Telemed Telecare.* 2005;11(suppl 1):39–41.

20. Van Voorhees BW, Ellis JM, Gollan JK, et al. Development and process evaluation of a primary care Internet-based intervention to prevent depression in emerging adults. *Prim Care Companion J Clin Psychiatry.* 2007;9:346–355.

21. Gofin R, De Leon D, Knishkowy B, Palti H. Injury prevention program in primary care: process evaluation and surveillance. *Inj Prev.* 1995;1:35–39.

22. Abramson JH, Gofin R, Hopp C, Gofin J, Donchin M, Habib J. Evaluation of a community program for the control of cardiovascular risk factors: the CHAD program in Jerusalem. *Isr J Med Sci.* 1981;17:201–212.

23. Abramson JH, Gofin J, Hopp C, Schein MH, Naveh P. The CHAD program for the control of cardiovascular risk factors in a Jerusalem community: a 24-year retrospect. *Isr J Med Sci.* 1994;30:108–119.

24. Sgan-Cohen HD, Mansbach IK, Haver D, Gofin R. Community-oriented oral health promotion for infants in Jerusalem: evaluation of a program trial. *J Public Health Dent.* 2001;61:107–113.

25. Gofin J, Gofin R, Abramson JH, Ban R. Ten-year evaluation of hypertension, overweight, cholesterol, and smoking control: the CHAD program in Jerusalem. Community syndrome of hypertension, atherosclerosis and diabetes. *Prev Med.* 1986;15:304–312.

26. Gofin R, Palti H, Adler B. Time trends of haemoglobin levels and anaemia prevalence in infancy in a total community. *Public Health.* 1992;106:11–18.

27. Gofin R, Adler B, Palti H. Time trends of child development in a Jerusalem community. *Paediatr Perinat Epidemiol.* 1996;10:197–206.

28. Bratt JH, Foreit J, De Vargas T. Three strategies to promote sustainability of CEMOPLAF clinics in Ecuador. Centros Médicos de Orientación y Planificación Familiar. *Stud Fam Plann.* 1998;29:58–68.

29. Jackson C, Fortmann SP, Flora JA, Melton RJ, Snider JP, Littlefield D. The capacity-building approach to intervention maintenance implemented by the Stanford Five-City Project. *Health Ed Res.* 1994;9:385–396.

30. D'Amour D, Ferrada-Videla M, San Martin Rodriguez L, Beaulieu M-D. The conceptual basis for interprofessional collaboration: core concepts and theoretical frameworks. *J Interprofessional Care.* 2005;19:(suppl 1): 116–131.

31. Cook DA. Models of interprofessional learning in Canada. *J Interprofessional Care.* 2005;19:(suppl 1):107–115.

32. Pan American Health Organization. Renewing primary health care in the Americas. March 2007. http://www.paho.org/english/AD/THS/Primary HealthCare.pdf. Accessed February 2009

33. World Health Organization. The World Health Report 2008—primary health care (now more than ever). http://www.who.int/whr/2008/en/index.html. Accessed February 2009.

34. US Census Bureau. Health insurance coverage: 2007. http://www.census.gov/hhes/www/hlthins/hlthin07.html. Accessed February 2009.

35. Centers for Medicare and Medicaid Services. Federally Qualified Health Center fact sheet. http://www.cms.hhs.gov/MLNProducts/downloads/fqhcfactsheet.pdf. Accessed February 2009.

36. Sixty-Second World Health Assembly. Primary health care, including health system strengthening (WHA62.12, Agenda item 12.4, 22 May, 2009). http://apps.who.int/gb/ebwha/pdf_files/A62/A62_R12-en.pdf. Accessed June 2009.

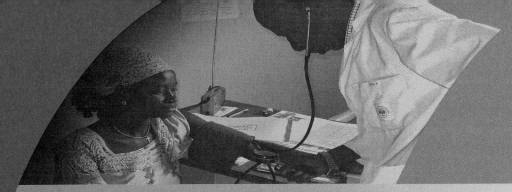

CHAPTER 5

Community-Oriented Public Health (COPH)

LEARNING OBJECTIVES

By the end of the chapter, learners will be able to

- understand and discuss the concept of community-oriented public health (COPH);
- elaborate on the functions of public health at the population and community levels;
- understand the differences between Community-Oriented Primary Care (COPC) and COPH;
- discuss the services involved in COPH;
- identify COPH practices;
- understand the needs for capacity building in COPH.

CHAPTER OUTLINE

KEY TERMS

capacity building
community-oriented primary care (COPC)
community-oriented public health (COPH)
community-oriented public health functions
community-oriented public health services
population-based public health

Box 5-1 Case study: Project renewal

The municipality of city J decided to address the recovery of certain neighborhoods within the city. The neighborhoods were characterized by poor housing and overcrowding. The population was mainly composed of immigrants who were living in the city for about 10 years and had a low educational level and a higher unemployment rate than the rest of the city. The population was aging because the younger generations were moving to other parts of the city or to other cities. To improve the situation and realize the potential of the neighborhood, the Municipal Health Department, together with the Department of Social Services, created Project Renewal, which included enlarging the existing homes and promoting small enterprises for the local people. A special health program for the elderly population was programmed to address vision and hearing problems, oral health, and mobility. The program was operated by the city's health department in collaboration with other services. Community participation was stimulated, and several committees were set up that, together with professionals, decided on health and social policies.

INTRODUCTION

Population health, whether at the local, state, or national level, is the domain of public health. As the confines of populations are increasingly expanding and communications and new technologies provide a global dimension to populations, public health's sphere of action is also expanding. Nevertheless, defined populations continue to be the focus of attention for most public health actions. In community-oriented public health (COPH), the community level is the focus of attention.

> ## Box 5-2
> ## Definition of COPH
>
> COPH is the discipline that applies population health principles in the context of the community's health. It deals with the identification and analysis of the health status and its determinants in a particular community, group of communities, or geographic region. It is followed by interventions addressing the community's health needs and their determinants through promotion, and prevention actions through multidisciplinary and intersectoral cooperation. COPH reinforces the social justice and social accountability dimensions of public health.

COPH is not only realized through the actions of the health sector, but also by other agencies and organizations, with the community's involvement. Intersectoral cooperation, as well as the actions of professionals from different backgrounds, are at the core of COPH activities. By definition, COPH is community based and acts through different settings where people live, study, work, receive care, or spend their leisure time. In this chapter we elaborate on the target populations in COPH, the functions of COPH, the differentiation from population-based public health and community oriented primary care (COPC), and the capacity-building needs in COPH.

THE TARGET POPULATION IN COMMUNITY-ORIENTED PUBLIC HEALTH

The target population for COPH is an identifiable entity, a community, or groups of communities in which its members and the providers of public health services identify. It encompasses all members of the community, regardless of insurance status or their enrollment in a specific insurance or health scheme. The community can be located in a rural or urban area, and it can vary in size from a neighborhood, a ward, or a statistical area. Larger divisions, such as cities, counties, or districts, could constitute the target community, depending on the decision makers' area of action or the public health intervention required.

For example, a COPH program in Barcelona, "Health in the Neighborhoods," addresses health issues and their social determinants within the context of the Catalan government program of gentrification of dilapidated neighborhoods (see Case Study 11). In coordination with municipalities and primary care centers, the program aims to improve the residents' life conditions and facilitate social cohesion; it addresses priority health needs identified by the population and other stakeholders.

The New York City Department of Health and Mental Hygiene targeted impoverished neighborhoods (encompassing several statistical areas) that have a high burden of disease for the development of prevention activities related to nutrition, childhood asthma, teen pregnancy, physical inactivity, and newborn health.[1] In the neighborhoods, the department deployed multidisciplinary teams led by a physician that included members with expertise in epidemiology, program development, and community activities.

Water fluoridation is another example where a local health department is responsible for implementing an intervention to improve a population's dental health. While other actions can be performed by individuals or health services (such as using or recommending fluoridated tooth paste, or fluoride supplements), water fluoridation addresses the community level.

A well-defined community in COPH serves several purposes (see Table 5-1). These purposes include the following: (1) *For its members and organizations*, the community provides a natural framework for interaction with individual or institutional contacts. It is through these contacts that community members can express their health needs, services are provided and interventions can be channeled. Local health services, NGOs, community administrations, and schools bear responsibility for specific activities for their members, constituents, pupils, or populations they serve or represent. Health departments can thus channel their activities or interventions through these institutions. (2) *For public health professionals and institutions*, a well-defined community provides the framework for the measurement and assessment of the community's health status and needs, as well as their determinants. It also allows for the provision of an appropriate answer or program for the community at large or any of its high-risk subgroups. The identification of the denominators for all of the measurements entails using census data or carrying out surveys for the specific place if information is not already available. (3) *For policy makers* whose mandate is to decide on policies at different levels, the ultimate implementation may include providing certain services or enacting and enforcing regulations and laws at the com-

TABLE 5-1 The Purpose of Defining the Community in COPH

Stakeholders	Purpose
Community members and community organizations	To offer a framework to express community needs and define the target for the delivery of interventions
Public health professionals and institutions	To measure health needs and their determinants in a specific place and deliver programs for the community at large or its subgroups
Policy makers	To decide on health policies, provide services, and enforce regulations and laws in certain populations

munity level. This can be realized through local health departments, health services, or other health-related organizations that cooperate with one another or act independently.

COMMUNITY-ORIENTED PUBLIC HEALTH FUNCTIONS

A community's health status is the expression of biological processes and their determinants interacting with the social, physical, cultural, economic, or political environment at the personal or ecological level (see Chapter 1). COPH attends to community health through public health functions implemented by public health departments and other institutions at the community level.

Essential Public Health Functions and Services

International and national organizations, such as the Pan American Health Organization (PAHO)[2,3] the regional office of the World Health Organization (WHO), have defined the essential functions of public health. In the United States, the Centers for Disease Control and Prevention (CDC)[4] and other organizations have defined essential public health services.[5,6] PAHO defines essential public health functions as "the indispensable set of actions under the primary responsibility of the state, that are fundamental for achieving the goal of public health which is to improve, promote, protect, and restore the health of the population through collective action."[3]

A comparison of the CDC's public health services and PAHO's public health functions show both similarities and differences (see Table 5-2). Both organizations identify functions related to health assessments, such as diagnosis and monitoring (CDC 1, 2; PAHO 1) and health surveillance (PAHO 2); health education, promotion, and participation (CDC and

PAHO 3, 4, 5); policy and enforcement (CDC and PAHO 5, 6); health services equity and its evaluation (CDC 7; PAHO 7, 9); workforce development (CDC and PAHO 8); and research (CDC and PAHO 10). PAHO adds a function related to the reduction of the impact of emergencies and disasters on health.

Essential Community-Oriented Public Health Functions

Similarly to the essential public health functions, COPH functions can be defined as shown in Box 5-3.

The COPH functions (Table 5-3) are implemented for defined communities. Thus, COPH is an effective method for implementing traditional public health functions at the community level.

A strategic plan for health education and promotion activities is the basis for the development and implementation of health interventions. This should be done according to sound

Box 5-3 Definition of COPH functions

COPH functions are a set of actions, which are the responsibility of local health departments or health agencies, that are carried out to improve, promote, protect, and restore the health of the community through collective action. These actions can be delivered by institutions other than (or in cooperation with) health agencies, such as social services, housing departments, or police and fire departments, among others.

TABLE 5-2 Public Health Services and Functions—CDC and PAHO

	CDC	PAHO
1	**Monitor** health status to identify community health problems	**Monitor**, evaluate, and analyze health status
2	**Diagnose and investigate** health problems and health hazards in the community	**Surveillance, research, and control** of the risks and threats to public health
3	**Inform, educate, and empower** people about health issues	**Health promotion**
4	**Mobilize** community partnerships to identify and solve health problems	**Social participation** in health
5	**Develop policies and plans** that support individual and community health efforts	Development of **policies and institutional capacity** for public health planning and management
6	**Enforce** laws and regulations that protect health and ensure safety	Strengthening of public health **regulation and enforcement** capacity
7	**Link** people to needed personal healthcare services and assure the provision of healthcare services when otherwise unavailable	**Evaluation** and promotion of equitable access to necessary healthcare services
8	Assure a competent **public health and personal healthcare workforce**	**Human resources development** and training in public health
9	**Evaluate** effectiveness, accessibility, and quality of individual and population-based healthcare services	**Quality assurance** in personal and population-based healthcare services
10	**Research** for new insights and innovative solutions to health problems	**Research** in public health
11		Reduction of the impact of **emergencies and disasters** on health

data and available resources based on the evidence of effectiveness from the literature. Strategic planning may include services and institutions, other than those specifically related to health, that may be needed for a comprehensive approach in dealing with health problems. Exposure to lead or environmental pollution, for example, requires the intervention of agencies that deal with the environment. The use of child car restraints and bicycle or motorcycle helmets involves transportation departments and the police to enforce laws. The sustainability of actions needs to be assured during planning.

National or state health policies need to be applied in local communities. It is the function of COPH to adapt these policies locally, on the basis of the local situation and priorities and considering the culturally diverse groups of the population and at-risk populations.

The functions related to community health assessments, whether they take the form of a community diagnosis or community health surveillance, are the basic steps to define the community's needs and to study trends over time. The assessment should include identification of inequities in services provision and health status inequalities.

The development, implementation, and evaluation of interventions are natural and needed steps following the assessment of community health needs. Preparedness and rehabilitation plans should also be in place because it is at the community level where national policies will be applied. Even global emergencies—such as influenza A (H1N1), known as swine flu, which appeared in April 2009—ultimately need a COPH approach. As H1N1 started spreading across nations from the original cases in Mexico, the World Health Organi-

TABLE 5-3 The Functions of COPH

Strategic planning	Plans are developed and intervention alternatives and available resources are examined to best address priority health issues in the community. This is based on data and evidence of good practice to assure the sustainability of interventions. The health service can include different sectors and agencies in the planning process for a comprehensive approach to address the health issues. Planning can be expanded to include nonhealth agencies for disaster efforts and existing health hazards, such as lead exposure, asthma irritants (pollution, cockroaches, etc.), or hearing loss (noise level in industry or music).
Adapting policies to the local level	National policies are adapted according to the specific community's needs and the local scene and culture.
Community health assessment	Existing data sources are identified or new information is gathered to determine the community's health status and its determinants, needs, and assets. Health surveillance is performed, and an analysis is completed of equitable service provision, gaps in provided services, and health inequalities.
Development, implementation, and evaluation of interventions	The development, implementation, and evaluation of interventions is done according to set priorities for prevention, promotion, and maintenance of the community's health. Preparedness plans are developed in case of man-made or natural disasters.
Service-oriented research	Service-oriented research is the basis for health assessments, intervention programs, and planning. It identifies and monitors inequities in healthcare services and health status.
Capacity building	Capacity building assures a trained workforce based on appropriate competencies that address health literacy, cultural competence, behavioral science and methodology, inequities and inequalities, and team building.
Coalition building	Partnerships are created among health services, other services and institutions, and community members to pool human and economic resources.

zation promptly issued its first report on global preparedness and reached its highest level of alert within a short time span.[7] Many countries followed the WHO recommendation, and adequate measures were put in place. Although H1N1 was declared a pandemic, the WHO made specific recommendations for communities, such as advice on the use of masks and other preventive measures in community settings, as well as prevention and mitigation in communities with few resources.

To get sound data, service-oriented research is needed. This will provide a baseline assessment for the programs and their evaluation. The research should also have the ability to detect high-risk groups, inequities, and inequalities, which all need to be addressed.

To attend to all these functions, an appropriate workforce is necessary. Capacity building should prepare the workforce not only in the methodologies needed, but it should also consider the knowledge and understanding of local community characteristics. The competencies should be built accordingly, and issues such as health literacy, culture and health, behavioral sciences, and quantitative and qualitative methodologies (among others) should be addressed. In addition, coalition building to address multifaceted community health problems is essential to face the complex and multifactorial health problems that affect a community.

COPH activities can be initiated by a health department or other health agency for a specific community, multiple communities, or larger populations when specific problems have been identified or health policies are being applied (see Figure 5-1). This follows a top–down approach and will express the COPH functions as determined by the health agency. The degree of community participation in the process may vary. Conversely, problems can be identified by local health clinics that develop COPC practices (see Case Studies 13 and 14) or by community members who organize themselves to approach the health agency. This will then be followed by measuring the needs and designing a program in collaboration with other agencies, in accordance with the type of program developed. This is the bottom–up approach, which can be facilitated by the specific policies of the health agency to stimulate communities and support them in the development of COPH programs, as in the case of Barcelona (see Case Study 11).

COMMUNITY-ORIENTED PUBLIC HEALTH AND POPULATION-BASED PUBLIC HEALTH

Public health, by definition, is population based, although it is not necessarily community oriented because the community boundaries may not be relevant for public health levels of action. Public health services are identified with organizations, such as health departments, ministries of health, public health agencies, and the CDC. Although their functions impact the lives and occupations of people and their environment, providers are not usually known to the public or directly related to it. Even though public health institutions may direct their actions to specific communities, there are distinctions between the traditional population-based public health focus and the community-oriented public health focus, as shown in Table 5-4.

FIGURE 5-1 The top–down and bottom–up development of COPH

Top–down (begins with department of health or public health agencies)

Health agency identifies problem (traffic accidents, lead poisoning)

Health agency performs assessment

Health agency develops intervention program

Program implementation through health and other agencies

Program implementation through health and other agencies

Health agency develops program

Health agency performs assessment

Community organizes to approach the health agency

Community (members, health services) identifies problem (traffic accidents, lead poisoning)

Bottom–up (begins with community)

TABLE 5-4 Focus of Population-Based Public Health and Community-Oriented Public Health

	Population-based public health	Community-oriented public health
Needs assessment and definition	Not always performed; usually aggregated data for the whole nation or minimal information for specific areas; performed according to political will	For a specific community, health status, behaviors, and determinants are assessed; usually initiated by local services
Priorities	Decided at national, district, or local levels; may or may not be based on a health assessment of population or local services	Decided at the community level with community participation
Interventions	Decided as policies; overall assigned budget or no targeted budget	Targeted and tailored to the specific community
Services	Overall recommendation of service delivery; no specific service recommendation for action	Community health services and partnership with other health-related services and organizations
Community participation	Variable, usually limited	Seeks to integrate community members and organizations in all activities
Sustainability	Organized as projects; seldom integrated into services	Program integrated into the community service

In population-based public health, public health policies might be enacted or applied according to what is deemed to be adequate for a population without an appropriate needs assessment. Because the level of action could be for a government office, the nation as a whole, or an entire school health system, what may be relevant for a specific population or school may not be needed or may not be a priority in another community. Frequently policies are reactive more than proactive, and proper planning is lacking. Health assessments completed through surveys may encompass large populations and cover the entire nation. This provides a wealth of information regarding health status, behaviors and trends, and availability and accessibility of health services and programs. Assessments may also highlight inequities and disparities. However, they might be provided as aggregate information and might not address particular issues that are relevant to specific communities. In addition, the information may not include a sufficient number of people in a particular community to provide a meaningful health assessment.

In COPH, given that the community is defined, a health needs assessment is warranted to develop and evaluate interventions or for surveillance and monitoring. In this health assess-ment, knowledge of the community facilitates the inclusion of relevant health status determinants, which are essential for intervention program development and ultimately for its success.

Priorities for action in COPH need to be determined to make the most efficient use of resources for addressing community health problems. This might not be the case in traditional public health where decisions might be based on extraneous factors or interests in which the population was not consulted or does not have a say. In COPH the process is based on the local needs assessment; it follows selected criteria and involves the community.

In the framework of traditional public health, interventions for a certain condition are based on policy recommendations to be implemented at different levels and for diverse populations. An overall budget might be assigned to the interventions to be distributed in the country, districts, or other areas, or the budget might be based on grants that have to be obtained for the specific purpose. In COPH the intervention is geared toward a specific community and is tailored to its socioeconomic and cultural characteristics. Procuring an appropriate budget might be the responsibility of the local service or organization.

The services that will deliver the intervention may not be specified, and the recommendations may be unclear because they could vary greatly in different contexts. In COPH, because of close contact with the community and its services, the delivery of the interventions are carried out through appropriately identified venues, such as primary care facilities, schools, or other health-related institutions.

Community participation might be variable or not be considered in public health, but it is an integral component of COPH. This can be realized at different levels and at different degrees, from compliance with advice or recommendations to full partnership in decision making. The integration of community members at levels other than the community level might be variable.

The potential for sustainability is better realized when the programs are integrated into community services with a bottom–up approach of COPH than when they are designed with a top–down approach with limited resources.

COMMUNITY-ORIENTED PUBLIC HEALTH SERVICES

Health departments or public health agencies are especially well positioned for the delivery of COPH. Within their roles of policy development and implementation and their capabilities for priority identification and setting health goals, health departments can provide the leadership, resources, incentives, and direction for local communities to address their priority health issues. The opportunity or mandate for coalition building and creation of community partnerships are additional features that enable the implementation of public health at the community level. The New York City health department has created district public health offices to target specific communities with prevention activities.[1] There have been successful experiences in the Partnership for the Public's Health (PPH) in California, where local health departments and community partners acted on capacity building, community health improvement programs, and policy and systems changes. Sustainable changes were made in most participating communities.[8]

At the practice level, services that are provided in the community are the venues for COPH. School health services are one of these venues for incorporating COPH. These services cater to the majority of school-age children and are provided by different types of frameworks, such as school clinics and school health centers. Activities carried out in these settings include, among others, immunizations, screening, health surveillance, health education, first aid centers, advice, and referrals. A school health program developed by the CDC suggests that health services are one component of the program; other activities, such as physical education, nutrition services, coun-

seling and psychological services, and keeping a healthy school environment, are realized through the school setting as a whole. Parents and community involvement are considered to be resources for an effective response to the health needs of students.[9]

Hospitals, which traditionally provide individual care in outpatient clinics and their wards, are also developing a community orientation. The community orientation is considered to be the organization-wide generation, dissemination, and use of information to address the community's health needs.[10,11] Although some of the motivation for this community orientation is related to monetary gains (through tax exemption), there is genuine interest in tackling the community's health needs and their determinants. The degree of nonprofit hospitals' community orientation increases when they are part of a network and when their locations are in areas that are accustomed to community-oriented activities. Challenges for disseminating a hospital's community orientation is not only organizational, but also part of the intrinsic understanding of the goals and priorities of the institution balanced against demonstrable and tangible gains in the community's health and well-being. An example of community-oriented services of hospitals is provided in Case Study 6 on the Parkland Health & Hospital System in Dallas, which developed a plan for Dallas County based on a COPC approach and partnered with diverse community organizations.

Primary care services are one of the main settings where COPH is provided to the public. The integration of clinical individual care and public health activities (through prevention, promotion, treatment, and rehabilitation activities) has great potential to deal with community health problems. It also provides opportunities for reducing the fragmentation of health services and for offering a continuum of care for community members.

Community-Oriented Public Health and Community-Oriented Primary Care

One example of integration of clinical care and public health is community-oriented primary care (COPC) (see Chapters 3 and 4). COPC is characterized by addressing the needs of all members of a defined community (the healthy and the sick), and it includes health promotion activities, provision of preventive care, and treatment and rehabilitation. A comparison of the characteristics of COPC and COPH is provided in Table 5-5.

The target population in COPC can be geographically based or defined through membership in an insurance plan. It is usually of small dimension (i.e., a neighborhood) and centered on a primary care service. The unit of care can be indi-

TABLE 5-5 Comparison of COPC and COPH

	COPC	COPH
Population and area covered	Defined community; usually small, centered in a primary care clinic, geographically defined, or based on registration to a primary care service	A community or a number of communities, regardless of insurance status
Setting	Primary care clinic	Varies according to the health problem and the type of intervention
Service providers	Primary care (healthcare team) with a bottom–up approach; coordinated actions with other sectors	Public health departments or agencies; top–down approach; could include primary care (multiple) and other health services and sectors
Interventions	Promotion, prevention, treatment, rehabilitation	Promotion, prevention
Financing	Taxation, insurance, special fees	Health department or other health agency budget
Community participation	Yes	Yes

viduals or families, and the larger community is also considered in understanding the health status and its determinants to enable intervention. The target population in COPH is usually a community or a number of communities, irrespective of the healthcare providers, the insurance provider, or status.

The setting in COPC is defined as a primary care clinic. In COPH, however, the setting varies depending on the health problem addressed and the type of intervention needed.

The service provider in COPC is a primary care team, usually through a bottom–up approach, that provides the service based on the health needs of the specific community. In COPH, the ministries of health, health departments, or health agencies are the ones that deliver the services, usually through a top–down approach (which could also include primary care clinics and other health services and sectors). In both COPC and COPH, intersectoral cooperation is needed.

The interventions delivered in COPC usually cover the natural history of a disease or condition, thus including comprehensive care through health promotion and prevention, treatment, and rehabilitation. In COPH, the interventions only address promotion or prevention.

The financing of COPC programs are integrated into the health service budgets, which could be based on taxation, an insurance program, special fees, or other means, according to

the type of service. In COPH, financing depends on the health department or other agency budgets.

Community participation is common to both COPC and COPH and may vary in degree, according to the community's characteristics and the service or program provided.

Multidisciplinary Teams and Organizations in COPH

Health services are not the only organizations attending to the community's healthcare needs. This is due not only to the high costs of health care, but it also reflects the complexity of health issues and their determinants. Health services alone are limited in their capacity to offer solutions and alternative paths for interventions, and they need the cooperation of other sectors and organizations, both public and private.

The present obesity epidemic, for example, needs to be addressed by health services in coordination with other sectors. Healthy eating habits and physical activity are ultimately an individual responsibility. But for people to consume healthy and nutritious foods, they should be accessible in neighborhood groceries; people need to be educated on nutrition; facilities for physical activity should be available, such as bike paths and safe routes to walk to school; policies in schools and public places should be enacted to encourage healthy eating; businesses should be involved, providing information on healthy choices and promoting those products; and finally, the media should stimulate eating healthy foods and physical activity.

CAPACITY BUILDING FOR COMMUNITY-ORIENTED PUBLIC HEALTH

To be successful, COPH requires public health and healthcare professionals who are focused on communities and who have been educated and trained to work together. Unfortunately, one or both of these essential ingredients are often missing. Let us take a look at the current state of clinical health professions education and interprofessional collaboration and suggest options for improvement.

Medical and Nursing Professionals

Healthcare professionals acquire their knowledge and skills, and, more comprehensively, their competencies in continuous education after graduation. For physicians, traditional schools of medicine usually follow the biomedical model proposed by Flexner in his report of 1910,[12] which is in the German tradition; medical education has a strong biomedical scientific basis and hands-on bedside clinical training. However, Flexner, who was not a doctor but an educator, realized 15 years later[13] that "scientific medicine in America—young, vigorous and positivistic—is today sadly deficient in cultural and philosophic background." A review article in the *New England Journal of Medicine* in 2006 asserted that "more emphasis should be placed on the social, economic, and political aspects of health care delivery."[14]

To this day, most schools follow the Flexnerian model, and very few medical schools have community-based teaching. Although epidemiology and public health are part of the curriculum, community-based learning is not frequent, or it is at best limited. The combination of the theoretical basis of population health obtained in the classroom with community-based application is considered a successful combination for training future physicians.[15]

In the late 1970s, community-oriented medical schools started using innovative curricula, mostly based on problem-based learning (PBL), which integrated the basic sciences and clinical applications using novel teaching methods, and they took medical education outside the hospital walls. In 1979 the Network of Community-Oriented Educational Institutions for Health Sciences, was founded under the auspices of the World Health Organization (WHO), with members , from developing and developed countries.[16] These institutions flourished over the years and encompassed about 150 institutions 30 years later. In 2002 the Network partnered with the WHO Towards Unity For Health (TUFH) project. The new organization, The Network: Towards Unity for Health, which has an official relationship with the WHO, has created a platform to develop a more practice-oriented focus in teaching.[17]

Specialty training, such as family medicine, prepares professionals for the care of individuals and families in the community. However, community medicine, which would extend their field of action and influence, may not be a component of the curriculum. If it is, it may often be part of the curriculum in name but not in practice.

Of note, the residency program in social medicine at the Montefiore Medical Center in New York City for family physicians, internists, and pediatricians has been sustainable for nearly 40 years. Its curriculum has a community orientation and integrates social medicine and clinical practice. Its graduates are well-positioned for leadership in their professions.[18] Also, since 1993 in Spain, the residency program of Family and Community Medicine of the National Health System includes COPC training.[19]

The nursing profession provides more opportunities for community medicine teaching and training.[20] The practice of nursing in the community is not only more acceptable than in other professions, but it is also an integral part of the profession.

Public Health Professionals

Graduate public health professionals with master of public health (MPH) degrees are versed in population health, with strong methodology components in quantitative methods, such as epidemiology and biostatistics, as well as qualitative methods and behavioral sciences.[21,22] The principles and application of population health to specific communities, and practical community experience that the programs require, provide a robust basis for the understanding of community health and the practice of COPH. Practicum experiences, which are often community based, are now a required part of MPH programs in the United States.

Needs in Capacity Building for Healthcare Professionals

A desirable future of capacity building for COPH should strive for a curriculum that has both a community base and opportunities for different professions to share the same space both in the classroom and in the community. Interprofessional education (IPE) has been proposed and advocated by the WHO,[23,24] the US Institute of Medicine,[25] and by other organizations.[26] Although the Institute of Medicine emphasizes individual care and the improvement of care quality, others also consider the improvement of population health.[27]

Another capacity-building endeavor was developed by the Association of Teachers of Preventive Medicine (now called the Association for Prevention Teaching and Research, APTR)

Box 5-4 COPH at the community level

COPH brings traditional public health to the community level, addressing local needs and priorities and adapting and tailoring interventions to local realities. Thus, communities benefit from promotion and prevention activities that are specific to the community (or groups of communities). Through COPH, communities also benefit from the adaptation of national or regional policies that seek to apply them in accordance to the realities of the community.

The challenges that communities face regarding health problems and their determinants need well-coordinated and specific interventions. Although there is much to be accomplished regarding improvements in community health, and the task requires well-coordinated health services, COPH is favorably positioned and has the tools to affect community changes and address the wide scope of community health and health care.

that convened the Healthy People Curriculum Task Force. The task force includes representatives of healthcare professions (such as allopathic and osteopathic medicine, nursing and nurse practitioners, dentistry, pharmacy, and physician assistants) to develop the Clinical Prevention and Population Health Curriculum Framework.[28] The framework contains four components: evidence base for practice; clinical preventive services and health promotion; health systems; and health policy and community aspects of practice.

For COPH, interprofessional learning is necessary to develop a common understanding and goals for community health improvement. Simultaneously learning about the diversity of populations, the social determinants of health, the assessment of needs and culturally sensitive interventions, communications and health literacy, team building and leadership, coalition and partnership building, and working together in the field provides an opportunity for a lifelong practice of partnership and integration of health care.

SUMMARY

COPH is the discipline that blends population health principles in the context of the community's health. COPH is achieved not only through the actions of the health sector, but also by other agencies and organizations, with the community's involvement. The COPH functions include strategic planning; adapting policies to the local level; health assessment; development, implementation, and evaluation of interventions; service-oriented research; capacity building, which is interprofessional by nature; and lastly, coalition building.

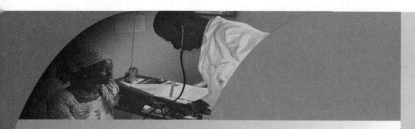

Discussion Questions

- Are state populations a target of COPH?

- How can COPH functions be distinguished from public health functions that are not community oriented?

- Are all health services adequate for COPH?

- Is COPC a particular example of COPH?

- Can professionals in different fields be trained on COPH with a similar curriculum?

Review Questions

- What are the suitable populations for COPH?

- What are the COPH functions?

- What are the differences between COPH and population-based public health?

- What are the services that could develop COPH?

- What are the needs in capacity building for COPH?

REFERENCES

1. Goodman A. President Obama's health plan and community-based prevention [editorial]. *Am J Public Health.* 2009;99:1736–1738.

2. The Partnership for Maternal, Newborn & Child Health. Essential public health functions as a strategy for improving overall health systems performance. http://www.who.int/pmnch/topics/health_systems/paho_who_ephf2007/en/index.html. Accessed May 2009.

3. Pan American Health Organization, World Health Organization. *Public Health in the Americas: Conceptual Renewal, Performance Assessment, and Bases for Action.* Washington, DC. PAHO–WHO; 2002.

4. Centers for Disease Control and Prevention. 10 essential public health services. http://www.cdc.gov/od/ocphp/nphpsp/essentialphservices.htm. Accessed May 2009.

5. American Public Health Association. 10 essential public health services. http://www.apha.org/programs/standards/performancestandardsprogram/resexxentialservices.htm. Accessed May 2009.

6. Public Health Functions Project. Public health in America. http://www.health.gov/phfunctions/public.htm. Accessed May 2009.

7. World Health Organization. Global alert and response (GAR). http://www.who.int/csr/don/2009_05_01/en/index.html. Accessed May 2009.

8. Cheadle A, Hsu C, Schwartz PM, et al. Involving local health departments in community health partnerships: evaluation results from the partnership for the public's health initiative. *J Urban Health.* 2008;85:162–177.

9. Centers for Disease Control and Prevention. Healthy youth! Coordinated school health program. http://www.cdc.gov/HealthyYouth/CSHP/. Accessed July 2009.

10. Proenca EJ, Rosko MD, Zinn JS. Community orientation in hospitals: an institutional and resource dependence perspective. *Health Serv Res.* 2000;.35:5(pt 1):1011–1035.

11. Shortell SM, Washington PK, Baxter RJ. The contribution of hospitals and health care systems to community health. *Annu Rev Public Health.* 2009;30:373–383.

12. Flexner A. *Medical Education in the United States and Canada: A Report to the Carnegie Foundation for the Advancement of Teaching.* New York, NY: Carnegie Foundation for the Advancement of Teaching; 1910.

13. Flexner A. *Medical Education: A Comparative Study.* New York, NY: MacMillan; 1925.

14. Cooke M, Irby DM, Sullivan W, Ludmerer KM. American medical education 100 years after the Flexner report. *New Eng J Med.* 2006;355:1339–1344.

15. Chamberlain LJ, Wang NE, Ho ET, Banchoff AW, Braddock CH 3rd, Gesundheit N. Integrating collaborative population health projects into a medical student curriculum at Stanford. *Acad Med.* 2008;83:338–344.

16. Schmidt HG, Neufeld VR, Nooman ZM, Ogunbode T. Network of community-oriented educational institutions for the health sciences. *Acad Med.* 1991;66:259–263.

17. Kaufman A, van Dalen J, Majoor G, Carrasco FM. The Network: Towards Unity for Health. 25th anniversary. *Med Educ.* 2004;38:1214–1217.

18. Strelnick AH, Swiderski D, Fornari A et al. The residency program in social medicine of Montefiore Medical Center: 37 years of mission-driven, interdisciplinary training in primary care, population health and social medicine. *Acad Med.* 2008;83:378–389.

19. Gofin J, Foz G. Training and application of community-oriented primary care (COPC) through family medicine in Catalonia, Spain. *Fam Med.* 2008;40:196–202.

20. The history of public health and community health nursing. In: Stanhope M, Lancaster J, eds. *Foundations of Nursing in the Community. Community-Oriented Practice.* Elsevier; 2005.

21. Council on Education for Public Health. *Criteria for Accreditation of Graduate Schools of Public Health.* Washington DC: Council on Education for Public Health; 2005.

22. Association of Schools of Public Health. *Accreditation of Public Health Education Programs.* St. Moritz, France: Association of Schools of Public Health; 2005.

23. World Health Organization. *Learning Together to Work Together for Health. Report of a WHO Study Group on Multiprofessional Education of Health Personnel: The Team Approach.* Geneva, Switzerland: World Health Organization. Technical Report Series. 1988;769:1–72.

24. Yan J, Gilbert JH, Hoffman SJ. World Health Organization study group on interprofessional education and collaborative practice. http://www.who.int/hrh/professionals/announcement.pdf. Accessed August 2009.

25. Greiner AC, Knebel E, eds. *Health Professions Education: A Bridge to Quality.* Washington, DC: Institute of Medicine, National Academies Press; 2003.

26. Barr H. Interprofessional education in the United Kingdom. Some historical perspectives 1966–1996. http://www.cipel.ac.uk/links/documents/InterprofessionalEducationintheUK-SomeHistoricalPerspectives.pdf. Accessed August 2009.

27. Health Canada. Interprofessional education for collaborative patient-centred practice. http://www.hc-sc.gc.ca/hcs-sss/hhr-rhs/strateg/interprof/index-eng.php. Accessed August 2009.

28. Allan J, Barwick TA, Cashman S, et al. Clinical prevention and population health: curriculum framework for health professions. *Am J Prev Med.* 2004;27:471–476.

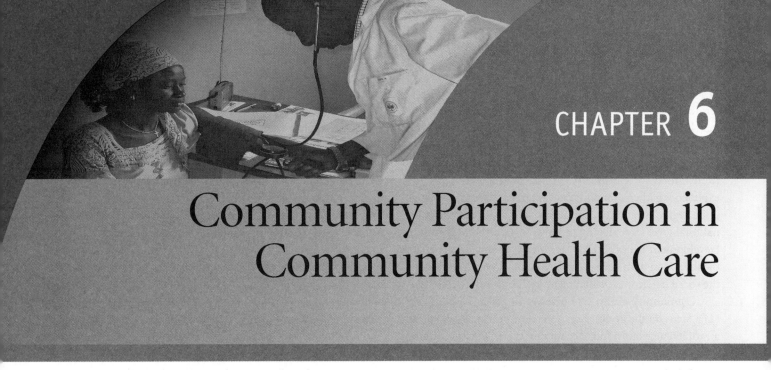

CHAPTER 6

Community Participation in Community Health Care

KEY TERMS

community health care   community participation
community involvement

INTRODUCTION

Community participation has been implemented by health services since the 1940s, as exemplified by Kark in Pholela, South Africa,[1] and Geiger in the United States in 1960.[2] However, it was not until after the 1978 Alma-Ata International Conference on Primary Health Care that community involvement was considered to be one of the pillars of the primary health care approach developed by the World Health Organization (WHO).[3] The rationale for including the concept as a pillar was that greater and more effective community participation in health services could bring better care for the population and ultimately lead to better health. Thirty years after the Declaration of Alma-Ata, the complexity of the different types and purposes of community participation determined the need to continue efforts to reinforce participation and learn from the experience gathered in different contexts. A current challenge is the degree assigned to community participation at the international level in achieving progress toward the Millennium Development Goals (MDGs) regarding, among others goals, the reduction of maternal and child mortality and addressing the social determinants that relate to the aims of the MDGs.[4]

Community health care involves two main dimensions: (1) a focus on the health care of the community as a whole or any of its subgroups; and (2) community participation aiming to maintain or improve the health and health care of community members. The first dimension depends on the health service's mission and strategies. The second dimension depends on the community's willingness and decision to be involved in promoting their health and health care.

Participation in health care and especially in community health care should be considered a principle and not merely an input to a project or activity. As a principle, participation implies a relevant dimension of community life and community organization. The principle, the right to health and the right to health care in any community, is an expression of social justice toward the fulfillment of maintenance and improvement of the public's health. A community's participation in its own health care has been a topic of discussion throughout the last decades.[5-11] Proposals and strategies to assess and increase its feasibility and applications have been on the agenda of national and international health organizations.

In this chapter we will analyze different definitions related to community participation; the purpose and role of community participation in community health care; and the spectrum, types and determinants of community participation. A framework will be presented for the development of community participation in community health care, including monitoring and evaluation.

DEFINITIONS

Conceptually and operationally, community involvement is an integral component of community health care. However, community involvement is not always included in community health care activities. Community participation and community involvement are frequently used interchangeably in the literature. Throughout this chapter, unless specified otherwise, we will generally refer to *community participation* as the most commonly used term.

In some definitions of community, the dimension of community participation may be implicit because it involves having a sense of belonging and a collective perception of needs and priorities; it is "the ability to assume a collective responsibility for community decisions."[12] Community participation has been described by Kahssay and Oakley[7] as "a means," a process of people cooperating with projects, and as "an end," a goal in itself. This includes individuals who voluntarily agree to participate to assure cooperation with certain service activities or when participation is carried out in collaboration with institutions outside the local setting. However, Morgan[8] describes collaboration differently: "A utilitarian effort to use community resources and to decrease costs."

Rifkin described community participation as "a dynamic process which enables local people, through involvement and experience, to gain access and control to health care resources."[13] As related to empowerment, "community participation [is] a way of giving people power over their health choices; a means in itself; as active and based on community initiatives; as a process whereby communities are strengthened in their capacity to control their own lives and make decisions outside the direction of professionals and authorities and evaluated by qualitative methods."[13]

When the community is defined as being registered in a healthcare service, the feeling of sharing, as proposed by Willmott and Thomas,[14] may not be relevant for community participation. Members registered in a healthcare service or health plan do not usually share collective actions or have a collective voice toward the common good and the extent and type of participation. This might hamper participation.

The various definitions point to the different levels of participation. The definitions may also reflect the different disciplines, perspectives, and ideological backgrounds of the authors and the different experiences in community participation at the time the definitions were formulated.

Box 6-1 Community participation

Community participation in health care could be considered as the activities performed by community members (individually or in groups) intended to improve the community's health, the health care, or the organization of services.

FACTORS INFLUENCING PARTICIPATION

Community participation will vary depending on the context where the initiative is taking place. It may depend on several factors, such as the economic level of the community; the geographic location (urban, rural); the sociocultural and political context; and the organization of the health institution and its population coverage. The degree of participation by a community in an urban area might be facilitated by the proximity of the community members' residences in relation to the service, especially when the community is defined by its geographic location or if its members belong to one service location. In rural areas, participation will depend on the distance between the community members' residences and the service. The sociocultural aspects, such as the degree of organization and the presence and effectiveness of leadership, may influence the degree of participation.

A community's culture should be seen as the natural context where activities for community health improvement will be adapted and developed.

In addition to the local culture, which may determine whether the community considers participation to be for the common good, other local characteristics play a role in the acceptance, or rejection of participation in community activities. For example, socioeconomic context, low literacy rates, general neglect, social discrimination, and dependence on authorities through generations may hinder participation.[15] The political context in which these communities operate (if there is a participatory culture or environment, or if participation is seen as interfering) may influence how a community perceives its role.

LEVELS OF DECISION FOR COMMUNITY PARTICIPATION: LOCAL, REGIONAL, NATIONAL

Community participation can be expressed as a local endeavor resulting from the relationship between community members and the local health service or a proposed activity by the regional or national level. Whether it is a locally initiated activity or a proposed policy, this could generate benefits for both the community and the services.

The local initiative represents an expression of involvement beyond the individual interest. It might be generated by the common feelings of belonging, ownership, or the particular cultural values of the community (helping others). It may also derive from a feeling of trust toward the health services and the active promotion of participation by the healthcare team. In a review of several case studies in different countries, Morgan[8] confirmed the value of the local grassroots context on influencing participation.

In some instances the decision to establish a community participation environment is made at the regional or national level and is influenced by the strategies of international donors. This might be referred to as a vertical approach in contrast to a grassroots initiative. The scope and success of such a vertical approach will depend on (1) whether participation involves a relatively large proportion of the members; (2) whether the opinions and willingness for involvement of the team and community members have been considered; (3) whether the proposed participation takes into consideration the specific characteristics of the community, such as education, cultural values, and beliefs; (4) whether there is political will and logistic and organizational support; and (5) whether community participation contributes to the success and sustainability of the policies from the national or regional level.

When community participation results from a vertical approach, and especially when donors dictate the policy to follow, a similar blueprint is often adopted in different socioeconomic contexts, cultures, and countries. Applying a general blueprint may affect the success of community participation when the specific local socioeconomic and cultural factors and customs are not considered. Moreover, needs identified by the local community may be different from those determined by external agents.

LEVELS OF PARTICIPATION

Different levels of participation have been recognized. Rosato et al. observed that an ongoing assessment of interventions to improve maternal and child health aimed at community participation from women and their families established a differential meaning of participation, mobilization, and empowerment.[4] Mobilization was defined as "a capacity building process through which communities, individuals, groups, or organizations plan, implement, and evaluate activities on a participatory and sustained basis to improve their health and other needs, either on personal initiative or stimulated by others." The review suggests that there are differences in the effect of mobilization—working through changes in behavioral risk factors (home-care practices) or through changes in socioenvironmental risk factors by developing the capacities of communities to be empowered and make choices. Several studies in this review suggest evidence that mobilization is an effective method for promoting participation and empowering communities.[16,17]

Empowerment is described as a goal in itself when the community takes responsibility for actions related to their own health and health care that eventually could develop into community organization and development. Community empowerment aims to emphasize the concept of health as a right and encourages communities to strive for affordable and accessible health care. Empowerment may also give the community the opportunity to demand transparency and accountability of all parties involved in their health care. Empowerment, which entails a high degree of involvement, requires an in-depth and long-term investment that may constitute an important challenge for both the healthcare team and community members. With regard to involvement in the decision making process, empowerment requires knowledge about the organization and the health service's function.

Empowerment may run the risk of being misinterpreted. In some cases the concept and the term are promoted and applied, but empowerment might actually be used for cheap human resources in places with scarce means.[18] Community health care should consider empowerment as a process that may start by having community members serve as resources and moves toward their engagement in active and shared responsibilities with the healthcare service.

The different levels of participation, each of which implies a higher degree of involvement, are presented in Table 6-1.

TYPES OF COMMUNITY PARTICIPATION

Community participation could be a one-time activity or a continuous process geared toward a sustainable improvement of the community's health. Table 6-2 shows several types of community participation at the individual and the collective levels.

In community health care, participation may begin at an individual level with a specific activity that eventually could develop into collaborative, collective-oriented participation. Considering community participation as a process, moving from the individual to collective levels, may relate to the two patterns of community participation: *issue-oriented participation* (focused on a single health-related issue) and *collaboration-oriented participation* (oriented to broader determinants of health), as were identified in a qualitative analysis of 34 community health partnerships.[19]

The type of community participation may also depend on the purpose of a specific activity. For example, a suggestion of community participation in a health impact assessment (HIA) faced the following dilemma. The HIA needed to be completed in a short time to adjust to established timelines, but the community was not ready (with the necessary knowledge, skills, or willingness) to respond. Therefore, it was suggested to delegate the HIA to small groups of experts.[20] In this case, community participation could still have a role in the preliminary preparatory stage of HIA, and later, when community members gain expertise, they can fully participate in the process.

COMMUNITY PARTICIPATION IN COMMUNITY HEALTH CARE

Community health care promotes community participation as an integral component for the organization and functioning of health services. In community health care, community participation is not an instrument, but rather a strategic component that promotes and facilitates the dialogue among community members and health and other community services.

TABLE 6-1 Levels of Participation

Community participation	Participation by a community member or members in isolated and nonspecific activities related to a healthcare service
Community involvement	An active role of sharing in healthcare activities
Community collaboration	A combination of the two previous levels
Community mobilization	The involvement of community groups or organizations that are working together toward a common goal
Community empowerment	A process resulting from an acquired knowledge and consciousness by individuals or groups that participate in decisions regarding their own and their communities' health and lives

TABLE 6-2 Individual and Collective Community Participation

Individual level	• Providing community information to health services • Accepting and complying with a prescribed approach • Being a member of a healthcare committee related to the health service in the community • Promoting discussion of local problems • Volunteering for a nonhealth, yet directly related, function in the health services, such as being a guard at the facility • Engaging in specific health service activities, such as recruiting community members to participate in health discussions, lab tests, and performing measurements (blood pressure, weight, and height) during screenings and surveys • Initiating health projects • Being a member of the health service's board of directors • Having specific responsibilities as a member of a health services board
Collective level	• Grouping together patients who share a particular disease for self-care training • Engaging in group discussions on issues related to the organization of services • Taking shared responsibility for recruiting community members to health services intervention, such as street groups encouraging neighbors to attend health education sessions • Discussing and deciding on health priorities • Developing proposals for specific health programs • Monitoring the quality of health services • Determining community priorities • Allocating community resources

Elements to Enhance Community Participation

Elements to consider for enhancing community participation for community health care are presented in Table 6-3.

Among those elements, the *definition of community and community members* is necessary to establish a common understanding among the community members and the healthcare professionals. The definition will not exclude or discriminate socially and economically marginalized people.

Mutual respect could be considered a requirement in community participation. Similarly, a *common understanding* of the different roles played by community members and the healthcare team, as well as the clarification of expectations from the outset, is essential to develop trust. This will facilitate starting and continuing the process.

The *commitment* of the healthcare team, manifested in the incorporation of community participation as an integral component of its activities, and the community's commitment are essential for a sustainable process. This will depend on their capabilities and concerns. It is necessary to be aware that a group of people in the community may be willing to be in-

volved only in one issue or problem that affects them personally, but not in community-wide issues or an ongoing basis. In addition, vested interests in participation may exist when there are personal or political gains. The identification of these issues and a clear definition of the purpose and common goals paves the way for successful and sustainable participation.

Both the activities and decisions made by community members and the healthcare team require ongoing *monitoring*. This will facilitate the analysis of the process and alert the team about modifications that are needed.

Communication and feedback are imperative for group interaction and coherence in the process. This contributes to an understanding of common goals and a discussion about differences, and it leads to transparency in the interactions among those involved.

Potential Situations Created in the Process of Community Participation

Participation in community health care should be considered a process. As such, it may create new situations for the healthcare

TABLE 6-3 Elements to Enhance Community Participation

Definition of community and community members	A clear definition of the community that includes all its members should be developed.
Mutual respect and understanding	Both the healthcare team and the community must adhere to mutual respect and understanding of their different culture, roles, and expectations.
Team's commitment	Participation should be explicitly incorporated in the healthcare team's plan of activities.
Community's commitment	Community members, community groups, and their institutions must be encouraged to participate in accordance with their capabilities and concerns.
Monitoring	Decisions taken and activities planned and implemented need to be monitored to identify obstacles and facilitate changes.
Communication and feedback	Communication must be facilitated between the healthcare team and the community for defining common goals and discussing differences.

professionals, the community, or both. These should be identified so they can be addressed in the field, if necessary, to facilitate a smooth-running process (see Table 6-4).

COMMUNITY PARTICIPATION AND COMMUNITY COALITIONS

Coalitions are established by individuals or groups within a community to create a mechanism of partnership toward a common goal. This coalition needs to have maximum sector representation and diversity, thus reflecting the different expertise available. The power generated by a coalition may transcend the benefits if community members or organizations participate on their own for the improvement of the community's health and health care.

Community coalition is widely used to promote citizen participation in public health.[22] For example, a 23-partner coalition in New York, including social services, housing, faith-based organizations, child healthcare and primary care providers, and the city health department, engaged in a community-wide immunization program. Children enrolled in the program were 53% more likely to be up to date and receive timely immunizations than children in the usual care group. This was assessed to be due to increased coordination between stakeholders and the sense of community ownership.[23]

In some circumstances, a community coalition is made of organizations only, which may not include individuals living in the particular community. The constituency of a coalition in relation to a particular community should be explicitly stated to avoid confusion or misunderstanding as related to its scope. In the absence of community members, the understanding of community needs and functioning by the coalition may reflect the interests of the organizations, but it may not reflect community interests. The success of creating a coalition will be influenced by the political environment and existing policies at national and regional levels.

PARTICIPATION SUSTAINABILITY IN COMMUNITY HEALTH CARE

Participation might be considered an input to a specific project, yet when participation is viewed as a process integrated into health care, it has the potential to increase sustainability of the service activities and of participation itself. Sustainability in participation requires a commitment from all involved parties, as does having a supportive environment. If participation is implemented as a cheap resource (a product), the potential of sustainability is reduced. When health activities are based on a true partnership, sustainability is more feasible.

ROLE OF STAKEHOLDERS IN COMMUNITY PARTICIPATION

Health care alone can't provide the remedies to problems at the community level, whether the problems are health or the

TABLE 6-4 Potential Situations Created in the Process of Community Participation

Overexposure	In certain communities in which innovative health care is being developed, members may be overexposed to the training of healthcare professionals, repeated surveys, or exposure to the media. To avoid harm to community members and their relationship with the health service, careful planning and negotiation are required.
Paternalism	The healthcare team may act in a patronizing way toward the community, making clear the differences in knowledge and trying to impose their way with their "good professional techniques." This may provoke resistance and mistrust and has to be dealt with by both the professionals and community members.
Differences in expectations	The partnership between healthcare professionals and community members, whether individually or as part of organized groups, creates an environment of mutual expectations. The different expectations of professionals and the community may result in failure of commonly proposed activities. Healthcare professionals must be cautious about implementing a "cosmetic value of participation"[21] or making the proposed activities "look good" without incorporating authentic community involvement. Mutual expectations have to be clarified from the outset.
Imbalance of power	An imbalance of power can be expressed if the professionals claim absolute responsibility on health matters or by the internal structure of forces within the community. Health matters might be initiated by the community and shouldn't be ignored by the healthcare team. Specifically, the professionals may play the role that their institutions wish to impose, but within the community the presence of political leaders may impose attitudes not concordant with the spirit of community health among all community members.

determinants of health. Other agencies and social sectors that work in and provide their services to the same community, referred to as stakeholders, are important to consider in community participation.

The stakeholders' involvement needs to consider their degree of familiarity with the day-to-day life of the community; to what degree the community recognizes the stakeholders as representatives or partners; and whether the stakeholders are able to employ a culturally competent approach. Although the stakeholders have a common purpose (having a vested interest in the outcome of their involvement), each one contributes a specific role in the maintenance, improvement, and sustainability of community participation. The identification and analysis of their specific roles could enhance the content and features of community participation in health services. The stakeholders' involvement reinforces the idea that their collective contribution could have better results on health and health care than their separated and isolated actions (see Table 6-5).

A special consideration should be given to international donors in the promotion of community participation. Their involvement in encouraging participation should avoid imposing their view of community health needs. Donors should work in close coordination with the local stakeholders while promoting participation in health activities. If international donors impose their identification of needs, the community's willingness to participate may be affected to such an extent that it could be obliterated.[24]

COMMUNITY HEALTH WORKERS' ROLE IN COMMUNITY HEALTH CARE: PROMOTORAS AND OTHER INITIATIVES

One expression of community participation is provided by community members who are motivated about healthy living and have acquired basic health care skills. They may provide a link between the health service and community members. The concept of community health workers (CHWs) was an

TABLE 6-5 Potential Role of Stakeholders in Community Participation

Policy makers within the healthcare delivery system	• Establish and maintain an explicit policy of close relationships with the local health services. • Act in coordination with local health services. • Provide logistic support to community participation activities. • Contemplate bottom–up proposals (initiated by local community members).
Healthcare managers	• Consider and support community participation as part of the functions of the health services. • Encourage and facilitate the involvement of community members in health services functions in coordination with policy makers. • Allocate resources to allow the coalition to occur. • Emphasize the accountability and transparency dimension of their work.
Healthcare professionals	• Accept and engage in training to acquire the knowledge and skills to work with the community. • Discuss, organize, and decide who among the team members (nurses, physicians, social workers, community health workers) are more appropriate to be the liaison with the community, according to their training and role. • Encourage and coordinate community members' participation in activities.
Academic institutions	• Include community participation in the curriculum of healthcare professionals as an integral component. • Promote and organize community-based curriculum activities in the teaching of health sciences professionals. • Collaborate in the training of community members on service-related activities. • Collaborate in the evaluation of participation.
Communities	• Encourage community members to exercise the right to be actively involved in their health care. • Encourage community members to acquire skills that could be useful in health services activities and in community work. • Express their willingness to participate by accepting roles in health services activities.

important development from the WHO's International Conference on Primary Health Care in 1978 at Alma-Ata.[3] After the conference many countries adopted the CHW model, but these programs were questioned regarding the empowerment of CHWs. It was maintained that there were limitations in their work because of socioeconomic and political constraints and a lack of support from healthcare professionals.[25] Recently, more specific types of CHWs have become an important link between the healthcare system and community members. One of these developments is the *promotoras*, which work in Latin America and within the Latino population in the United States.

Community health care could also benefit from another community member, the *peer educator*.[28,29] Peer educators are community members who experience a certain condition (e.g., diabetes) and are willing to share information and their experiences with other community members who are afflicted with a similar condition. Because peer educators may have the same cultural background and a much better understanding of the problem, they may be more willing to be involved. Peer educators require a selection process by the health service based on, among other characteristics, personality, willingness to learn, and the degree of acceptance by the person in need.

Given the trend of increasing numbers of chronic patients and the shortage of primary care professionals, various types of community healthcare workers may constitute an important contribution to health care.

Box 6-2 Promotoras

Promotoras are female community health workers, also referred to as health advocates, lay health advisors, lay health workers, Latina community health workers, peer counselors, and neighborhood workers. They are salient members in community participation.[26] Promotoras are responsible for raising health awareness by providing information and health education and increasing efforts to involve community members and stakeholders in community activities.

Although promotoras primarily focus on individual activities, they also include community-wide activities. In a recent community-focused initiative targeting women at risk for HIV infection on the US–Mexico border, the promotoras' roles were to motivate and encourage women to seek preventive services. Their activities also included involvement in the women's social networks. For this work, the promotoras are also called *animadoras* (motivators).[27] In this activity the animadoras were able to not only encourage women to use the services, they also were able to assess the population's main barriers in the prevention of HIV.

OPPORTUNITIES AND BARRIERS TO COMMUNITY PARTICIPATION

Community Health Care aims to promote and engage in community participation and needs to identify and assess the opportunities (to consider them) and barriers (to overcome them) that may be present in the community.

For Professionals

Biomedical training that is focused on the hospital and the hierarchy, or top–down, approach of medicine may be a potential obstacle for physicians regarding community participation. Healthcare professionals may have a negative or indifferent attitude toward participation and may have difficulties in accepting community members' opinions regarding health matters and health care. Some professionals may not have received training regarding the sociocultural context effects on health and the importance of community participation or how to address it. This may discourage its application in their practice.

A study that aimed to determine the importance physicians assign to public roles showed that community participation was rated as important by more than 90% of the respondents.[30] A study on primary care physicians' commu-

nity-related training suggests that training can positively influence their involvement in working with the community in health-related activities.[31]

As part of the primary healthcare strategy in New Zealand, primary health organizations (PHOs) were created to develop community participation and assess its benefits to the community and the healthcare organization. A tool kit called Community Participation: A Resource Kit and Self-Assessment Tool for PHOs was developed for healthcare professionals. A pilot study in primary care settings showed that the tool kit was relevant, and evidence of a commitment to engaging with communities was seen, while also showed concern about the time required for these activities in the privately owned general practices.[32]

There are professionals who may be reluctant to be engaged in community participation. In addition, if professionals are precluded from this process by national or regional authorities, the prospects for community participation are scarce. Community participation requires that healthcare professionals have knowledge, skills, and supportive attitudes. The specific skills are communication, conflict management, community organization, and cultural sensitivity (see Table 6-6). Although having these skills may facilitate the health services promotion of community participation, their absence could become barriers. This, however, can be overcome by training.

For Community Members

The opportunities and barriers for community members' participation relates to their personal and social contexts (whether they are residents or registered members of a healthcare organization). The opportunities would be related to the local environment of collective work or having personal or social relationships with community members who are already involved. Opportunities may also be determined by specific characteristics of the population or sectors of the population, for example time availability from retired community members or mothers of young children who have a common need. A close relationship with a healthcare team member could also be a trigger for community members to be involved not only in their health care, but community health care as well.

The type and level of participation should be acceptable to community members and healthcare professionals alike, and it should be adequate and appropriate to their skills. Sharing results and demonstrating success enhances the community's willingness to participate. When communities are not well organized, the prospects of participation are limited. The barriers to community participation could be hampered by the fact that volunteer work may be time consuming and

TABLE 6-6 Necessary Skills for Professionals Involved in Community Participation

Communication	Communication skills need to address communications with populations or individuals who have diverse cultural or ethnic backgrounds. Community members may or may not be versed in health issues and could have differing interests and goals regarding their own or their community's care. Knowing the local language may facilitate communication.
Conflict management	Community members' opinions related to their participation in the function of health services may create conflicts. They may be caused by previous relationships or as a consequence of their involvement in community participation. Conflict management skills help to create consensus among community representatives and between community representatives and the healthcare team. Clarity on goals and strategies minimizes the likelihood of conflict. Mutually agreed-upon protocols for interaction also facilitates group dynamics.
Community organization	Healthcare professionals need to identify formal and informal groups that may be involved in the process of organizing the community for the development of better social and environmental conditions. This function can be delegated to members of the team who were trained for that purpose.
Cultural sensitivity	Professionals and community members may come from different cultures. Therefore the recognition of the customs, values, and beliefs of the community members is required.

unrewarding or by the lack the necessary knowledge or skills. This could be solved by offering incentives and training.

PROFESSIONALS AS COMMUNITY MEMBERS

Healthcare or other related professionals who have skills and experience in community activities may have a unique contribution to community development.[30] This is possible if the professional considers his or her role to be that of a resident who is interested in the welfare and progress of the community, and conversely if the community views the professional as a true and equal partner (see Box 6-3).

CASE STUDIES ON THE DEVELOPMENT OF COMMUNITY PARTICIPATION

The following experiences suggest that establishing specific links between healthcare professionals and community members, whether initiated by community members or the health service, may positively affect the community's health status and produce some organizational changes in health services.

Health Educator Home Visits to Promote Survey Participation

The healthcare team in a community health center in Jerusalem, Israel, developed a community diagnosis of cardiovascular risk

factors as a basis for a COPC program on the control of related risk factors. To increase participation in the community diagnosis, nurses provided the names of 12 residents who were well-known in the community to be visited by a health educator. The health educator visited each one of the residents, explained the purpose of the survey to them, and stressed the need for their involvement. A snowballing technique followed, in which the health educator solicited the participants to invite 12 acquaintances in the neighborhood to their house so they could convey the importance of participating in the survey and eventually becoming involved in activities at the health center. Additional home meetings were facilitated, and the survey had a response rate of 86%. Part of these residents became involved in community activities related to the health center.[33]

Increasing Trust in the Health Center by Responding to Community-Specific Interest

A health center in Boston, Massachusetts, aimed to reactivate community involvement by having their primary care services develop a working partnership with community members. Physicians from a COPC residency program gathered the community perspectives regarding local health problems.[34] The health center staff identified HIV/AIDS and substance abuse as significant health problems. However, the community identi-

Box 6-3 Case study: Neighborhood Health Committee Development

In a Jerusalem neighborhood with a population of 45,000, with a local community administration composed of volunteers, a participant resident with community medicine expertise was invited to be the chairman of the health committee. The first task of the committee was to recruit a group of residents (professionals and nonprofessionals). The initial activities consisted of defining the objectives of the health committee. There were two proposals: (1) to help resolve some of the deficiencies in the healthcare delivery system, and (2) to work on health promotion activities. These two clearly different proposals were a reflection of the composition of the committee. Some of the members had complaints about the neighborhood health services, and others addressed more general health issues. After a long process of learning and building trust, the committee decided to concentrate on the latter. With time, they were able to recruit more residents and organized various activities of health promotion, mainly related to women's health, which were sustained over time. Among the lessons learned was that the professional community member created an environment of relevant content, interest, and motivation for other community members. After the founding professional resident left the committee, the other members continued the work, which developed into a framework for continuous knowledge improvement and new developments of health activities.

fied an unclean environment as a significant problem. A one-day street cleanup activity elicited participation from many residents. Learning from that activity, the center's staff changed its organizational approach to targeting streets rather than the community as a whole. Seven residents began functioning as street leaders, and the community's trust in the health center increased. Later this was associated with an increased use of healthcare services.

Community Health Outreach to Identify Health Risks and Resources

In a Jerusalem community with elderly people living alone, cases of respiratory ailments were frequent during the winter cold weather. Nurses from the local health center were taking care of the elderly population through a home care program. During their scheduled home visits, nurses noticed that most of the elderly people living alone were experiencing problems with their home heating. The healthcare team suggested that the nurses identify neighbors to assist the elderly residents. These recruits visited their elderly neighbors' homes daily and assisted in maintaining the home temperature by bringing fuel or switching the heating on and off at set hours. This activity was associated with reduced respiratory morbidity among the elderly people.

EVALUATION OF COMMUNITY PARTICIPATION

Although a variety of community participation experiences exist, evaluations of their effectiveness is limited, mainly due to the lack of preplanning. The vagueness in the definition of the community and the lack of consistency in methodology makes drawing conclusions difficult. Additionally, most of the evaluations refer to the process, rather than the outcomes, and short-term rather than long-term results.

An evaluation of community participation is necessary to provide the required evidence of beneficial results to health institutions, policy makers, and the community itself. The evaluation measures should address the effects of the health service's organization, the team and community's satisfaction, and the impact on the health and well-being of the community. It should incorporate quantitative and qualitative measurements to identify the factors that influence participation among the different groups in the community, the scope of mobilization of local resources (number of people, time, expertise), and sustainability with or without external funds because institutions that receive help from donor organizations are encouraged, and sometimes required, to evaluate the process and outcomes of community participation.

A systematic review of 42 papers in the English literature between 1966 and 2000 suggests that involving patients in health care has contributed to the production of new or improved sources of information for patients and improved accessibility to services. In addition, new services were reported, including advocacy, initiatives for employment, and preventing the closure of hospitals. As illustrated by that review, community participation was related to the organization of health services, but no health outcomes were reported.[35]

An example of an evaluation is provided by the National Health Service (NHS) in the United Kingdom, which requires primary care trusts (PCTs) to widen participation in planning and decision making and engage with service users and local communities. For that purpose, local statutory and voluntary community-building partnerships were developed. This development necessitated the use of instruments to measure the work done by community participation in health care. In this context, a self-assessment tool was developed to evaluate the involvement and allow organizations to assess their progress and identify areas for improvement.[36] The method was piloted in two PCTs, which revealed its usefulness.

A FRAMEWORK FOR THE DEVELOPMENT OF COMMUNITY PARTICIPATION IN COMMUNITY HEALTH CARE

The development of community participation in community health care is facilitated when a framework exists. Table 6-7 shows the elements to be considered by health services and community members who are interested in engaging community participation.

This framework should not be considered static. It offers the option of considering additional elements and new components, whether they are proposed by the team or by community members. The community may consider extending their involvement to include a community development dimension. This possible expansion would be related to the socio-economic, cultural, and political contexts in which the community exists. The community members' awareness of this possible expansion may encourage them to engage in more active roles in the health service.

TABLE 6-7 Framework for the Development of Community Participation in Community Health Care

Elements	By healthcare professionals	By community members
Assessment of team willingness to involve the community in the functions of health services	• Assess knowledge of and attitudes toward involvement • Promote internal organization to identify the need and to discuss and facilitate involvement • Suggest recruitment of community members	• Preliminary assessment by community members selected by the team and by community leaders • Internal discussions to promote and organize the assessment • Acceptance to be part of the participation process • Community may challenge the healthcare team by requesting involvement in health services delivery
Capacity building	• Carry out before and throughout community participation • Assess knowledge on community structure and organization to develop skills • Understand the socio-economic-political context • Develop conflict-solving skills • Develop skills to coordinate services	• Assess health knowledge and skills on community work • Provide skill-building training that may increase members' self-confidence and abilities for participation at different levels • Recognize and analyze the different levels of participation, from isolated volunteer work to empowerment
Communications	• Organize ongoing communication with the community • Share relevant health information with the total community • Provide information about current and planned activities	• Facilitate communications within the community • Independently collect data and gather information • Provide feedback to healthcare team about service's activities
Organizational support	• Develop institutional policy to maintain its role in community healthcare services • Reinforce the bottom–up approach by the team • Provide logistic support • Promote dialogue between the health service institution and the team	• Encourage and facilitate the creation of community groups to engage in community activities • Identify existing internal community resources, such as willingness to participate, special skills, professionals, time

continues

TABLE 6-7 Framework for the Development of Community Participation in Community Health Care—continued

Elements	By healthcare professionals	By community members
Environmental support by other sectors in the community	• Identify other sectors in the area that could be ready to partner and coordinate actions • Recruit stakeholders and institutions • Organize coalitions	• Identify links with external organizations and pursue collaboration • Become involved with other sectors to change physical environment for safety and create facilities to promote physical activities • Be part of coalitions related to local health services
Accountability	• Organize and demonstrate transparency in team activities • Provide feedback regarding decisions and allocation of resources	• Share information and organizational features with the total community • Involve community members in decisions related to allocation of resources
Evaluation of participation	• Assure evaluation planning in advance • Design reliable, simple, and practical records • Include measurements of community involvement, changes in the organization of services, and state of health	• Suggest components of evaluation • Assure evaluation of satisfaction • Promote the value of evaluation within the community
Sustainability of community participation as part of health services	• Maintain internal discussions on the benefit of community participation • Promote planning to assure that community health projects could develop as components of programs and then be integrated into community health services	• Assure community participation after financial support is terminated • Promote internal discussions regarding the role of participation in the sustainability of community health care

MONITORING ACTIVITIES THROUGHOUT THE DEVELOPMENT OF COMMUNITY PARTICIPATION

Monitoring is an integral component in the development of community participation. It assesses the progress in the development of community participation and alerts the team to needs for change and improvement. In Table 6-8, monitoring activities based on the previously presented development framework are presented.

The applicability of these monitoring activities need to be decided according to the stage of community participation and the degree of partnership between health services and the community. Skills in carrying out this process need to be assessed for both the professionals and the community. These may be acquired, or monitoring could be performed by a trusted individual or group. The community participation monitoring activities could promote and facilitate the evaluation of the impact of participation on the community health status.

SUMMARY

As one main dimension of community health care, community participation plays an important role in the organization and functioning of community-oriented health services. Participation is expressed at different levels and dimensions. It could range from volunteer work in certain health services activities to being part of the discussions and decisions on resource allocation and priorities and consensus on goals and strategies. Community participation could be a result of a local initiative or by decisions taken at the national, or regional levels. When participation results from decisions by both the community and the organization, optimal results can be obtained. Frameworks for the development and monitoring of community participation in community health care are proposed as a vehicle to facilitate the work of healthcare team members and to ensure sustainable improvements in the community's health status.

TABLE 6-8 Monitoring Throughout the Development of Community Participation

Steps of development	Dimensions by healthcare professionals	Dimensions by community members
Assessment of team willingness to involve the community in the functions of health services	• Number, type, and participants at assessment meetings • Results of assessment • Plan for recruitment and retention	• Documentation of community member meetings • Were the leaders interviewed? • Were internal discussions held about the team's promotion of involvement? • Did the community organize health activities by themselves? • Community readiness and preparedness to participate
Capacity building	• Teaching objectives, content, and methodology • Measurement of knowledge acquired • Degree of satisfaction with training	• Level of knowledge and skills on community work • Degree of satisfaction with training • Assess level of participation by members of the community
Communication	• Type of communication used (amount and content), with community members and with institution	• Are there mechanisms for sharing experiences within the community? • Level of awareness in the community of the objectives and strategies of the services
Organizational support	• Is there an institutional policy regarding participation? • Type of logistic support to facilitate effectiveness	• Were community groups organized? • Did the community assign relevant roles within the community?
Environmental support	• Plan for recruitment of other sectors • Coalition formation	• Were people invited to be part of a coalition? How? • Degree of satisfaction with the involvement of other sectors
Accountability	• Records kept to retrieve data to be used in accountability • Built-in mechanisms to assure a process to elaborate and provide data to the community and the institution • Meetings organized specifically to provide feedback	• Community perception about mechanisms of accountability by the team • Degree of acceptance of participation at the total community level

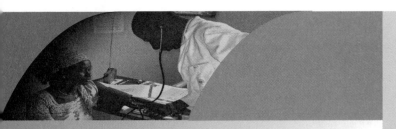

Discussion Questions

- To what degree is the healthcare system responsible for involving the community in community health care? Why?

- How much volunteerism is a desirable and adequate expression of community participation?

- Is community mobilization an adequate strategy in healthcare system reform?

- What are the potential obstacles for community members to accept their neighbors as active agents of behavioral change?

Review Questions

- Which strategies encourage community mobilization?

- What type of resources may community members provide? Why?

- What are the components of the framework for developing community participation in community health care?

- What should be the main elements to evaluate community participation?

REFERENCES

1. Kark SL, Stuart GW. *A Practice of Social Medicine.* Edinburg, Scotland: E&S Livingstone; 1962.

2. Geiger JH. Community-oriented primary care: a path to community development. *Am J Public Health.* 2002;92:1713–1716.

3. World Health Organization. *Primary Health Care: Report of the International Conference on Primary Health Care.* Geneva, Switzerland: World Health Organization; 1978.

4. Rosato M, Laverack G, Grabman H, et al. Alma-Ata: rebirth and revision. 5. Community participation: lessons for maternal, newborn, and child health. *Lancet.* 2008;372:962–971.

5. Bracht N, Tsouros A. Principles and strategies of effective community participation. *Health Promot Int.* 1990;5:199–208.

6. Zakus JDL, Lysack CL. Revisiting community participation. *Health Policy Plan.* 1998;13:1–12.

7. Kahssay HM, Oakley P. *Community Involvement in Health Development: A Review of the Concept and Practice.* Geneva, Switzerland: World Health Organization; 1999.

8. Morgan L. Community participation in health: perpetual allure, persistent challenge. *Health Policy Plan.* 2001;16:221–230.

9. Chitambo BR, Smith JE, Ehlers VJ. Strategies for community participation in developing countries. *Curationis.* 2002; 25:76–83.

10. Lawn JE, Rohde J, Rifkin S, Were M, Paul VK, Chopra M. Alma-Ata 30 years on: revolutionary, relevant, and time to revitalize. *Lancet.* 2008;372: 917–927.

11. Lehmann U, Van Damme W, Barten F, Sanders D. Task shifting: the answer to the human resources crisis in Africa? *Hum Resour Health.* 2009;21:7–49.

12. Suliman A. Effective refugee health depends on community participation. *Carnets Enfance.* 1983;2:2.

13. Rifkin SB. Paradigm lost: toward a new understanding of community participation in health programs. *Acta Tropic.* 1996;61:79–92.

14. Willmott P, Thomas D. *Community in Social Policy.* London, England: Policy Studies Institute; 1984. Discussion paper No. 9.

15. Dinat N, Ross L, Ngubeni V. The Soweto care givers network: facilitating community participation in palliative care in South Africa. *Indian J Palliative Care.* 2005;11:28–33.

16. Morrinson J, Tamang S, Mesko N, et al. Women's health groups to improve perinatal care in rural Nepal. *BMC Pregnancy Childbirth.* 2005;5:6.

17. Costello A, Azad K, Barnett S. An alternative strategy to reduce maternal mortality. *Lancet.* 2006;368:1477–1479.

18. Mitra D. Globalization's labor force status, and empowerment: a cross-national study. http://digitalcommons.uconn.edu/dissertations/AAI3276635. ETD Collection for University of Connecticut. Paper AAI3276635. Published January 1, 2007. Accessed November 2009.

19. Cheadle A, Senter S, Solomon L, Beery WL, Schwartz PM. A qualitative exploration of alternative strategies for building community health partnerships: collaboration versus issue-oriented approaches. *J Urb Health.* 2005;82:638–652.

20. Parry J, Wright J. Community participation in health impact assessment intuitively appealing but practically difficult. *Bull World Health Organ.* 2003;81:388.

21. Chambers R. Paradigm shifts and the practices of participatory research and development. In: Nelson N, Wright S, eds. *Power and Participatory Development: Theory and Practice.* London, England: Intermediate Technology Publications; 1995:30–42.

22. Butterfoss FD. Process evaluation for community participation. *Ann Rev Public Health.* 2006;27:323–340.

23. Findley SE, Irigoyen M, Sanchez M, et al. Effectiveness of a community coalition for improving child vaccination rates in New York City. *Am J Public Health.* 2008;98:1959–1962.

24. Chowdhury M. Community participation in health care. *Bull World Health Organ.* 2004;82:881.

25. Werner D. The village health worker—lackey or liberator. *World Health Forum.* 1981;2:46–68.

26. Reinschmidt KM, Hunter JB, Fernández ML, et al. Understanding the success of promotoras in increasing chronic disease screening. *J Health Care Poor Underserved.* 2006;17:256–264.

27. Ramos RL, Green NL, Shulman LC. Pasa la voz: using peer driven intervention to increase Latinas' access to and utilization of HIV prevention and testing services. *J Health Care Poor Underserved.* 2009;20:29–35.

28. Karwalajtys T, McDonough B, Hall H, et al. Development of the volunteer peer educator role in a community cardiovascular health awareness program (CHAP): a process evaluation in two communities. *J Community Health.* 2009;34:336–345.

29. Simmons D, Voyle J, Rush E, Dear M. The New Zealand experience in peer support interventions among people with diabetes [published online ahead of print March 2, 2009]. *Fam Pract.*

30. Gruen RL, Campbell EG, Blumenthal D. Public roles of US physicians. *JAMA.* 2006;296:2467–2475.

31. Steiner BD, Pathman DE, Jonnes B, Williams ES, Riggins T. Primary care physicians' training and their community involvement. *Fam Med.* 1999;31:257–262.

32. Neuwelt P, Crampton P, Crengle S, et al. Assessing and developing community participation in primary health care in Aotearoa New Zealand: a national study. *N Z Med J.* 2005;118:1218. htpp://www.nzma.org.nz/journal/118-1218/1562/. Accessed November 2009.

33. Abramson JH, Gofin J, Hopp C, Schein MH, Naveh P. The CHAD program for the control of cardiovascular risk factors in a Jerusalem community—a 24-year retrospect. *Isr J Med Sci.* 1994;30:108–119.

34. Klevens RM, Cashman SB, Margules A, Fulmer HS. Special contribution: transforming a neighborhood health center into a community-oriented primary care practice. *Am J Prev Med.* 1992;8:62–65.

35. Crawford MJ, Rutter D, Manley C, et al. Systematic review of involving patients in the planning and development of health care. *Br Med J.* 2002; 325:1–5.

36. South J, Fairfax P, Green E. Developing an assessment tool for evaluating community involvement. *Health Expect.* 2005;8:64–73.

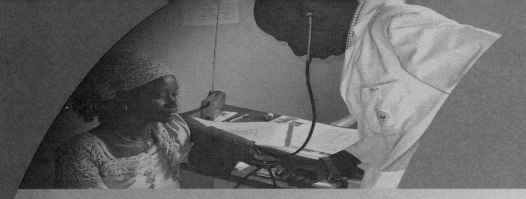

CHAPTER 7

Integration of Health Services in Community Health Care

LEARNING OBJECTIVES

By the end of the chapter, learners will be able to

- recognize the presence and meaning of the divide between clinical individual care and public health;
- identify fragmentation of health services;
- identify factors related to fragmentation of health services;
- describe and analyze appropriate approaches of health services integration;
- identify the role of stakeholders in health services integration;
- discuss and analyze the process and levels of health services integration for the development of community health care.

CHAPTER OUTLINE

KEY TERMS

fragmentation of health services

integration in community health care

integration of health services

INTRODUCTION

Health care in different countries and contexts is often characterized by fragmented services. Fragmentation of health services refers to having multiple healthcare providers for different health needs, as opposed to receiving overall health care at one location. As a consequence little, if any, continuity of care exists, even though providers take care of the same community.

Fragmentation is reflected in growing disparities in the delivery of health services among different subgroups of a population.

Medicine (clinical individual care) and public health (population care) are two disciplines with unique focuses that require different professional skills. Both are complementary and compelled to respond to the same population's health needs and demands, but they act through different channels. However, medicine and public health can be coordinated and integrated.

In this chapter, we analyze the current situation of the fragmentation of health services in community health care, mainly between medicine and public health. The chapter explains the negative effects of fragmentation and the challenges it poses for the community's health and health care. The chapter also discusses approaches for integration of health services.

FRAGMENTATION OF HEALTH SERVICES AS A BARRIER TO CONTINUITY OF CARE

Continuity of care constitutes one of the features of primary care, but is also needed in relation to other levels of care, and with public health, to assure that community members will receive appropriate care.

Horizontal and Vertical Levels

The fragmentation of health services is present at both the horizontal and vertical levels. The horizontal level refers to health services that are at the same level of care, whereas the vertical level describes the different levels of care, such as hospitals and community health services. Fragmentation at the horizontal level is demonstrated by separation of the following services:

- clinical individual care and public health services
- preventive and curative care
- services provided by specialists and generalists
- biomedical and psychosocial models of care
- public and private sectors

An individual or a family seeking care often needs to visit different healthcare professionals at various locations. They therefore may need to make various financial arrangements and spend time to arrange various appointments and travel, with a potential loss of working hours. The individual or family, as well as the healthcare system, must bear these increased costs. Additionally, little or no communication channels exist among the health services to exchange relevant individual or family health information. Consequently, duplication in the use of services, such as laboratory tests, may exist and become a burden for the individual, family, or healthcare system.

Furthermore, the emphasis on biological mechanisms of a disease might be more frequently considered in this type of setup. That emphasis diverts attention away from the behavioral, social, economic, cultural, and environmental factors that may be related to a health condition, all of which are inherent to community health care.

Between vertical levels of care, a separation exists when there are no established mechanisms for referrals between hospitals and community health services. Patients are usually discharged from hospitals without a specific plan for the continuation of care to be implemented by primary care professionals and healthcare providers in the community. Patients may not receive pertinent information about follow-up consultations.

The Schism Between Medicine and Public Health

Two of the most important components of any defined community healthcare approach are its medicine and public health dimensions. The former is focused on individual patient care and consultation; the latter is focused on population-oriented health issues. In addition, medicine primarily addresses diagnosis and treatment of diseases, whereas public health primarily addresses health promotion and disease prevention. The differences were not only based on professional perspectives and skills, but also on the institutional and social environment. While medicine is mainly concerned with the physical health of the individual patient, public health addresses the health of populations and its behavioral, social, and economic determinants.[1]

Furthermore, the separation may be associated with the traditionally defined framework of the public health discipline. Detels and Breslow[2] defined public health as "the process of mobilizing local, state, national and international resources to ensure the conditions in which people can be healthy." Winslow[3] defined public health as "the science and art of preventing disease, prolonging life, and promoting physical health and efficiency through organized community efforts." However, suggestions to redefine public health have been proposed because the definitions might be too open to interpretation, and also in order to emphasize the public, and the need to use evidence in public health actions.[4]

In some countries the separation of disciplines is expressed as individual clinical care or medical care and public health. This is not a semantic difference; the distinction reflects differing points of view of the healthcare professions because medicine may be considered only physicians' work. This denomination is also a reflection of particular characteristics of health services functions, where a lack of physicians exists in various regions of the world and clinical care is provided by other healthcare professionals.

Because the divide between medicine and public health is expressed mainly at the primary care level, medicine and primary care (focused on clinical curative care) or primary health care (comprehensive approach to health and health care) are commonly mistaken as synonymous. Some may even regard primary health care as more closely related to public health, especially because primary care providers may offer promotion and prevention services.

Specialty care, provided by physicians who have completed advanced education and clinical training in a specific area of medicine, is often regarded as the epitome of medicine.[5] The increasing number of specialists compared to the decreasing number of general practitioners in primary care plays a role in the fragmentation of health services. The system is acting on the parts, without giving attention to the whole. The ongoing debate of an ideological and organizational nature about the intrinsic important role expressed by each one of the two disciplines may help to narrow the gap between medicine–individual health care and public health. This is particularly relevant where professionals and organizations agree to recommend a community orientation of primary care.[6,7]

A World Health Organization (WHO) international Delphi study[8] and the US Department of Health and Human Services[9] formulated the Essential Public Health Functions (EPHF). These functions include analysis of health status, surveillance, health promotion, social participation, development of policies, strengthening of regulations, promotion of equitable access, human resources development, quality assurance research, and reduction of impact of emergencies and disasters on health. Among these functions are those performed by individual healthcare services, such as analysis of health status and health promotion. Concomitantly, individual health care could be considered part of public health functions when they are able to produce population-wide benefits.[10]

THE NEGATIVE EFFECTS OF FRAGMENTATION

The fragmentation of healthcare services primarily affects the quality of health care manifested by duplication of services and, consequently, waste of resources, lack of communication among various professionals, and increasing health status gaps among different groups in the community.

The delivery of primary care in the United States is implemented through three major disciplines: family medicine, general internal medicine, and general pediatrics. This is a fragmented model and thus has not contributed to the improvement of overall health in the US population.[11] Additionally, specialists who provide care in ambulatory settings are also assuming the functions of primary care providers (routine and preventive care), which further contributes to the fragmentation of services.[12]

To compound the issue, financing and the delivery of care is provided by a variety of distinct and competing organizations. Almost no relationships exist among them, and there is poor information exchange and different incentives that affect quality and costs.[13]

Enthoven states, "fragmentation of services is affecting the lives and the well-being of many Americans, as well as contributing to the excessive level and unsustainable growth rate of expenditures on health care."[14] One example relates to adolescent care. A report on adolescent health in the United States indicates that services and providers for teens are fragmented, resulting in gaps in care. Most adolescents can't access specialty services in mental health, sexual health, oral health, or substance abuse treatment. These gaps are more pronounced in populations that are vulnerable to risky behavior and those that are poor.[15]

The effects of fragmentation are present across the globe in different countries and organizational frameworks. Countries with universal health care may expect to have more fragmentation because of organizational changes in primary care coupled with a trend of fewer professionals pursuing primary care, such as in Finland's social security system.[16] In an analysis of the healthcare systems in Canada, the United Kingdom, France, and Germany,[17] these nations expressed dissatisfaction with the organization of their delivery of healthcare systems. Although these countries' healthcare system components aspire to integrate, fragmentation still persists. Observations in healthcare services in these countries showed a substantial overuse of services and management that allowed physicians and hospitals to practice medicine without appropriate regulations. These countries are recommending reorganization of services to become more efficient.

An assessment of the current situation of health services in Latin American countries[18] identified the following negative effects of fragmentation: debilitation of the public sector, inequity, greater out-of-pocket expenditures, a medical-oriented model of care, high costs, and inefficiency from duplications of actions. In an effort to improve this situation, proposals have been developed for the creation of Integrated Health Care systems in several countries in the region.

In Africa, a study of economic effects on the organization of health services in Tanzania, Ghana, and South Africa identified a large number of separate funding mechanisms and a wide range of healthcare providers paid from different funding pools.[19] This creates a financial burden for patients who do not have the ability to pay for their health care.

In developing countries, there is fragmentation in the way healthcare system strengthening activities are conducted. There are usually various projects and donors working to improve the delivery of care. However, each donor supports, for example, the national HIV/AIDS program in different ways. This is done without coordination or accountability and for short periods of time. Activities are usually interrupted before the system has been able to integrate them.

THE FACTORS RELATED TO FRAGMENTATION

A proposal for the integration of services requires the identification of factors related to the continuation of fragmentation in a specific context. The following analysis may assist in identifying and reducing those factors and result in a more rational organization of health services. The domains and factors related to fragmentation are (1) health policy, (2) human resources, education, and training, (3) economic resources, (4) health information, and (5) community perceptions and priorities (see Table 7-1).

Health Policy

Decisions to maintain separation: Specific decisions made by healthcare authorities (top–down) at the central level (national, regional, or district) on maintaining separation in the organization of services may create tension with local health services and teams that are not consulted about the changes. Tension may also exist among the local, clinical, and community levels with the national level, as seen in the new healthcare organization policy for personal healthcare services in the United States. These services are claiming an orientation toward integrated primary care and assuming responsibility for the care of populations.[20]

Reorganization of services: The introduction of a reorganization process for activities at the clinical level, without appropriate consultation with and preparation by local teams, may constitute a new threat for organizations and individual professionals, which contributes to fragmentation.

Priority setting: Differing priorities by the institution, such as organizing services for cost containment, may result in

TABLE 7-1 Factors Related to Fragmentation

Health policy	Human resources, education, and training	Economic resources	Health information	Community perceptions and priorities
Decisions to maintain separation at the central level	Different career paths for healthcare professionals	New approaches, such as integration may require extra resources	Lack of information infrastructure	Perceptions of medical and public healthcare professionals' roles
Reorganization of services without consultation	Shortage and migration of healthcare professionals	Fee-for-service remuneration	Separated health information sources	Varying community expectations about medical and public health practice
Priority setting	Educational initiatives without a policy of service innovation	Lack of incentives toward integrated care	Poor quality of health information	Binding forces with personal physicians
Separate funding	Training programs that do not include integrated systems	Differing salaries at various institutions	No mechanism of data sharing	Anonymous public healthcare practitioners
Decentralization of health services	Time allocation	Institutional higher revenue	Individual vs. population level information	Priority to maintain personal care

a delay of prioritized integration activities previously decided at the clinic level.

Separate funding: Separated funding streams and entrenched bureaucracies for different service components make the integration of community health care difficult.

Decentralization: The decentralization of health services in different communities may have various resource allocations. Communities that have adequate or extra resources tend to be innovative in meeting the needs of the population through the introduction of integrated services; in communities that are poor in resources, the introduction of changes might be limited.

Human Resources, Education, and Training

Career paths: Community health approaches involve a variety of healthcare professionals who have pursued different career pathways. Typically, primary care practitioners with minimal training in population health, as well as public health doctors and nurses who are less familiar with day-to-day patient consultations, are barriers for an integration proposal. The reluctance to change may be present in professionals of both fields, and it may also play a role in the barriers to adopt a community healthcare approach. The difficulty in converting to a proactive attitude in a health practice after training and practicing in a reactive mode may slow the adoption of the integrative approach.

Shortage and migration of healthcare professionals: Countries experience shortages of healthcare professionals. In the United States this shortage is more acute at the primary care level, and in developing countries it is evident across all levels of care. One of the reasons for these shortages is that medical graduates prefer other specialties (which are better compensated). In developing countries, mainly Africa and Southeast Asia, migration to developed countries accentuates the shortage.

Educational initiatives: The impact of educational innovations that integrate clinical medicine and public health are enhanced when a comparable health policy of service innovation with political and economic support exists.

Training programs: Both in public health and in medicine, there is a need to adequately prepare students to practice in an integrated system. For medical students, training requires the inclusion of individuals in the family context and the larger economic, social, and cultural contexts. Moreover, students need to learn about how to develop partnerships with other professionals and institutions in the community. Shortell and Swartzberg suggest that med-

ical students should also acquire skills for the identification and emphasis of social determinants of health.[21] Public health students should be exposed to the organization and functions of primary care institutions and professionals. Interprofessional training could stimulate interprofessional care, which could improve coordination and reduce fragmentation, thus lowering costs and increasing patient safety.[22] In many developing countries, small numbers of doctors are trained for specialization. Nurses are trained by faith-based organizations to work at their hospitals, and training programs are not integrated. There is a very limited number of health technicians, such as lab technicians, and their training is not integrated either.

Time allocation: The time required for reorientation of health services in already overloaded practices may become a barrier in the planning and implementation processes of community health care.

Economic Resources

Extra resources: The introduction of an integrated approach demands extra resources in an already constrained budget. In the long term, the process of integration becomes more manageable and effective; however, it initially presents a challenge. Contractual, organizational, and financial difficulties might be manifested by professionals working at the community level, including universal coverage systems such as in the United Kingdom.[23]

Fee-for-service remuneration: The prevailing fee-for-service model constitutes an obstacle to integration.

Lack of incentives and rewards: The lack of economic support while changing or adding new functions could be an obstacle to motivate professionals to promote integration.

Differing salaries: Professionals' reimbursement could change because the integration of various institutions may require creating competitive or equal salaries.

Institutional higher revenue: The maintenance of fragmentation with duplication of procedures might be preferred by health institutions to maintain and increase their revenue.

Health Information

Information infrastructure: Health information constitutes an essential component of care. It requires an adequate system to allow for patient care and community health information.

Separated health information sources: Separated sources, usually in paper-based records, produce duplication, affecting the quality of care and the patients' safety.

Poor quality: Medical records in a fragmented system without built-in quality control may be incomplete or lack reliable or valid information.

Data sharing: Electronic health records enable data sharing, which potentially facilitates integration between services and continuity of care.

Different type of information: Data should serve the purpose of specific data needed in individual care and provide relevant information at the community level.[24] The existing different type of information at individual and at population level require changes in the organization of data collection and analysis.

Community Perceptions and Priorities

Role perception: Most individuals perceive the role of medical care in terms of treating diseases or symptoms, and the meaning and role of public health is either unknown or not clearly understood.

Expectations: The public may expect that personal physicians provide all necessary care. They may have difficulty recognizing the value of integrating public health activities in their care.

Binding forces: The very close relationship between individuals and their personal medical doctors creates binding forces and opinions that might not favor or support integration.

Anonymous providers: Public health activities are perceived as promotion and prevention, creating a loose connection with unidentified professionals in the distant public health services. Although separate public health departments or public health programs provide important services, it is often more anonymous by nature and is not always recognized or appreciated by the community.

Priorities: Individual members in the community may give priority to maintain the same personalized care received instead of a new type of care that is unknown and creates uncertainty.

THE MEANING OF INTEGRATION

The meaning of integration varies among healthcare professionals and organizations. The application of the term in a generic or undefined manner lessens its merit, meaning, and the conceptual framework for integration. Above all, it is necessary to describe the content of integration, providing a specific mention of its components and not merely a convenient shorthand term to describe a health program. Integration of medicine and public health may be conceptualized as a multidimensional process, combining complementary approaches into a coherent whole.

Integration is a multifaceted concept that comes from the Latin root word *integer*, that is, to complete. *Integrated* is defined as organic parts of a whole or reunited parts of a whole.[25] According to Merriam-Webster OnLine,[26] integrate means "to form, coordinate or blend into a functioning or unified whole." Conceptually, we consider the whole to be health and the parts to be the biological determinants of health, the healthcare system, and the socio-cultural-economic and environmental determinants (see Figure 7-1).

Batterham et al.[27] point out that integration could be conceptualized as a process (of the two related concepts of patient care and public health) with an integrated structure. The introduction of integration in any type of health service implies a reorientation of the existing organizational, functional, and professional tasks and requires coordination between institutions and local healthcare teams.

APPROPRIATE APPROACHES FOR INTEGRATION IN COMMUNITY HEALTH CARE

Although increasing advocacy and proposals for integrated community health programs or services are developing, the application of integration lags behind. Health services reform in different countries are giving emphasis to increasing accessibility and lowering the cost of medical care. These changes, not including coordination among health services, may not have an impact on the existing fragmentation.

Taking into account the benefits of integration of medicine and public health, the current separation challenges healthcare practitioners and healthcare organizations to consider options to change the situation (see Figure 7-2).

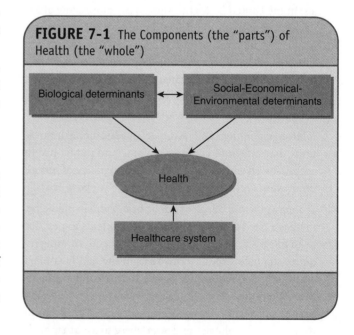

FIGURE 7-1 The Components (the "parts") of Health (the "whole")

FIGURE 7-2 Integration Options

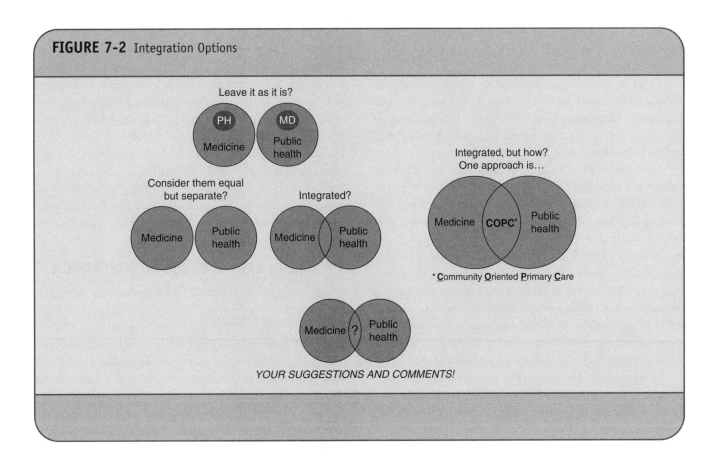

Three questions need to be answered to identify and promote integration alternatives that are conducive to a community healthcare approach:

- Is integration needed?
- What are the proposed approaches and their expected effectiveness?
- How feasible is it to integrate medicine and public health?

Is Integration Needed?

The need for integration is manifested when the system emphasizes biological processes and medical care at the expense of health promotion and the recognition of the socioeconomic and political determinants in the health–illness continuum. These realities have negative effects on health and healthcare services, leading to deterioration in quality of health care and increasing costs, which may lead to inequities.[28]

Lasker[29] states that in spite of the fact that the separation between medicine and public health existed for decades, their relationship should be reexamined. The recognition that the two sectors are under economic and performance pressures and that neither primary care nor public health can accomplish their missions alone should drive the need for integration. The stark differentiation between medicine and public health is no longer applicable in health, and integration has also been advocated as a human rights issue.[1]

What Are the Proposed Approaches and Their Expected Effectiveness?

Evidence suggests that integrating primary care and public health in diverse socioeconomic situations and health services systems has a positive impact on the public's health.[30–32] The following paragraphs describe some examples of effective integration of medicine and public health. Effectiveness was measured mainly by positive changes in health outcomes and the organization of care.

The community-oriented primary care (COPC) approach (see Chapters 3 and 4) integrates primary care and community medicine. The approach calls for responsibility for the health care of a defined population based on the assessment of its health needs; it sets priorities, plans for, and implements programs to address the identified needs.[33–44] In this respect, COPC is considered to be public health that is integrated into the local clinical level. It has shown effectiveness in changing risk factors for cardiovascular diseases and improving infant mortality, growth and development of children, and health behaviors, among others (see Chapter 3).

Other integration approaches that have shown effectiveness include Medicine and Public Health Initiative,[45] Planned Approach to Community Health (PATCH),[46] Healthy Communities,[47] Community–Campus Partnerships for Health (CCPH),[48] and the UNICEF Act, Analyze, Access (AAA) program.[49]

Further examples of healthcare integration include health services in developing countries. In Sri Lanka, the integration of family planning and maternal health-related services into primary health care[50] was based on several strategies implemented within and outside the health sector. The integration has shown a substantial decrease in maternal mortality. Also, the integration of leprosy services into the primary healthcare services resulted in improved logistics and promoted changes in the attitudes and training of healthcare workers. This was supported by an intensive advertising campaign to inform the population. This integration determined a more efficient process of diagnosis, treatment, and management of the disease.[51]

In Bolivia, Haiti, and Bangladesh, the census-based, impact-oriented (CBIO) approach[52] based on COPC methods demonstrated an effective intervention of infant, children under five, and maternal mortality.

In Costa Rica, the structural reform in the national healthcare system strengthened the primary healthcare services and included approaches of integrated care.[53] The reforms evolved with a political will to support the approach and resulted in the improvement of health conditions in the country. The integrated structures were more evident at the management level than at the practice level.[54]

How Feasible Is It to Integrate Medicine and Public Health?

The feasibility of integrating medicine and public health should be analyzed alongside models that are explicitly oriented to the integration and the experience of interventions that have already been implemented.[34–41,46,52]

With respect to models of integration, Lasker[29] describes four movements related to individual patient care that are emerging into a broader sociophysical environment—social medicine, COPC, preventive medicine, and initiatives to increase the population perspective in medical education. Regarding the content and scope of both social medicine and preventive medicine, a combination of curative and preventive actions are implied, although the actions may not be referred to as social medicine or preventive medicine.[55,56] The feasibility of the COPC approach is also analyzed in the literature as previously described[31,35,43,44] and in Chapters 3 and 4. Also, the

primary healthcare approach—developed after the Declaration of Alma-Ata, which incorporated clinical care (treatment and rehabilitation) with public health (promotion and prevention)—constitutes a movement with relevant experience and applications.[57] Medical education implies a long-term investment, requiring complex and comprehensive measures to evaluate its effect in the organization of services.

The application of each model in the specific local reality needs to take into account the human and economic resources, available facilities, conformity with health policies (local, regional, and national), the healthcare team members' attitudes (interest, motivation, and cooperation), and cultural milieu (citizen–society relationship and democratic spirit).

THE ROLE OF EPIDEMIOLOGY IN INTEGRATION

Epidemiology is a key element in integration and an important element in the development of a community health approach. Before the 1900s, clinical medicine and public health interventions were related; however, after the evolution of both disciplines, epidemiology was considered a public health discipline. The teaching of epidemiology became included in schools of public health. Its exit from medical schools with the subsequent separation from mainstream medicine was one of the main causes of the gap between medicine and public health.

In the second half of the 20th century, when the emphasis of epidemiology shifted from the macroenvironment (environmental and population level) to the microenvironment (individual level) with the study of personal characteristics and behaviors, it returned to a renewed relationship with the clinical professions. Moreover, the development of clinical epidemiology and molecular epidemiology tended to bring issues of public health closer to clinical medicine.[58]

An illustration of epidemiology's role in the integration of medicine and public health is in the complementary use of epidemiological and clinical skills in primary care. General practitioners and family physicians are frontline gatherers of information about their patients', families', and community's health needs. Although the physicians often apply their family- and community-related findings only to the individual patient, potential application exists at the community level. For example, the findings could be used for a needs assessment when clinical medicine and public health are integrated into practice. Epidemiological methods also provide tools for the appropriate evaluation of the effectiveness of alternative community interventions that practitioners plan to implement.

Ibrahim discusses the increasing awareness of integrating medical delivery systems and managed care organizations that stems from the value of population-based health principles in medical and public health practice.[59] The principles relevant to an integrative approach include (1) community and clinical epidemiology perspectives, (2) evidence-based practice, and (3) emphasis on prevention and outcomes. The implementation of these principles requires the organization of a management information system (MIS), which is a basic element in the development of integrated community health care. MIS requires skilled personnel or expert support.

The isolated use of epidemiological methods by medical systems to assess the quality of patient care does not constitute integration between medicine and public health, and thus it may not relate to the integrative component of a community healthcare approach.

VALUES TO CONSIDER IN THE DEVELOPMENT OF INTEGRATED COMMUNITY HEALTH CARE

In the last years, literature related to the delivery of health care has included the following values and priorities that should guide any type of healthcare services: equity, quality, relevance, and cost-effectiveness. Equity means to reduce any form of discrimination based on age, race, sex, religion, ethnicity, and socioeconomic status. Quality refers to satisfactory responses to meet an individual's health concerns. Further, relevance means that the most important problems must be tracked first. Lastly, cost-effectiveness compares the cost of a health intervention with the expected health outcome.

The presence or absence of these values is closely related to the different ways health services are organized. To promote and incorporate these values, it is necessary to have practical experience, an attitude derived from scientific knowledge, and firm convictions.[28] Equally important, the values must be considered in the context of the social, economic, cultural, and political context of the specific population.[60] These values should be considered in conjunction with conditions that have already been discussed in this chapter: (1) a common concern for the population, (2) a shared health information system, (3) an organizational approach to integrate interventions, and (4) a partnership with stakeholders.

THE ROLE OF STAKEHOLDERS IN SERVICE INTEGRATION

The medical sector alone cannot adequately deal with the social determinants of the community's health. Thus, integration requires the active involvement of disciplines, institutions, and other sectors that provide services to the community. It is therefore necessary to consider the following roles of stakeholders:

- Who among the stakeholders is directly involved in taking care of the community's health needs?

- What are the approaches used by stakeholders that promote the health of the public more effectively than merely technical and administrative coordination of medicine and public health activities?
- How should stakeholders deal with inequalities in health, health determinants, and human rights?

The integration of health services should include partnership among five stakeholders: (1) healthcare policy makers, (2) healthcare managers, (3) healthcare professionals, (4) academic institutions, and (5) community members. Each group of stakeholders has a defined role in the development of integration and in their involvement in community health care.

The Role of Healthcare Policy Makers

Whether integration of primary care and public health is implemented at the local, regional, or national level, health policy is necessary to enforce a sustainable reorientation of health services. The relationship between healthcare policy makers and politicians should answer the increasing demand for rational organization in the delivery of health care. The allocation of resources is dependent on explicit health policy; therefore, the policy decisions could be a catalyst for the framework to be followed by other stakeholders.

To promote integration it is important that policy makers not only make decisions on organizational levels, but also consult and reach consensus with all involved stakeholders regarding strategies and plans to promote healthcare delivery integration.[61] An example of integration at the regional level is provided in Catalonia, Spain, where policy makers took steps to promulgate a law for the integration of public health and primary care (see Case Study 11).

The Role of Healthcare Managers

Healthcare managers are responsible for organizing, allocating financial resources, and managing health services. Because the healthcare managers' priorities are coverage, access to care, and the cost-effectiveness of their services, the proposal of an integrated service should be based on rational, economically feasible, and accountable systems.

The Role of Healthcare Professionals

Because of the number of disciplines involved with specific skills and responsibilities, the role of healthcare professionals should be formally established for the development and practice of an integrated approach. Clinical professionals have been trained with a focus on curative medicine and tertiary care, and an integrated system would require them to also perform activities related to prevention and promotion at the community level. In this respect, the motivation of the professionals, as well as an adequate remuneration system and incentives, may be as important as specific training.

An additional element in stimulating professionals for new roles is the recent change in the attitudes of international professional organizations. The World Organization of Family Doctors' (Wonca) Durban Declaration[6] describes the need for family physicians to extend their fields of action from individuals and families to incorporate communities. In addition, the Wonca guidebook *Improving Health Systems: The Contribution of Family Medicine* analyzes the different roles of family medicine in the implementation of primary health care, which features elements needed for the integration of primary care and public health.[62] The COPC approach is clearly emphasized throughout the book.

There are two different trends among family physicians: (1) physicians who emphasize clinical and communication skills as the central issue in their contribution to primary care and (2) physicians who emphasize that family medicine should extend its field of action toward a community orientation.[44] In the latter case, the family physicians could fulfill the leadership roles in working toward the integration between medicine and public health. Preventive medicine physicians in the United States could also take a role in an integration approach by working with populations, as well as with individual patients, and being involved in reviewing and planning health services.

The involvement of other healthcare professionals in the integration of medicine and public health are of paramount importance. Nurses typically have close relationships with patients and other people in the community. They have an important role in narrowing the gap between individual and community care. In Manchester, England, the involvement of health visitors, district nurses, school nurses, and nurse practitioners in a health needs assessment process in a primary care setting is an example of integration, where an interface between primary care and community development is accomplished through a public health approach.[63] An orientation toward community actions with an integrative approach has been suggested for physician assistants in the United States.[64] Among social workers in healthcare settings in Spain, there is a modest change in their focus on intervention from the individual social care level to the community level.

The Role of Academic Institutions

Because of academic institutions' functions in education, research, and service delivery, institutions of medicine, nursing, and public health studies have the potential to address complex issues related to the process of health services integration. This poses a challenge to traditional teaching programs and attitudes of academic leaders. Thus, the educational strategy for integration requires a cultural and attitudinal change at the academic level. The increasing interest in public health and development of liberal arts and pregraduate education[65] is of crucial relevance for the attitudinal change of future healthcare professionals.

Community-based medical education can be considered a means for addressing the fragmentation of services and therefore should be part of the training of health sciences professionals (medical, nursing, and public health).[66,67] The development of the Network of Community-Oriented Educational Institutions for Health Sciences (today called The Network: Towards Unity for Health), including schools of medicine worldwide, provided an essential bridge toward education on integration of health services.[68] From the beginning of their studies, students in those institutions are made aware of a community's health needs by working in community-based settings and learning about the appropriate interventions to deal with the identified health needs.

This type of practice increases the social accountability of academic institutions. It requires a commitment that must be reflected not only in a different training location (community based) but, more specifically, in a community-oriented approach that provides students with field experiences in recognizing populations' health needs. When students work *with* the community, not only *in* the community, this provides a better understanding of the health–illness process and may create a sense of belonging to the community.[66] This may motivate students and create positive attitudes toward integrated health care that could be maintained throughout their careers.

The Role of Community Members

In an integrated community health approach, the community should be considered a partner, not just a consumer. Thus, this approach entitles the community to rights and responsibilities. In that sense, the other stakeholders need to consult and discuss with community members for suggestions, priorities, and special needs. Concomitantly, when the community is willing to participate, it must have or acquire a suitable organization to facilitate its partnership in the whole process, in protecting its rights, and in ensuring an active involvement in all relevant collaborative activities.

Institutions and professionals often hold considerable power in society, and communities hold little power, especially in impoverished areas. Therefore, the integration must consider a greater participatory role of the community in health and health-related interventions to establish more balanced involvement and power. This imbalance of power constitutes an important source of disparities in health status in different societies.

THE FIVE STAKEHOLDERS' COMMITMENT

Proposals for integration among the five stakeholders should consider the opportunities and the constraining factors in forging the partnership, not only for an increase of communication but also for an appropriate commitment of each one of them, moving from ad hoc arrangements to long-term commitments. It is also important to consider that integration at local and regional levels or by providers at the national level is almost impossible without the organizational commitment of the health services and the political commitment of the public health authorities and of appropriate economic resources.

THE MEASUREMENT OF INTEGRATED HEALTH CARE

Healthcare system reform toward integration requires the availability and assessment of measurements of organizational changes. An established agreement on how to measure the conceptual application and methodological framework of the process of integration is necessary for its monitoring and evaluation. According to Devers et al.,[69] integration measures can be considered in three areas:

- measures of precursors: the organization and functions of services and the involved health services' attitudes toward measurements
- intermediate outcomes: the coordination of activities and functions during the process of integration
- immediate and long-term outcomes: a systematic provision of continuum of care, improvement of the community's health status, and an increase in the team's and community's satisfaction

A systematic review of publications that cover structural, cultural, and procedural aspects of integration uncovered 24 different methods to measure integrated healthcare delivery.[70] The data sources for the methods reviewed were questionnaire surveys (most commonly used), automated registered data, or a combination of methods. Structural and procedural aspects were often included, and cultural aspects were rarely used.

THE INTEGRATION PROCESS

From the community's viewpoint, the integration of services may achieve meaningful results that are not possible if services act in a fragmented or separated manner. The integration may form through the combination of activities, processes, or structures of those services. To deal with the separation in healthcare systems, Lasker[71] emphasizes the power of collaboration in which individual clinical services, together with population-based strategies, could improve both the quality and access of care to influence the community's health status. On the basis of a national survey of more than 500 cases, Lasker analyzed and categorized various experiences as they related to public health and medicine. The latter broadly included primary care and hospital care. The experiences, considered to be *synergies*, were based on the combination of resources and skills and also structural arrangements. These arrangements were related to coalitions, contractual arrangements, administrative coordination of activities, advisory bodies, intraorganizational exchange of expertise, and informal (ad hoc) arrangements. These combinations allowed benefits larger than what could be obtained by each partner separately.[72]

Additionally, a literature review of 114 papers about collaboration between primary care and public health was carried out by the Canadian Health Services Research Foundation. It included countries in North America, western Europe, Australia, and New Zealand.[24] Papers were classified by type of model according to Lasker's synergies categorization. The most common type reported was synergy III, which relates to the application of a population perspective to medical practice.

FOUR INTEGRATION LEVELS FOR THE DEVELOPMENT OF COMMUNITY HEALTH CARE

We suggest four progressive levels of integration of primary care and public health to promote and organize community health care (see Table 7-2).

These four suggested methods of integration require the identification and analysis of the negative effects of fragmentation and an understanding of the benefits of integration. They also require the willingness of the different actors involved in the health services organizations to accept changes in specific activities and to recognize the value of contributions from other organizations that serve the same community.

SUMMARY

Fragmented health services are expressed mainly by the separation of medicine and public health, as well as multiple healthcare providers, as opposed to receiving comprehensive health care. Among the main negative effects of fragmentation are the lower quality of health care, duplication of services, waste of resources, and lack of communication among service providers. These effects are felt in different countries and organizational contexts. Factors related to fragmentation include health policy, human and economic resources, health information

TABLE 7-2 Four Integration Levels in the Development of Community Health Care

Coordination at the clinical interface	Health services should coordinate functions to assure continuity of care at different levels, provide primary care with appropriate referrals to hospitals, follow-up with discharged patients, and take further actions at the community level.
Coordination between primary care and public health	Specific activities and services between primary care and public health institutions that are responsible for the same population should be co-ordinated. For example, in an immunization program, the primary care practitioners provide the required vaccinations, with logistic support and information at the population level given by public health practitioners and services.
Integration of primary care and public health services	Primary care teams should jointly engage in providing individual health care and public health initiatives. The COPC approach should be used to integrate medicine and public health in an organizational structure that is based on a unified process. In this approach, the team takes responsibility for a total defined population, carries out an assessment of health needs at the population level, sets priorities, and plans and implements programs to address the identified needs.
Integration of different levels of service organizations and intersectoral coordination	The COPC team should develop intersectoral links in a region or district, as well as with other health services to provide health care for the region's population.

systems, and community perceptions of the roles of the medical profession and public health.

As a multidimensional process, integration aims to consider the biological determinants of health, the socio-cultural-economic determinants, and the health system as parts of health care, which is referred to as the whole. Several approaches for the integration of health services, like COPC, have demonstrated their feasibility and effectiveness.

Integration requires the collective efforts of stakeholders, such as policy makers, healthcare managers, healthcare pro-fessionals, academic institutions, and community members. Four expressions for the development of integrated community health care are suggested, including coordination at the clinical interface, coordination between primary care and public health, integration of primary care and public health services, and integration of different levels of service organizations and intersectoral coordination.

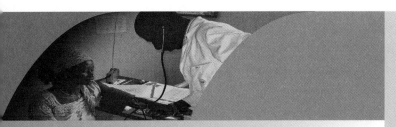

Discussion Questions

- How do the determinants of health influence the fragmentation of health services?

- How can medicine–individual clinical care and public health disciplines influence each other to contribute to better health care?

- Is it possible to develop community health care without integration of health services? If yes, how? If no, why?

- What could be the role of healthcare professions students in the development of health services integration?

Review Questions

- How is fragmentation expressed in health care?

- What are the differences between medicine–clinical individual care and public health?

- What are the factors related to fragmentation?

- What are the appropriate approaches to integration in community health care?

- What are the four integration expressions in the development of community health care?

REFERENCES

1. Gruskin S, Tarantola D. Health and human rights. In: Detels R, McEwen J, Beaglehole R, Tanaka H, eds. *Oxford Textbook of Public Health*. 4th ed. New York, NY: Oxford University Press; 2002;311–335.

2. Detels R, Breslow L. Current scope and concern in public health. In: Detels R, McEwen J, Beaglehole R, Tanaka H, eds. *Oxford Textbook of Public Health*. Vol. 1. 4th ed. New York, NY: Oxford University Press; 2002:3–20.

3. Winslow CEA, The Untilled Fields of Public Health. *Science*. 1920: 51:23–33.

4. Heller RF, Heller TD, Pattison S. Putting the public back into public health. Part I. A re-definition of public health. *Public Health*. 2003;117:62–65.

5. Schroeder SA, Sandy LG. Specialty distribution of US physicians—the invisible driver of health care costs [editorial]. *N Eng J Med*. 1993;328:961–963.

6. Wonca. Health for all rural people: the Durban Declaration. http://www.rudasa.org.za/download/durbandec.pdf. Accessed July 2009.

7. Gofin J, Foz G. Training and application of community-oriented primary care (COPC) through family medicine in Catalonia, Spain. *Fam Med*. 2008;40:196–202.

8. Bettcher DW, Sapirie S, Goon E. Essential public health functions: results of the international Delphi study. *World Health Stat*. 1998;51:44–54.

9. Public Health Functions Project. Public health in America. http://www.health.gov/phfunctions/public.htm. Accessed July 2009.

10. Developing Healthy People 2020. Third meeting: June 5 and 6, 2008. http://www.healthypeople.gov/HP2020/advisory/FACA3Appendix7.htm. Accessed July 2009.

11. Halvorsen JG. Perspective: united we stand, divided we fall: the case for a single primary care specialty in the United States. *Acad Med*. 2008;83:425–431.

12. Valderas JM, Starfield B, Forrest C B, Sibbald B, Roland M. Ambulatory care provided by office based specialists in the US. *Ann Fam Med*. 2009;7:104–111.

13. Cebul RD, Rebitzer JB, Taylor LJ, Votruba ME. Organizational Fragmentation and Care Quality in the U.S. Healthcare System. *Journal of Economics Perspective*. 2008;22:93–113.

14. Enthoven A. Integrated delivery systems: what they do; why we need them; and how to get there from here. Presented at: The Petrie-Flom Center for Health Law Policy, Biotechnology and Bioethics, Harvard Law School; June 13–14, 2008. http://www.law.harvard.edu/programs/petrie-flom/workshops_conferences/Conferences/Fragmentation/ProgramFINALi.pdf. Accessed August 2009.

15. The National Academies. Adolescent health services: missing opportunities. http://www.bocyf.org/ahc_brief.pdf. Published December 2008. Accessed August 2009.

16. Kokko S. Towards fragmentation of general practice and primary healthcare in Finland. *Scand J Prim Health Care*. 2007;25:131–132.

17. Brown L. Comparing health systems in four countries: lessons for the United States. *Am J Public Health*. 2003;93:52–56.

18. Vásquez ML, Vargas I, Unger JP, Mogollón, Ferreira da Silva MR, Paepe P. Integrated health care networks in Latin America: toward a conceptual framework for analysis. *Rev Panam Salud Pública*. 2009;6:360-367.

19. McIntyre D, Garshong B, Mtei G, et al. Beyond fragmentation and towards universal coverage: insights from Ghana, South Africa and the United Republic of Tanzania. *Bull World Health Org*. 2008;86:871–876.

20. Starfield B. Public health and primary care: a framework for proposed linkages. *Am J Public Health*. 1996;86:1365–1369.

21. Shortell SM, Swartzberg J. The physician as public health professional in the 21st century. *JAMA*. 2008;300:2916–2918.

22. Retchin SM. A conceptual framework for interprofessional and comanaged care. *Acad Med*. 2008;83:929–933.

23. Cornell SJ. Public health and primary care collaboration: a case study. *J Public Health Med*. 1999;21:199–204.

24. Martin-Misener R, Valaitis R. A scoping literature review of collaboration between primary care and public health. A report to the Canadian Health Services Research Foundation April 21, 2009. http://fhs.mcmaster.ca/nursing/docs/MartinMisener-Valaitis-Review.pdf. Accessed August 2009.

25. Kodner DL, Spreeuwenberg C. Integrated care: meaning, logic, applications, and implications: a discussion paper. *Int J Integr Care*. 2002;2:e12. www.ijic.org/publish/articles/000089. Accessed August 2009.

26. Merriam-Webster OnLine. www.merriam-webster.com. Accessed July 2009.

27. Batterham T, Southern D, Appleby N, et al. Construction of a GP integration model. *Soc Sci Med*. 2002;54:1225–1241.

28. Boelen C. *Towards Unity for Health: Challenges and Opportunities for Partnership in Health Development. Working Paper*. Geneva, Switzerland: World Health Organization; 2000.

29. Lasker RD. The collaborative imperative. In: Medicine and public health: the power of collaboration. New York, NY: New York Academy of Medicine; 1997 http//www.eacsh.org/pdf/MPH.pdf. Accessed July 2002.

30. Hart T, Thomas C, Gibbons B, et al. Twenty-five years of audited screening in a socially deprived community. *Br Med J*. 1993;302:1509–1513.

31. Abramson JH. Community-oriented primary care-strategy, approaches, and practice: a review. *Public Health Rev*. 1988;16:35–98.

32. Harvey P. The impact of coordinated care: Eyre Region South Australia 1997–1999. *Aust J Rural Health*. 2001; 9:69–73.

33. Longlett SK, Kruse JE, Wesley RM. Community-oriented primary care: critical assessment and implications for residents' education. *J Am Board Fam Pract*. 2001;14:141–147.

34. Geiger HJ. Community-oriented primary care: a path to community development. *Am J Public Health*. 2002;92:1713–1716.

35. Epstein L, Gofin J, Gofin R, Neumark Y. The Jerusalem experience: three decades of service, research, and training in community-oriented primary care. *Am J Public Health*. 2002;92:1717–1721.

36. Gillam S, Schamroth A. The community-oriented primary care experience in the United Kingdom. *Am J Public Health*. 2002;92:1721–1725.

37. Tollman SM, Pick WM. Roots, shoots, but too little fruit: assessing the contribution of COPC in South Africa. *Am J Public Health*. 2002;92:1725–1728.

38. Pickens S, Boumbulian P, Anderson R, Ross S, Phillips S. Community-oriented primary care in action: a Dallas story. *Am J Public Health*. 2002;92:1728–1732.

39. Rhyne RL, Hertzman PA. Pursuing community-oriented primary care in a Russian closed nuclear city: the Sarov-Los Alamos community health partnership. *Am J Public Health*. 2002;92:1740–1742.

40. Brown TM, Fee E. "Palliatives will no longer do": the deep roots and continuing dynamic of community-oriented primary care [editorial]. *Am J Public Health*. 2002;92:1711–1712.

41. Mullan F, Epstein L. Community-oriented primary care: new relevance in a changing world. *Am J Public Health*. 2002;92:1748–1755.

42. Illiffe S, Lenihan P. Integrating primary care and public health: learning from the community-oriented primary care model. *Int J Health Serv*. 2003;33:85–98.

43. Kark SL. *The Practice of Community-Oriented Primary Care*. New York, NY: Appleton-Century-Crofts; 1981.

44. Foz G, Gofin J, Montaner I. Atención primaria orientada a la comunidad: una visión actual. In: Martín Zurro A, Cano Pérez JF, eds. *Atención Primaria—conceptos, organización y práctica clínica*. 6th ed. Madrid, Spain: Elsevier; 2008.

45. Glasser J. Medicine and public health initiative (MPHI) in a nutshell 2008. http://www.mphi.net/?page_id=34&lang=en-us. Accessed July 2009.

46. Gage County-PATCH/health lifestyles. www.beatricene.com/patch/. Accesed April 2010.

47. Noris T, Pittman M. The healthy communities movement and the coalition for healthier cities and communities. *Public Health Rep*. 2000;115:118–124.

48. Community–Campus Partnerships for Health. Transforming communities and higher education. http://www.ccph.info/. Accessed July 2009.

49. UNICEF. Act, analyze, access program (AAA). 2008. http://www.unicef.org/rightsresults/files/HRBDP_Urban_Jonsson_April_2003.pdf. Accessed July 2009.

50. Fernando D, Jayatilleka A, Karunaratna V. Pregnancy-reducing maternal deaths and disability in Sri Lanka: national strategies. *Br Med Bull.* 2003;67:85–98.

51. Kasturiaratchi ND, Settinayake S, Grewal P. Processes and challenges: how the Sri Lankan health system managed the integration of leprosy services. *Lepr Rev.* 2002;73:177–185.

52. Perry H, Robison N, Chavez D, et al. Attaining health for all through community partnerships: principles of the census-based, impact-oriented (CBIO) approach to primary health care developed in Bolivia, South America. *Soc Sci Med.* 1999;48:1053–1067.

53. Bertodano I. The Costa Rican health system: low cost, high value. *Bull World Health Org.* 2003;81:626–627.

54. Barrett B. Integrated local health systems in Central America. *Soc Sci Med.* 1996;43:71–82.

55. Leaf A. Preventive medicine for our ailing health care system. *JAMA.* 1993;269:616–618. http://jama.ama-assn.org/cgi/reprint/269/5/616. Accessed July 2009.

56. Porter D. How did social medicine evolve, and where is it heading? *PLoS Med.* 2006;3:e399. http://www.pubmedcentral.nih.gov/picrender.fcgi?artid=1621092&blobtype=pdf. Accessed August 2009.

57. Pan American Health Organization. *Health in the Americas.* Washington, DC: Pan American Health Organization; 2002.

58. Adami HO, Trichopoulos D. Epidemiology, medicine and public health. *Int J Epidemiol.* 1999;28:S1005–S1008.

59. Ibrahim MA, Savitz LA, Carey TS, Wagner EH. Population-based health principles in medical and public health practice. *J Pub Health Manag Pract.* 2001;7:75–81.

60. Boelen C, Glasser J, Gofin J, Lippeveld T, Orobaton N. Towards unity for health: the quest for evidence. *Educ Health.* 2007;20:2–9.

61. Bergman H, Beland F. Commentary on: the future of health care in Canada. *Int J Integr Care.* 2002;2. www.ijic.org/publish/articles/000086/. Accessed July 2009.

62. Boelen C, Haq C, Hunt V, Rivo M, Shahady E, World Organization of Family Doctors. *Improving Health Systems: The Contribution of Family Medicine—A Guidebook.* Singapore: Bestprint Printing Company; 2002.

63. Horne M, Costello J. A public health approach to health needs assessment at the interface of primary care and community development: findings from an action research study. *Prim Health Care Res Dev.* 2003;4:340–352.

64. Gofin J, Cawley JF. The physician assistant and community oriented primary care (COPC). *Perspect Physician Assist Educ.* 2004;15:126–128.

65. Riegelman R. Undergraduate public health education: past, present, and future. *Am J Prev Med.* 2008;35:258–263.

66. Gofin J. Planning the teaching of community health (COPC) in an MPH program. *Public Health Rev.* 2002;30:293–301.

67. Waterstone T, Sanders D. Primary health care teaching: some lessons from Zimbabwe. *Med Educ.* 1987;21:4–9.

68. The Network: Towards Unity for Health. What is The Network: Towards Unity for Health? www.the-networktufh.org. Accessed July 2009.

69. Devers KJ, Shortell SM, Gillies RR, Anderson DA, Mitchell JB, Erickson KL. Implementing organized delivery systems: an integration scorecard. *Health Care Manage Rev.* 1994;9:7–20.

70. Strandberg-Larsen M, Krasnik A. Measurement of integrated health-care delivery: a systematic review of methods and future research directions. *Int J Integr Care.* 2009;9:e01.

71. Lasker RD, Weiss ES, Miller R. Promoting collaborations that improve health. *Education forHealth.* 2001;14:163–172.

72. Lasker RD, Abramson DM, Freedman GR. *Pocket Guide to Cases of Medicine and Public Health Collaboration.* New York, NY: New York Academy of Medicine; 1998.

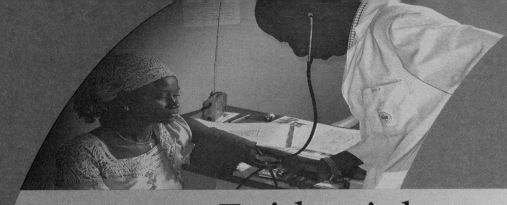

CHAPTER **8**

Epidemiology as a Tool for Community Health Care

J. H. Abramson

INTRODUCTION

Epidemiology is the basic science of community health care. Without epidemiology as one of its foundations, community health care is a fiction or a mere aspiration or a well-meaning activity not necessarily directed at the community's major needs, with an uncertain or (at best) a guessed or hoped impact on health. Epidemiological information of some kind (whether less exact or more exact, whether narrow or wide in its scope) is essential if community health care is to be useful and effective, and if it is to be demonstrably useful and effective. This requires the use of epidemiological methods.

The affinity between community health care and epidemiology is clear. By definition, community health care is directed at a specific population or specific populations. And by definition, epidemiology is the study of the distribution and determinants of health-related states or events in a specific population or specific populations and the application of this study to the control of health problems.

THE SCOPE OF EPIDEMIOLOGY

There are sometimes misconceptions about the scope of epidemiology. Epidemiology is of course not only the study of epidemics. Nor is it concerned only with the occurrence and distribution of diseases and deaths. It embraces disabilities and behavioral and other problems that are not necessarily defined as diseases and which, like diseases, might be the foci of preventive, therapeutic, or rehabilitative community programs. It can also extend to the study of positive health, such as physical fitness, longevity, mental and social adjustment, and healthy growth and development, which might be the foci of promotive community programs. In fact, back in the 5th century BC, Hippocrates, who is often considered the father of epidemiology, was concerned with the epidemiology of health rather than the epidemiology of disease.[1] And epidemiology is concerned not only with disease and health states, but also with their determinants, which may be risk factors or protective factors, or factors that modify the effects of risk factors or protective factors.

These determinants are specified in the *Dictionary of Epidemiology*'s definition of epidemiology[2] as "all the physical, biological, social, cultural, and behavioral factors that influence health." Studies of air pollution, smoking habits, concepts of disease causation, or mother–child relationships that are conducted because of interest in their health implications can be classified as epidemiological studies, even if they do not specifically appraise associations with health. In his classic writings on the uses of epidemiology, Morris[3] extends the scope of epidemiology to studies of health services and their operation. He also writes of experimental epidemiology, and a respected epidemiology textbook[4] calls clinical trials (which are conducted in clinically selected subgroups of a population) "epidemiological studies evaluating treatments."

Epidemiology can thus be construed as embracing every influence on health and health care. Regrettably, some epidemiology textbooks ignore this broad interpretation, confining their consideration of determinants to those that can be measured at an individual level, such as serum cholesterol concentration and smoking habits, and paying little attention to the social, cultural, and environmental context or to health care or the healthcare system.

EPIDEMIOLOGICAL INFORMATION

Community health care requires two types of epidemiological information: information about the specific community and information (generally not based on that community) concerning the specific problems on which care may be focused—their predictors; their manner of diagnosis; their causes, natural history, and consequences; and the effects of therapeutic, preventive, or promotive interventions. The latter body of knowledge permits the practice of *evidence-based community health care*, analogous to evidence-based medicine ("the conscientious, explicit, and judicious use of current best evidence in making decisions about the care of individual patients"[5]) and evidence-based public health ("a public health endeavour in which there is an informed, explicit, and judicious use of evidence that has been derived from any of a variety of . . . research and evaluation methods"[6]).

EPIDEMIOLOGY IN COMMUNITY-ORIENTED PUBLIC HEALTH AND COMMUNITY-ORIENTED PRIMARY CARE

In accordance with the distinction made in this book between *community-oriented public health* (COPH) and *community-oriented primary care* (COPC), we will give separate consideration to the use of epidemiology in these two modes of community health care.

COPH refers to a focus on local communities when implementing a public health program, not necessarily through the medium of primary healthcare practices, but generally taking account of differences among communities in their needs, resources, and other features. COPC refers to an integrated form of practice in which practitioners of primary health care (doctors, nurses, health educators, managers, and others) not only deal with the needs of individuals and families; they also try to treat the community as a patient by appraising the health needs of the population and establishing community health programs to deal with these needs in a systematic way, whether in the clinical framework or by way of educational and other outreach activities. COPC integrates the care of individuals with the care of a community as a whole or its various subgroups.

COPH programs are generally operated by public health authorities, health maintenance organizations, primary care trusts, or other agencies that provide services to large regions, whereas a COPC program is generally conducted in the framework of a general or family practice, a local community clinic or health center, or a community hospital.

A COPH program that is implemented in a number of primary care practices may, of course, share the features of COPH and COPC. The features of COPH and COPC may also be shared if a group of primary care practices, say in the same city, embark on a joint, broad (citywide) COPC program in collaboration with the city's public health department.

Community health care can be seen as a cyclic process, with procedures analogous to those in the clinical care of an individual patient,(see Chapter 4, Table 4-1) namely examination, diagnosis, treatment, follow-up, and reassessment (followed, if necessary, by a repetition of the cycle). The COPC cycle is pictured in Chapter 4, Figure 4-1. The contributions of epidemiology in each phase of the cycle and illustrative examples are described in Chapters 2–5 and in the Case Studies. What follows here is a brief outline of some of these contributions.

DETERMINING THE COMMUNITY'S HEALTH NEEDS

Before determining a community's health needs, it is necessary to define the community. This may be easy or hard. In

COPH it may be easy if a geographic or administrative demarcation is used, and in COPC it may be easy if there is a defined population for whose welfare the practice is responsible. In other instances in COPC, the aggregate of people who seek care, or those who have sought care recently, or those who seek care repeatedly, or some defined group of them, may be regarded as the community for COPC purposes; or a family physician who does not have a list of registered patients might define the community as all the members of families of which any single member is an active patient.

Information may be required about the target population as a whole or about defined subgroups for whom programs are contemplated or provided, such as infants and their parents, people with a specific disease, or specific high-risk groups; different parts of the population may have different needs. In addition to this prime definition of the community as the target population for whose health care the practice is responsible, it may be decided to also designate for study the community of which the members of the target population (or a large number of them) form a part. For example, if a COPC practice serves part of the population of a town, it may be decided to seek information about the town as a whole to learn about available facilities and services, environmental hazards, patterns of leadership and communication, and other relevant ecological factors and to find census and other easily accessible data that can be applied (even with reservations) to the target population. This extension may also permit the collection of information required for the planning and evaluation of broader programs, possibly in cooperation with public health or other agencies, such as community health education projects that are not restricted to members of the practice's target population.

Census data, population registers, birth and death statistics, hospitalization data, service utilization data, registers of patients with cancer or other diseases, centralized pharmacy records, and other data banks are generally the main available sources of information in COPH; special surveys may also be contemplated. These sources may provide aggregate measures that are based on the attributes of individuals (such as disease or unemployment rates) or families (such as mean income), as well as global measures that are not (e.g., levels of environmental pollution, criminality, and safety in the community).

These sources may also be used in COPC. But in COPC, the primary care service's clinical records, if they have been maintained with care and especially if they have been computerized, can provide a great deal of additional data about the population's health state and other characteristics. Not only can they provide statistics, they can also pinpoint individuals

who, because of their health state, age, risk status, or other characteristics, merit special attention or the planning of special subgroup programs. In some instances, it may be possible to augment the data by incorporating survey questions or examinations into clinical routines or by conducting sample surveys in the community. In addition, because of their close and continuing relationship with the community, the COPC practitioners may have gotten to know the community. They may be aware, for example, of the community's aspirations and felt needs and of the beliefs and customary practices that may have an impact on health and participation in health programs, and they may know what facilities, services, key informants, community leaders, and community organizations could play a role in deciding on, planning, and applying these programs. The planning of community care programs requires qualitative as well as numeric information.

In both COPH and COPC, what is needed is information about the community's health problems and their determinants and consequences. This may be termed a *community diagnosis* that characterizes the community and its health status. Just as a diagnosis of a patient's state of health is a prerequisite for good clinical care, so a community diagnosis, leading to a needs assessment, provides a basis for the care of a community. This community diagnosis may be solely descriptive, or it may be analytic, exploring associations between, say, a disease and the risk factors prevalent in the community or between a disease and time lost from work.

The community diagnosis has no pretensions to completeness; it always deals with selected health problems and selected determinants, and sometimes with selected subgroups of the community, and it does not necessarily need to be very detailed. The choice of topics may be guided by prior knowledge of the community or a prioritization process, or it may be an expression of a national or institutional health policy that is not based on local findings.

The community diagnosis can serve at least three purposes. First, taken in conjunction with considerations of feasibility and cost and available evidence concerning the effectiveness of interventions, it permits decisions on the *case for action* directed at specific problems—what problems, which of their determinants, and which subgroups should be given priority? Although accurate information is obviously desirable for this purpose (and decisions are often postponed until additional information can be collected) it is sometimes regarded as sufficient to rely on epidemiological data concerning a community that is believed to be similar or pertains to a broad region that includes the specific community. Second (and especially if individuals requiring special attention have been pinpointed), the community diagnosis can help in the planning and implementation of the chosen intervention program or programs. And third (this is where accurate local information is definitely required), the community diagnosis provides baseline data for the subsequent measurement of changes to assess the effectiveness of the intervention.

EPIDEMIOLOGY AND COMMUNITY HEALTH PROGRAMS

Community health programs are interventions designed to deal with a community's main health problems. The program may focus on a single problem or on a *community syndrome*[7] of associated problems that are causally interrelated or have shared or related causes. The decision to plan a program to deal with a specific problem or set of problems is (or should be) based not on whim or an arbitrary policy decision, but on epidemiological information. Judicious decisions about priorities require the facts that a community diagnosis can provide about the extent of health problems (e.g., incidence or prevalence rates in different subgroups) and their effect in the community (e.g., complications, disability, mortality, and the proportions of cases of a disease that can be attributed to specific risk factors), and they also call on available epidemiological evidence concerning the importance of the problems and the effectiveness of programs designed to handle them. An understanding of the community's felt needs and demands, its readiness and capacity to participate in the program, and relevant attitudes and customary practices may also play a part; this may require formal or informal discussions with community leaders, other key informants, and community organizations. Information on the use and availability of time, manpower, and other resources inevitably plays an important part in decisions both about priorities and the manner of intervention.

A clear formulation of the program's objectives (i.e., its hoped-for outcomes, expressed in measurable terms) is a prerequisite for subsequent monitoring and evaluation of the program. Besides the desired end results (e.g., a reduced prevalence of hypertension), the objectives should specify targets for the activities designed to achieve these results (e.g., screening for hypertension, treatment of hypertensives).

While the program is in operation, built-in monitoring procedures that produce real-time records of the performance of planned activities make it possible to gauge progress and, if necessary, make changes. Monitoring usually relates not only to the activities of staff members, but also to compliance and the utilization of services by members of the community.

SURVEILLANCE AND PROGRAM EVALUATION

Ongoing surveillance continues the diagnostic process and keeps it up to date. This is especially applicable in COPC, whose clinical context offers special opportunities for data collection. Well-designed routines and records provide information that is useful both in caring for the individual and, when analyzed, at a group level. A good deal of the information needed for surveillance and for program evaluation (as for community diagnosis) can thus be collected in the course of clinical care, either as part of the ordinary diagnostic investigation and surveillance of patients or by adding tests and questions to clinic procedures.

The key questions that the evaluation should answer relate to the achievement of the desired effects specified as the program's objectives, and of course to the avoidance of undesirable effects. The desired effect is not necessarily a change in the community's health status; in some programs it is the performance by personnel of specified activities (such as immunization or case finding) whose impact on community health is taken for granted; in others, the desired effect may be, for example, a change in dietary, smoking, or other behaviors, or sanitary or other environmental changes, or the development of community organizations that will contribute to community self-help and community development.

No program can be considered successful until it has been evaluated and found to be successful. Merely doing it is no proof that it was worth doing. But it must be stressed that in this context, program evaluation is not a hypothesis-testing undertaking that examines causal relationships between interventions and outcomes, employing the established methods of clinical and program trials. The assumptions on which the program is based, for example that (according to evidence collected elsewhere) avoidance of sweetened carbonated drinks will reduce the prevalence of obesity in schoolchildren, are generally taken for granted and not tested. The evaluation results will therefore be useful to those running the program and to the decision makers who have to decide on its modification and continuance, even if others doubt the validity of the assumptions, and even though the findings may not be generalizable. This is the kind of evaluation that has been termed a *program review*,[8] in contrast to a *program trial*. It asks, "How well is this program working?" rather than, "Is this kind of program a good thing?"

RESEARCH OPPORTUNITIES

That said, community healthcare programs offer a rich field of opportunities for epidemiologic research. This is especially true in a COPC context, where may be there is expected to be special efforts to obtain and record valid and reliable information as part of the integration of community diagnosis into clinical activities. Possible research topics include studies of conditions that are not often seen outside a primary-care context, studies of diagnostic and case management methods in a primary-care context, and studies of the impact of family settings on health.

Of particular interest to advocates of community health care is the evaluation of COPH or COPC itself, in terms of effectiveness, cost, and patient satisfaction. Such studies of effectiveness are hypothesis-testing studies, that is, program trials that aim to produce generalizable knowledge about the value of a particular kind of program. They require especially accurate objective information in terms of validity and reliability, and they are much more ambitious than program reviews.

Before-and-after comparisons may be enough to point to the effectiveness of a program, particularly if the findings are replicated in different community settings, but for the evidence of a cause-and-effect relationship to be more convincing, the changes must be compared with those in a control community or communities not exposed to the program. This presents problems in COPC because whatever control community is selected, there will inevitably be differences (in health personnel as well as in community characteristics) between it and the community to which the program is applied, and it may be difficult to rule out the influence of confounding factors. When a single treated community is compared with a single nontreated community, randomization is worthless (and unlikely to be practicable) because there will be the same differences between the communities, however they are allocated.

Controlled trials of community health programs are easier in the COPH context, where a considerable number of communities or primary-care practices are available, so that they can be randomly allocated to treatment and control groups, and the outcomes can then be compared using methods appropriate for comparisons of randomized clusters.[9] The practices participating in such trials may be stratified before they are randomized or matched, for example to ensure a balance among practices of different sizes or in different ethnic communities.

FINAL QUIZ

Q. Is epidemiology the basic science of community health care?

A. Yes.

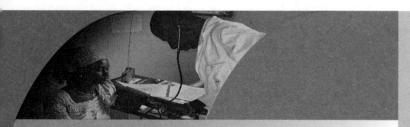

Discussion Questions

- Should all professionals involved in community health care have epidemiological training?

- How detailed should a community diagnosis be?

- Should intervention start only when the community diagnosis is complete?

Review Questions

- What kinds of knowledge does evidence-based community health care require?

- How do COPC and COPH differ, and what do they have in common?

- How can a COPC practice define the community it serves?

- What purposes may a community diagnosis serve?

- In a COPC context, how do program reviews and program trials differ?

REFERENCES

1. Galdston I. *The Epidemiology of Health.* New York, NY: Health Education Council; 1953.

2. Last JM, ed. *A Dictionary of Epidemiology.* 4th ed. Oxford, England: Oxford University Press; 2001.

3. Morris JN. *Uses of Epidemiology.* 3rd ed. Edinburgh, Scotland: Churchill Livingstone; 1971.

4. Rothman KJ, Greenland S, Lash TL. *Modern Epidemiology.* 3rd ed. Philadelphia, PA: Lippincott Williams & Wilkins; 2008.

5. Sackett DL, Rosenberg WMC, Gray JAM, Haynes RB, Richardson WS. Evidence based medicine: what it is and what it isn't. *Br Med J.* 1996;312:71–72.

6. Rychetnik L, Hawe P, Waters E, Barratt A, Frommer M. A glossary for evidence based public health. *J Epidemiol Community Health.* 2004;58:538–545.

7. Kark SL. *Epidemiology and Community Medicine.* New York, NY: Appleton-Century-Crofts; 1974.

8. Abramson JH, Abramson ZH. *Research Methods in Community Medicine: Surveys, Epidemiological Research, Programme Evaluation, Clinical Trials.* 6th ed. Chichester, England: John Wiley & Sons; 2008.

9. Murray IDM, Varnell SP, Blitstein JL. Design and analysis of group-randomized trials: a review of recent methodological developments. *Am J Public Health.* 2004;94:423–432.

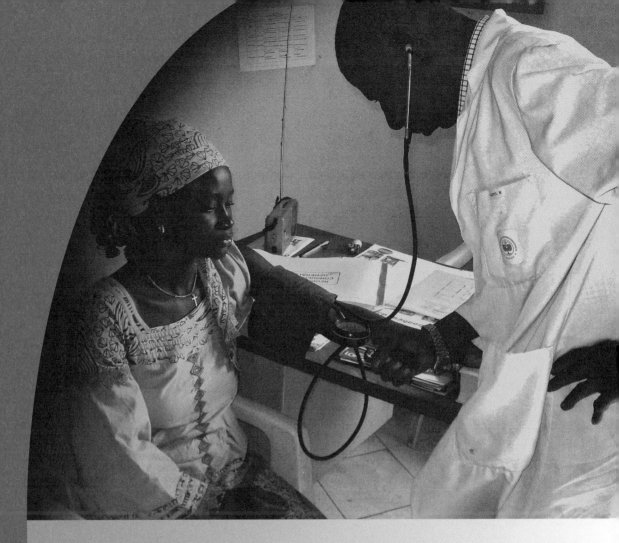

SECTION II

Global Application of Community Health Care: Case Studies

Preface to Case Studies

In this section readers are taken on a global grand round of community health across five continents.

Cases are presented for varied aspects of community health and health care. They encompass the health of children and adults in diverse environments and healthcare systems. Some of these cases present harsh physical and environmental situations, as well as social situations, that challenge not only the population but also health care, health workers, and health organizations. Others explore innovations in care delivery, from reorganization of the healthcare system with a community orientation to engaging the community in the process.

Through these studies, readers may identify the principles and methods analyzed in the chapters of this book and how they were adapted to the local context. Specific communities or groups of communities are the subjects of the cases that are related to academic institutions, the health system in a particular place, or the combination of both. They express new experiences and sustainable ones.

From each case there are many lessons to be learned.

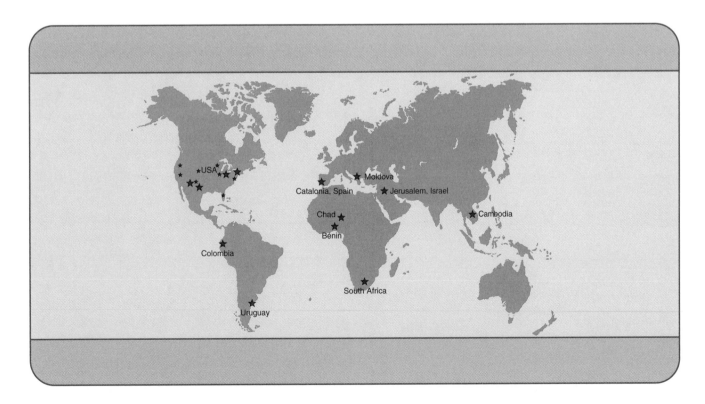

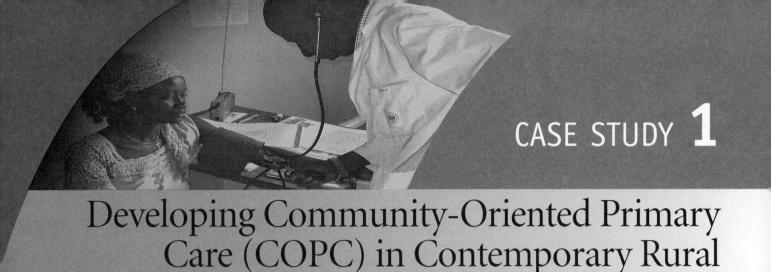

Developing Community-Oriented Primary Care (COPC) in Contemporary Rural South Africa: The Case of Stroke

Collin A. Pfaff, Stephen M. Tollman, and Kathleen Kahn

BACKGROUND

The Agincourt subdistrict of Bushbuckridge, Mpumalanga Province comprises rural communities situated in northeastern South Africa, 45 kilometers from the Mozambique border and adjacent to the Kruger National Park. It shares many of the features common to rural areas in the region, with poor roads and poor access to water. Electricity is supplied to most villages but not to all households. The area is densely populated, with 175 people per square kilometer. The area was historically part of the Gazankulu homeland and populated by Tsonga-speaking South Africans, and it was settled more recently by Mozambican refugees fleeing the civil war in the 1980s; residents of Mozambican origin now make up one-third of the population. The area has high unemployment. Many men, and increasingly women, are migrant workers with varying regularity of return visits. The few that are employed locally work in the public sector or in tourism or agriculture. The area is arid, making it unsuitable for subsistence farming, and thus many families rely heavily on old-age pensions or other non-contributory social grants provided by the government.

Western health care began in the area as a patchwork of hospitals and clinics set up by missionaries, but these were later taken over by the apartheid government in the 1970s and incorporated into the quasi-independent homeland administrations of Gazankulu and Lebowa. This resulted in gross inequality because homeland services were deliberately underfunded and often poorly managed. The democratic transition in 1994 introduced a district-based healthcare system with attempts made at redressing the past. Today healthcare facilities in the Bushbuckridge region consist of government-run primary healthcare clinics that are staffed by nurses. These clinics are supported by three district hospitals. There are several private practitioners working in the area. The community also commonly seeks help from traditional healers and faith healers from various churches.

The University of the Witwatersrand's School of Public Health in Johannesburg, South Africa began work in the area in 1982 through a small, independently funded Health Systems Development Unit (HSDU). This was an attempt to address some of the severe inequalities in health care in rural areas that was created by the apartheid regime. The work started with efforts to strengthen primary health care, particularly by training primary healthcare nurse practitioners. It also looked at ways of developing a district-based approach to healthcare provision. The project was influenced by the work on community-oriented primary care (COPC) by Sidney L. and Emily Kark, who had worked in a similar rural setting in Pholela, South Africa, more than 40 years earlier (see Chapter 3). The Pholela initiative involved a community health center paralleled by a community-based data surveillance system with regular community health surveys. Survey findings were used to inform new approaches to preventive and curative programs, such as child malnutrition and scabies. Applying these COPC principles, the HSDU team sought to establish a system to collect basic population and health data to identify priority health needs in the community, inform the development of interventions, and evaluate the impact of these interventions. Thus, a defined geographic area, covering rural villages such as Agincourt and incorporating a small network of clinics, was selected for regular health and sociodemographic surveillance.

Today the Agincourt surveillance site covers an area of 420 square kilometers and is home to 84,000 people in 26 villages. Lay field-workers produced hand-drawn village maps, and the project conducted the first community census in 1992.[1] This involved a door-to-door survey or census during which every household was visited, and every individual was enumerated and assigned a unique identification number. Routine vital events data, including all births, deaths, and in- and out-migrations, were collected. This census has been updated every year since. Special modules have been added to broaden its scope to address specific research priorities. Examples include temporary migration and labor force participation, healthcare utilization, food security, and education. Because only about half of deaths occur in hospitals, the verbal autopsy method was introduced to determine the probable cause of death by interviewing a close caregiver about the signs and symptoms of the terminal illness;[2] this was followed by rigorous assessment of the questionnaire by two or three physicians who were required to reach consensus. The hand-drawn maps have progressed to a sophisticated computer-based geographic information system that provides a platform for other research studies in the site. The Agincourt community has thus provided one of the few settings in sub-Saharan Africa where continuous longitudinal health data are available—data that span a period of major sociopolitical change and the emergence of the devastating AIDS epidemic.

THE HEALTH STATUS OF THE COMMUNITY

As surveys progressively accumulated vital health data, trends began to emerge revealing a community undergoing dramatic changes in patterns of health and disease. The death rate increased by 87% from 1992 to 2005, mainly due to a sixfold rise in infectious and parasitic diseases, particularly HIV and tuberculosis.[3] However, deaths from noncommunicable diseases also increased during the same period, particularly in adults older than age 65 years where deaths due to vascular disease increased by 65%. This emerging problem tends to be hidden by the overwhelming increase in deaths due to HIV/AIDS, but it clearly points to the fact that this community is in the midst of a profound health transition—communicable diseases are the main causes of ill health, accompanied by a concurrent rise in the rate and importance of chronic noncommunicable diseases.

Over time, the research was able to describe social trends in the community. Young women were migrating for work in rapidly increasing numbers. Many chronically ill migrant laborers were returning from the cities to their rural homes to die.[4] Older women were providing a significant source of financial, physical, and emotional support to sick adults and to fostered and orphaned children.[5] While the population was increasing, the household size was decreasing, with smaller percentages of children but similar percentages of the elderly and women. The number of households headed by women was increasing.[6]

Because the rise in cardiovascular-related events was an unexpected finding in this relatively remote rural setting, further research was conducted to investigate this trend more fully. With the population database of the Agincourt site, two additional screening questions were added to the 2001 annual census update in an effort to identify stroke victims. These people were then visited in their homes, and a detailed history and examination was done to validate a stroke diagnosis and to determine cardiovascular risk factors.[7] The study showed a prevalence of stroke of 300/100,000 people. The crude male:female ratio was 1:1.8. Although this prevalence was much lower than rates in high-income countries, it was double the rate found elsewhere in Africa. Also of concern was that two-thirds of these people needed assistance with at least one activity of daily living, which was higher than the rate in high-income countries.[8]

As part of the same study, issues around secondary prevention of stroke were examined.[9] Amongst 103 stroke survivors, 71% were found to have hypertension, but only eight were on antihypertensive medication, and only one of these had a blood pressure in the normal range; 83% were prescribed antihypertensive medication by a doctor or nurse when help was sought, but it was not continued; and only one patient was taking aspirin in spite of this being national policy. Thus, regardless of initial contact with the health service, there was very poor ongoing secondary care of stroke victims. On further enquiry, the cost of access to services and transportation, as well as a reluctance to take tablets that were not considered to help, were serious barriers. Stroke victims reported that when they were told their blood pressure was normal, they simply did not return to collect more medication.

Upon being interviewed, many people in this community differentiated between two similar illnesses, both causing strokelike symptoms: *xistroku* was caused by natural disease factors, and *xifulana* was human in origin and usually caused by those who were jealous or wanted to do harm.[10] To treat both causes, help was usually sought from a mix of allopathic practitioners, traditional healers, and church faith healers, although allopathic healers were usually consulted first.[9]

The same research team also interviewed a group of nurses. When asked about reasons for poor secondary care of stroke, they reported that drugs were frequently out of stock in the clinics and the equipment was faulty. A follow-up survey of all clinics in the study area found that none had fully functioning blood pressure measuring devices and that almost all the deficiencies were due to faulty valves or poorly functioning and wrong-sized cuffs, items that could be easily repaired or replaced at little cost.[11] Hypertensive drugs were always available in 50% of the clinics, but only one reported a regular supply of aspirin.

Further research in Agincourt to inform interventions included a cross-sectional risk factor survey of adults aged 35 years and older in the community.[12] More than two-fifths of participants were found to be hypertensive, but less than a quarter of them had used antihypertensive drugs in the previous week. Of the group currently on treatment, only half had a blood pressure lower than 140/90 mm Hg. More than a quarter of all men were smokers, although the quantities smoked were low. Obesity was found to be much more common in women than men. A quarter of participants had cholesterol higher than the highest desirable level, although the HDL to total cholesterol ratio was largely favorable. None of these participants were on treatment. Almost a third of those older than age 65 years had evidence of subclinical peripheral atheroma.

THE INTERVENTION PROGRAM

The principles of COPC involve a combination of public health and curative primary health care. In Agincourt, concerted effort has been made to gather local data to assess needs, set priorities, and generate context-specific social and cultural understanding. Considerable effort was devoted to training local health workers and managers. The project is now in a position to focus on more direct interventions in clinical care and services. Although the development of subdistrict health center–clinic networks was commenced, direct interventions have not recently been a prominent part of the project and need further development before the full elements of COPC are realized.

However, the research has, in several cases, informed specific interventions. The findings on stroke were communicated to the community in a unique way using applied theater to generate a community response.[13] Four of the research field-workers, who were residents in the community, developed a drama based on the research findings that was performed to groups of 30 to 100 people, typically under a tree. The story was of a man who collapsed while working in a field and was then taken to various healthcare providers. Much audience participation was encouraged by a joker who directed questions at them and invited them to come onto the stage and interact with the actors. At the end the field-workers asked the spectators what they thought of the dramatization and generated ideas for future interventions. One field-worker was amazed about how passionate people were about the dramatized situ-

ations, and another noted how involved people became in the process.

The research findings also had impact beyond the Agincourt community. Mpumalanga Province was selected to participate in a joint project supported by the World Health Organization (WHO) and the Flemish government to boost capacity for health promotion in addressing noncommunicable diseases. The Agincourt study findings were communicated to the provincial team, and they heavily influenced the development of a health promotion strategy to reduce the burden of excess mortality and disability from stroke and heart disease.

Three target sites outside of Bushbuckridge were initially selected. In each site, teams were formed and a situational analysis was done. The findings were presented in a series of workshops to health teams, nongovernmental organizations (NGOs), traditional healers, and community groups, where information on stroke and healthy eating was conveyed. Some of this was in the form of role play, inspired by the Agincourt applied theater approach. Use was also made of videos, active learning sessions involving pictures and discussion, and a physical exercise activity. The aim of these workshops was to increase the capacity of health promotion practitioners who worked in the community. In response to these workshops, a series of community events was initiated by the health promoters, including the establishment of community gardens, the formation of support groups, and awareness events such as fun runs, radio advertisements, and a mass education event. The confidence of the health promotion practitioners markedly increased. Several had the opportunity to attend university courses, an experience that was a dramatic benefit to other awareness programs they were involved in, such as HIV/AIDS and Integrated Management of Childhood Illnesses (IMCI).[14]

Overall it was thought that the project resulted in better integration of health promotion into the rest of the health service and improved community participation. Although the project has been rolled out to several other districts, it has lacked a rigorous monitoring and evaluation component to assess its real impact.

COMMUNITY PARTICIPATION AND INTERSECTORAL COOPERATION

From the very initial stages of setting up the Agincourt study site, the cooperation and support of the local community was a priority. An extensive series of discussions was conducted, and it was held by principle that all collected information and research findings would be shared. It was also agreed that all data entry would take place on-site and thus be visible to community members.

The LINC (Learning, Information, Dissemination and Networking with Community) office of the research unit is currently the community liaison, and it was specifically set up for this purpose. LINC trains field staff to give feedback presentations to community development forums, the community advisory group, and each village in the study area. These meetings often lead to lively discussions of the topic at hand. Fact sheets are distributed at the village level and often form the basis for discussions with community leaders. Interaction is also encouraged at planning stages of projects, and communities are informed about future census updates and research projects.

Since 2002, the LINC office has compiled directories of resources for health, development, and education that can be used by local communities. Because field-workers frequently encounter health and social needs during their household visits, they have information on all the available local services—government, NGO, and church based—and can make appropriate referrals.

The LINC office has also prioritized working with NGO partners and relevant government stakeholders, including health, welfare, education, and environmental affairs. These stakeholders have access to aggregated community-based data for use in planning and policy making. In some cases this has led to specific government responses (see Box C1-1).[1]

Box C1-1 Research to action: improving access to the child support grant

In response to information from the 2002 census on lack of access to the child support grant, a noncontributory social grant for those in need, local and provincial government departments developed several new initiatives. These included mobile campaigns with service providers in 20 villages where 8000 people applied for identity documents and birth certificates (documents required to access the grant); two *imbizos* (community workshops) to inform the community on available services; the employment of six government extension officers in the community to improve access; partnerships with the Mozambican consulate to assist former Mozambican refugees; and the establishment of a multidepartmental district task team to support orphans and vulnerable children. This is a productive example of community-acquired data advocating and then informing a specific service response.

LESSONS LEARNED

- Sharing information with a community empowers it to make decisions. The usefulness of this process has been observed in the increasing numbers of people who attend the community feedback sessions.
- Accountability to the community must be prioritized from the initial stages. This was evident in decisions on entry and storage of research data at the field site, as well as the careful process of community engagement and discussion prior to commencing any new study.
- The earlier programs of primary healthcare nurse training and subdistrict healthcare systems support gave credibility to the longer-term project of data gathering, whereas community returns are less immediate.
- Linking community-gathered data to policy development and practice remains a challenge. This process requires leadership and cooperation from both the project team and the government. As such, networks with local government and leadership are critical.

The COPC movement had its roots in South Africa. In spite of the groundbreaking start by the Karks at Pholela, the new initiative was crushed by the apartheid regime in the 1960s and has yet to become prominent in a truly significant way in postapartheid health policy.[15] This is in spite of a renewed focus on the district health system and government commitment to primary health care. The Agincourt research site is one example of a contemporary South African project inspired by the initial COPC principles. Collecting ongoing longitudinal health and sociodemographic data on a defined community provides information that can guide the development and improvement of local health and development services. Although the potential for translating this information into action, especially at a truly local level, and partnering with district health services needs to be more fully realized, there are some encouraging examples where this has taken place.

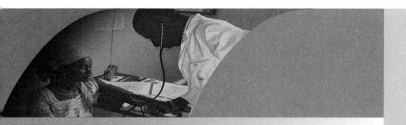

Discussion Questions

- In what ways is the Agincourt project a model of COPC? What areas of COPC does the project still need to develop?

- How did COPC shape the health priorities in this sub-district from what had previously been assumed?

- In what ways is the community involved in this project? In what ways could this be strengthened?

- Why has COPC, which has its roots in South Africa, struggled to realize its full potential? What needs to develop further before COPC can have its full impact?

REFERENCES

1. Kahn K, Tollman SM, Collinson MA, et al. Research into health, population and social transitions in rural South Africa: data and methods of the Agincourt Health and Demographic Surveillance System. *Scand J Public Health.* 2007;35(suppl 69):8–20.

2. Kahn K, Tollman SM, Garenne M, Gear J. Validation and application of verbal autopsies in a rural area of South Africa. *Trop Med Int Health.* 2000; 5:824–831.

3. Tollman SM, Kahn K, Sartorius B, Collinson MA, Clark SJ, Garenne ML. Implications of mortality transition for primary health care in rural South Africa: a population based surveillance study. *Lancet.* 2008;372:893–901.

4. Clark SJ, Collinson MA, Kahn K, Drullinger K, Tollman SM. Returning home to die: circular labour migration and mortality in South Africa. *Scand J Public Health.* 2007;35(suppl 69):35–43.

5. Schatz J. "Taking care of my own blood." Older women's relationships to their households in rural South Africa. *Scand J Public Health.* 2007;35(suppl 69):147–154.

6. Madhavan S, Schatz EJ. Coping with change: household structure and composition in rural South Africa 1992–2003. *Scand J Public Health.* 2007; 35(suppl 69):85–93.

7. SASPI Team. The prevalence of stroke survivors in rural South Africa: results from the Southern Africa Stroke Prevention Initiative (SASPI) Agincourt field site. *Stroke.* 2004;35:627–632.

8. Bonita R, Solomon N, Broad JB. Prevalence of stroke and stroke-related disability: estimates from the Auckland Stroke Studies. *Stroke.* 1997;28: 1898–1902.

9. SASPI Team. Secondary prevention of stroke—results from the Southern Africa Stroke Prevention Initiative (SASPI), Agincourt field site. *Bull World Health Organ.* 2004;82:503–508.

10. Hundt GL, Stuttaford M, Ngoma B. The social diagnostics of stroke like symptoms: healers, doctors and prophets in Agincourt, Limpopo Province, South Africa. *J Biosoc Sci.* 2004;36:433–443.

11. Connor MD, Hopkins T, Tollman SM, Thorogood M, Modi G. Blood pressure-measuring devices in rural South Africa: an audit conducted by the SASPI team in the Agincourt field site. *Cardiovasc J South Afr.* 2006;17:117–121.

12. Thorogood M, Connor M, Tollman SM, Hundt GL, Fowkes G, Marsh J. A cross-sectional study of vascular risk factors in a rural South African population: data from the Southern African Stroke Prevention Initiative (SASPI). *BMC Public Health.* 2007;7:326.

13. Stuttaford M, Bryanston C, Hundt GL, Connor M, Thorogood M, Tollman SM. Use of applied theatre in research dissemination and data validation: a pilot study from South Africa. *Health.* 2006;10:31–45.

14. World Health Organization. Integrated management of childhood illnesses (IMCI). http://www.who.int/child_adolescent_health/topics/prevention _care/child/imci/en/index.html. Accessed September 2009.

15. Tollman SM, Pick W. Roots, shoots, but too little fruit: assessing the contribution of COPC in South Africa. *Am J Public Health.* 2002;92:1725–1728.

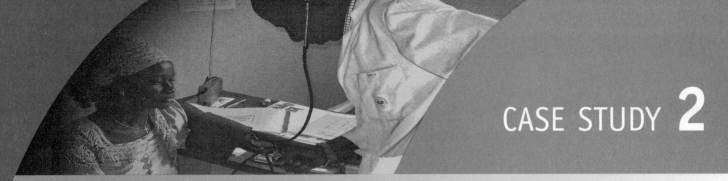

Community-Oriented Primary Care (COPC) and Refugee Participation in a Humanitarian Crisis: The Chad Experience

Camilo Valderrama

Any intelligent fool can make things bigger, more complex, and more violent. It takes a touch of genius—and a lot of courage—to move in the opposite direction.

Albert Einstein

BACKGROUND

The intensification of the conflict in Darfur in 2003 and 2004 forced the movement of more than 2 million Sudanese within and outside their country, making Sudan one of the countries with the largest number of forced migrants in the world.[1] Attacked or threatened by the Janjaweed militias, a paramilitary force supported by the Sudanese government, villagers from north Darfur, most of them belonging to the Zahagwa tribe, crossed the border to neighboring Chad. Thousands arrived to Bahai in northeastern Chad and settled under trees near the wadis.[a] After information was received about their arrival, an emergency team from an international relief organization, the International Rescue Committee (IRC),[b] did an exploratory mission in April 2004 to assess their needs.

The team—composed of water and sanitation, medical, and child protection emergency experts—was confronted with

---

[a]This Arabic term refers to a dry riverbed that contains water only during times of heavy rain.
[b]The International Rescue Committee, a nongovernmental organization, is a global network of first responders, humanitarian relief workers, healthcare providers, educators, community leaders, activists, and volunteers. It provides emergency relief, rehabilitation, protection of human rights, postconflict development, resettlement services, and advocacy for those uprooted or affected by violent conflict and oppression. For more information see http://www.theirc.org/about/.

a refugee and host population whose coping mechanisms were reaching their limit. In the first months, Bahai villagers from the same ethnic group as the refugees shared food and water with them. As more refugees crossed the border, water coming from the two wells in the village was not enough to meet the demands of villagers, refugees, and the animals they had managed to bring with them. Lying in the desert, hundreds of dead animals highlighted the severe scarcity of water being faced by both locals and refugees. Conflicts between the groups started to erupt. As the food reserves of the local population became exhausted, refugees started to sell or exchange the few possessions they had for food. The ones with no assets ate seeds that, in normal times, were used to feed goats and camels.

The only healthcare facility for the host population and refugees was a small healthcare post with one nurse, a midwife, and a nurse assistant providing curative and preventive activities, including antenatal care, the Expanded Programme of Immunization (EPI), and attention to uncomplicated deliveries. Consultations had increased, and drugs stocks were depleted. The nearest referral hospital for comprehensive emergency obstetric care was a 4-hour drive from the village. The only means of transportation for referrals were private vehicles, to which the refugees had no access.

In short, the IRC emergency team was confronting an unfolding humanitarian emergency. Does community-oriented primary care (COPC) and its participation principle have applicability in such context? This case study describes the challenges and lessons learned from a COPC process that was implemented by a team composed of international organizations, refugees, and local health authorities.

Participation, COPC, and the Humanitarian Link

In general, until recently humanitarian assistance looked at refugees as helpless victims stripped of their livelihoods and unable to cope with forced migration. Host populations were sidelined and resettlement arrangements were decided by government and humanitarian agencies. In the best cases, refugees were consulted regarding their survival needs. Decisions on the interventions and how to deal with those needs were left to emergency experts who knew better. In the late 1980s and mid-1990s, this mindset and approach started to be questioned with the imposing aid critique[2] and the do-no-harm approach[3] in 1999. In 2004, the inclusion of participation as one of the minimum standards in the Sphere Project Humanitarian Charter and Minimum Standards in Disaster Response set the stage for the active decision-making involvement of populations affected by disasters in the design, implementation, and evaluation of assistance programs.[4] In practice, however, the participation of these populations in decisions that affect their well-being continues to be neglected in many humanitarian operations.

In a humanitarian context where marked power asymmetries among international actors, refugees, and local health authorities exist, *decision ruling*, not only *decision making*, procedures need to be established before starting a participatory process as shown in other conflict-affected settings.[5] Decision-ruling procedures have to do with all stakeholders involved in a participatory process agreeing beforehand who will be involved in the decisions and in which decisions those representatives will be involved. Decision-making procedures have to do with agreeing on how, when, and where decisions will be made. When actors agree on these procedures, the power differences are reduced, making it possible for the voices of actors who are usually unheard to influence decisions in a forum created for this purpose.

To establish these procedures, a series of preparatory actions were taken. Firstly, it was important to understand the social organization of the refugee community that had settled in Bahai to identify its leaders, both formal and informal, and the way they had organized themselves to make decisions and act in this new and challenging environment. This was needed to ensure that representative voices of the interests of all the refugees were included in the COPC process and the decision-making procedures they had developed to solve their issues were taken into account. Key informants were identified, and semistructured interviews were conducted. Interviews were held in Arabic, the language spoken by most of the refugees, and translated to English by refugees who spoke both languages. Through triangulation of the different sources of information, it was possible to establish how the refugees had organized themselves after

their arrival, identify their leaders, and understand how decisions were being made in their new environment.

After their arrival, refugees had grouped themselves according to the village from which they had fled. They tried to recreate, as much as possible, their traditional governance structures to provide leadership and guidance. Where village leaders had joined their community, they continued to rely on their guidance and leadership. In refugee groupings where leaders had been killed or never reached the other side of the border, they elected a leader to represent their interests. Under the leader's guidance, they tapped into their own human and material resources to solve their most urgent needs; nurses and midwives who had been government employees in their villages and towns continued to provide health care to the sick and the pregnant women, and parents and teachers organized themselves to provide school classes for the children.

With a clear picture of the way refugees had organized themselves, a meeting was convened with the leaders to discuss and define the way the IRC and the refugee community could work together and the steps that needed to be taken to start tackling the health problems of the refugee community. Decision-ruling procedures were agreed upon. Decisions related to health would be left in the hands of the refugee health-care resources available in the community. These resources were to be identified by the refugee leaders to start the work. The IRC agreed to provide technical support to better inform decisions, as well as material support to implement decided-upon solutions to the problems that were encountered.

The leaders summoned all available refugee human resources who were working in health care. About 40 refugee healthcare workers came to the first meeting. They included nurses, midwives, and community health workers who, before the conflict, were working with the Ministry of Health in Darfur. As with the refugee leaders, decision-ruling procedures were jointly established among the refugees, local health authorities, and the IRC. When an agreement was reached, the COPC process was started.

THE HEALTH STATUS OF THE COMMUNITY

The first challenge the refugee–IRC team faced was to *define and characterize the community*. Mixed and contradictory reports existed of the number of community members. Estimates varied from 5000 to 20,000, and their location was not clear. It was possible to establish that refugees had settled around four wadis. To estimate the refugee population, the team decided to use participatory mapping.[c] Training and logistic resources

---

[c]Participatory mapping is any combination of participation-based methods for eliciting and recording spatial data.

and support to do the mapping was provided by the IRC team. Community health workers divided into four groups, and in 2 days it was possible to have a clear picture of the estimated number of families living under each of the trees. In this way the community was defined as the refugees living in the four wadis in the surroundings of Bahai, with a total of approximately 16,000 people.

With the locations identified and mapped and the approximate population number established, the next step was to characterize the community and assess its health problems. This was done using quantitative and qualitative methods. Sources of quantitative information included the healthcare center registers and registers from the mobile clinics that started at three sites soon after the participatory mapping took place. In addition, a survey was designed with the refugee healthcare workers with the objective of doing a census, establishing water sources and consumption patterns, and to establish mortality rates. Qualitative information was collected in each of the settlements through focus group with the community leaders and women and men from the communities.

Defining Health Problems and Selecting Priorities

The health problems and needs of the community were identified, and an analysis of the information was done with all members of the healthcare team. It was clear from the assessment and the healthcare center and mobile clinic data that the first priority to tackle was diarrhea because the number of diarrhea cases had increased, as had the number of deaths by this cause. It was decided that priority would be given to reduce the number of cases and deaths, as well as to increase the amount and quality of water for the refugee population.

Different options were discussed to reduce diarrhea mortality, which included adequate case management at the community and healthcare facility level and referral to the nearest hospitals for severe cases. Alternatives for the improvement in the quality and quantity of the water supply included actions in the short, medium, and long term. Short-term actions to improve quality included distribution and training in the use of flocculant-disinfectant water sachets;[d] medium-term actions included bringing in water tanks while a water system was being developed.

THE INTERVENTION PROGRAM

The intervention covered the previously defined community and focused on identified health needs. It was implemented by the team, which was composed of the healthcare staff of the government healthcare post and the refugee healthcare staff, including nurses, midwives, and community health workers. The activities took place through healthcare facility-based and outreach activities.

Implementation of primary healthcare (PHC) activities and public health (PH) actions to respond to the health needs of the refugees had to take into account and work with the existent healthcare system. At the same time it was needed to fill the existing gaps in services by establishing a temporary refugee healthcare system (RHS) that included refugee community healthcare workers, midwives, and nurses. The RHS relied on the support of the existent local healthcare services and facilities and the IRC to support both systems in terms of materials, human resources, and coordination while a refugee camp was established.

The PHC–PH program activities to address health priorities was done on the basis of mutually agreed-upon actions among the author, acting as the IRC emergency healthcare coordinator, the refugees' healthcare team, and local health authorities. The nature of the relationship was one of a partnership between the refugees and the IRC and between employers and employees, in which the actions carried out by the healthcare resources of the refugee community were compensated with weekly payments.

To reduce mortality and morbidity, attention was given to the successive stages in the natural history of diarrhea in this kind of environment. Mobile clinics with refugee nurses were established to provide curative services in the wadis, and drugs and supplies were provided to the local healthcare facility. A referral system from the wadis to the healthcare facility and from the healthcare facility to the referral hospital was established. Community health workers were trained in diarrhea case management following World Health Organization (WHO) guidelines and supplied with Oral Rehydration Salts (ORS). They were assigned a specific number of family trees for whom they were responsible to provide health education and train in the use of the water flocculation and purification sachets, treat mild cases of diarrhea, and refer severely dehydrated patients. In the meantime the water and sanitation expert was working on identifying and excavating wells to cope with the increasing water demand.

Each week the team, refugee nurses, midwives, community health workers, local health authorities, and the IRC healthcare coordinator met to *monitor progress of the activities* and *analyze the information* that was being collected on a weekly basis by the community health workers—the nurses in the mobile clinics and the local nurse in the Bahai health post—in their assigned family trees. Community health workers reported the

---

[d]The sachets contained powdered ferric sulfate (a flocculant) and calcium hypochlorite (a disinfectant), which was designed to remove particles from water and disinfect it.

number of deaths by diarrhea. Most of the deaths were happening at home among children whose mothers were not seeking health care. Actions included intensifying the distribution of the flocculant-disinfectant drinking water sachets, health education focused on the recognition of danger signs of diarrhea, distribution of ORS, and improvement of referrals to the mobile clinics by setting up a system of horse cars. Deaths by diarrhea started to drop slowly from an average of two deaths every week in the first month of the operation to no deaths in the following 4 weeks.

COMMUNITY PARTICIPATION AND INTERSECTORAL COOPERATION

Intersectoral cooperation was done at three levels. From the community side, community leaders wrote letters and visited the different agencies responsible for the well-being of refugees, including the United Nations High Commissioner for Refugees (UNHCR) and World Food Programme (WFP), as well as the United Nations Population Fund (UNFPA), asking them to respond to their needs. From the IRC level, reports were shared with different United Nations agencies at national and international levels. The media, including CNN, the BBC, and many others, visited the site. The IRC and the refugee community provided them with information on the refugee situation that was reported to the world and contributed to the acceleration of the agencies' response to establish a refugee camp and relocate refugees who were scattered in the wadis. Until 2009 the refugees continued living in the camp, waiting for the conflict to end so they could return to their villages.

    Intersectoral coordination also happened with donors regarding the submission of proposals to secure additional resources to maintain activities. In this case study, the submitted

proposal was based on the initial assessment and in consultation with refugees. However, refugees were not involved in the proposal design, that is, defining objectives, indicators, timetables, and budgets. This was due to time pressures and lack of available nongovernmental organization and IRC human resources to carry out or facilitate a participatory project design.

LESSONS LEARNED

- An understanding of the social organization and decision-making and ruling procedures of all actors in the COPC process must be gained before starting a participatory COPC process. Participation brings together actors with different interests that can be in conflict. Setting the rules of engagement beforehand contributes to constructively addressing conflicts that can emerge during the process.
- The assumption that time is a constraint for the active involvement of refugee communities in a COPC process in emergency situations is not an impediment for their participation if emergency workers have attitudes that allow them to facilitate and mediate participatory processes in emergencies.
- Sustaining the involvement of refugees in the long-term needs to be planned from the start. This experience proved the pitfalls of project models designed with heavy emphasis on upward accountability and little attention to actors' voices.
- Lastly, establishing decision-ruling and decision-making procedures in a COPC participatory process provides refugees, who are destitute citizens, with authority to decide on actions that will affect their well-being.

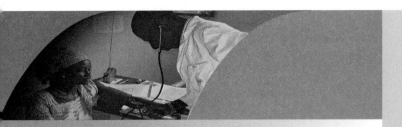

Discussion Questions

- How can a COPC practitioner working in emergency settings involve refugee communities without organized healthcare services in the decisions that need to be taken in the different steps of the COPC process?

- What skills are needed for a COPC practitioner to facilitate a participatory process in COPC?

- How can the project design of a COPC process be more participatory?

REFERENCES

1. Internal Displacement Monitoring Centre. Sudan: 4.8 million IDPs across Sudan face ongoing turmoil. http://www.internal-displacement.org/8025708F004CE90B/(httpCountries)/F3D3CAA7CBEBE276802570A7004B87E4. Accessed April 2009.

2. Harrell-Bond, BE. *Imposing Aid: Emergency Assistance to Refugees.* New York, NY: Oxford University Press; 1986.

3. Anderson, MB. *Do No Harm: How Aid Can Support Peace—Or War.* Boulder, CO: Lynne Rienner Publishers; 1999.

4. Sphere Project Humanitarian Charter and Minimum Standards in Disaster Response. Welcome to the Sphere Handbook, 2004 revised edition. http://www.sphereproject.org/content/view/27/84. Accessed February 2010.

5. Valderrama C. *Power and Participation in Rural Development: A Case Study from Mozambique* [DPhil thesis]. Brighton, UK: University of Sussex; 2008.

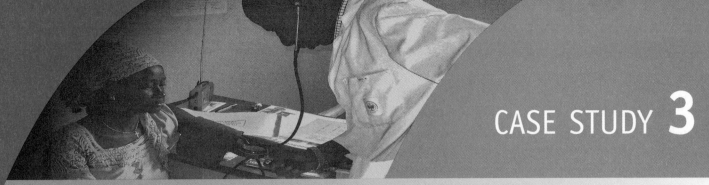

Multisector and Coordinated Intervention to Reduce Child Trafficking in Bénin, West Africa

Elizabeth Ponce, Alfonso Gonzalez, and Emilie Kpadonou

BACKGROUND

Bénin, with 6.7 million residents (58.3% rural, 44.8% aged 0–14 years), is a small country (112,622 square kilometers) in West Africa. It shares borders with Nigeria, Togo, Niger, and Burkina Faso. The official capital is Porto Novo, and Cotonou is the main city and seat of government. About 42 ethnic groups live in Bénin.[1] French is the official language, but it is spoken more in urban than rural areas. Fon, Adja, and Yoruba are the most popular vernacular languages in the south and Bariba, Dendi, Peulh, and Otamari in the north. The GDP per capita is US$513.3 of which 5.4% is for health. Animism is the most widespread religion, and it is practiced alone or with other foreign religions (Catholicism 27.1%, other Christianity 14.7%, Islam 24.4%, and others).[1] The main economic activity is agriculture, and cotton is the principal export product.

The healthcare system in Bénin is organized in a pyramidal structure at three levels: central or national, medium or department, and peripheral or communal as sanitary zones. At the peripheral level, primary care services are provided, including health promotion, immunizations, reproductive health, mother and child services, nutrition surveillance, and control of specific diseases (HIV, malaria, and tuberculosis). The coverage of the services is low in rural areas because of the need for out-of-pocket payments and lack of healthcare providers. Health insurance is almost nonexistent.[2] In 2004, Bénin had very few healthcare professionals (physicians 0.04 per 1000; nurses 0.84 per 1000, and community workers 0.01 per 1000).[3]

THE HEALTH STATUS OF THE COMMUNITY

In 2006, the total fertility rate was 5.6, and the infant mortality rate was 88/1000 live births, among the highest in the region. Life expectancy in the same year was 56 years. Just one-third of the adult population is literate, and from 2000 to 2006, more boys than girls were enrolled in school (60% and 47%, respectively).[4] Twenty-three percent of the children are underweight for their age, and malaria, diarrhea, and respiratory infection are the most prevalent problems among children. Child abuse, neglect, and child labor are frequent among children aged 5 to 14 years.

Child Labor and Child Trafficking

In 1999, the number of working children in the main cities (Cotonou, Parakou, and Porto Novo) was estimated at 480,000.[5] A study conducted in 2000 showed that about 99,000 rural children aged 7 to 16 years (8% of the total rural children) left their villages to work in another place in the country or abroad.[6] Twenty-six percent of children aged 10 to 14 years were working in 2002.[7]

According to Convention No. 182 of the International Labour Organization,[8] child trafficking (CT) is considered one of the worst forms of child labor. In Bénin there are two forms of CT: cross-border and internal trafficking. Bénin is a source, destination, and transit country for cross-border trafficking of children. Most of the children are abducted or leave home with intermediaries who sometimes give the parents a gift, a symbolic amount of money, a promise of educational opportunities, or other incentives. Almost no children are asked for their consent, and they leave their rural communities without documents. Children are trafficked into Cameroon, Democratic Republic of the Congo, Ivory Coast, Equatorial Guinea, Gabon, Ghana, Nigeria, Togo, the Persian Gulf States, and Lebanon; children from Burkina Faso, Niger, and Togo are sold into servitude in Bénin.[7] Child victims of cross-border trafficking often work as agricultural workers, domestic servants, market vendors, and commercial sex workers and in granite mines.

The magnitude of internal trafficking is evidenced by the great number of exploited children in the main cities of Bénin. These children can work from 10 to 20 hours per day, carry heavy loads, operate dangerous tools, and lack adequate housing, food, or drink. Most of their activities are related to selling in the streets (59.2% of girls), domestic work (6.7% of girls), and crafts and apprenticeship (73% of boys). About 43.5% of children work for members of their extended family, 28.4% for a third person, and 13.5% for their parents. None of these children go to school.[5]

THE INTERVENTION PROGRAM

In 1990, children as young as 3 years of age were found at the police station in Cotonou because they were lost and could not go back home. Because this situation persisted during the years, a 24-hour center with capacity for 30 children was created by the Swiss Foundation of Terre des hommes (Tdh) to protect and provide basic shelter, food, health care, and psychological support for those children. Most of the children were placed with families (relatives, acquaintances, or unknown people), and some of them experienced abuse, neglect, exploitation, or abandonment. For the first time, in 1999, some professionals raised concerns about internal and cross-border trafficking. From 1990 to 1999, children were referred to the center by the police of Cotonou, and in the context of this action 7203 children from different regions of Bénin and some from neighboring countries were recovered and reintegrated into their families.

In 2000, a multidisciplinary team in the Tdh was organized, and they decided to develop an intervention following the community-oriented primary care (COPC) approach. The team reviewed all biopsychosocial problems affecting children aged 5 to 14 years who were assisted by the center in the previous years to decide on priorities for intervention. All conditions were analyzed, and the following factors were taken into account: (1) the magnitude of the biopsychosocial condition; (2) the severity of the conditions; (3) the political, technical, and financial viability of managing an intervention through a coordinated strategy; and (4) the community's participation. Meetings between key persons of the center facilitated the analysis of the different situations and established the level of severity or vulnerability of the children. At that time, just one study about child labor in Bénin was available.[5]

As a result of the analysis, child victims of trafficking[9] were identified as the most vulnerable group, which was selected as one of the target populations of a new 5-year strategic plan from 2000 to 2004. The mission and vision of the organization related to CT were defined, and a comprehensive intervention was planned using a logical framework approach.[10] The overall aim was to reduce the frequency of CT in the communities of origin of recovered children in collaboration with multisectoral institutions. The objectives were to protect, rehabilitate, and reinsert victims; to prevent new cases by increasing awareness about CT and mobilizing the communities at high risk of trafficking; and to contribute to a coordinated national response and antitrafficking legislation. The city of Cotonou was identified as the main intervention community, followed by all villages where children victims of trafficking came from. The prioritization and planning process took about 4 months.

Before implementation, all members of the team, the beneficiaries, and the operational partners assessed resource availability and adequacy for the new program to be conducted from 2000 to 2004.[11] Following their recommendations, the structure and services were modified in response to the identified children's needs. Thus, a new building called Oasis Center, with a capacity for 60 boys and girls aged 5 to 14 years, was created and fully equipped. New professionals were hired, and holistic services were organized. The new multidisciplinary team was composed of a public health doctor, a medical doctor, a child psychiatrist, a nurse, a jurist, five social assistants, and 13 educators. From 2001 to 2002, a plan to reinforce the team's capacities was implemented.

Given the complexity and the number of people involved in CT (traffickers, victims, parents, employers) and actors fighting it (public officers, public institutions, international organizations, NGOs, leaders in the communities, etc.), three axes of intervention (alternative interventions strategies) were developed.

Axis 1: Direct Intervention or Tertiary Prevention

Axis 1, direct intervention or tertiary prevention, targeted parents, tutors, employers, and other stakeholders to reduce the recurrence of trafficking and rehabilitate the victim to prevent cascading negative outcomes. The expected results were that (1) children would be recovered and protected; (2) after 3 months, all children would be reintegrated into their families, which offer the minimal conditions for the safety of the child; and (3) an increased number of children would be reinserted to school or an apprenticeship after 1 year of intervention, with good nutritional status and good physical and mental health.

In 2001, a database of all individuals' files was created, with information related to the child and his or her family and employers. Data regarding 404 beneficiaries was collected and analyzed to assess the characteristics of child victims of trafficking, and the analysis was used to improve the quality of the services. The results showed that most of the children victims of trafficking were referred by the police, 70% were girls, 70% were aged 9 to 12 years, and 95% were from rural areas. About 68% of rural girls had never been in school, 35% were exploited as domestic servants, and 40% were domestic servants and also sellers on the streets. Most of the children were victims of physical abuse (72–78%) and emotional abuse (72–75%) by their employers. One girl was a victim of sexual abuse. About one-fifth did not have birth certificates. Most of the children (64%) were ill with malaria, respiratory infections, skin problems, or physical lesions when they arrived at the Oasis Center. Many Béninese boys who were exploited in Nigerian granite mines were undernourished and affected by schistosomiasis.[12] Almost half of the children (46.7%) were happy to find protection at the center, especially those who were victims of cross-border trafficking (93%), but some were very sad (14%) or fearful (3%). Their parents were married (44%), divorced (21.2%), or separated (7.5%); or the children were orphans (15.6%). Most of the mothers were illiterate and very poor (less than US$20 per month). In many cases the parents were also placed, trafficked, or abused as children.

The main activities that were implemented to improve the conditions of the children were as follows:

- coordination with former and new partners for *referral of victims*
- *protection and rehabilitation of victims* at the Oasis Center, respecting the victims' rights and attending to their individual needs (listening, affection, nutrition, shelter, clothing, health and psychological support, cognitive stimulation, social support, psychomotor stimulation, ateliers of preapprenticeship, juridical protection, leisure activities, etc.)
- *identification of the parents and employers* and their *sensitization*
- development of an *individual plan* for each child for reintegration and reinsertion into his or her family and *follow-up* for at least 1 year (home visitation and parenting education approaches)
- *coordination* with local services (health, education, and social) to respond to the child's needs and with local NGOs to respond to the parents' needs (alphabetization, microcredit, etc.)
- issue *birth certificates*

Axis 2: Community Intervention

Axis 2, community intervention, prevented new cases of trafficking in the villages of origin of reintegrated children through *primary prevention* (raising awareness of entire communities) and *secondary prevention* (mobilizing particular villages and families at high risk of CT). As expected, the communities of origin became sensitized about CT, and communities at high risk developed an effective system of prevention and control of CT.

The main activities of Axis 2 were as follows:

- development of *awareness campaigns* in all communities where trafficked children were reintegrated
- *contact all local authorities* to involve them in child protection issues and *create a system of protection*
- identify children at high risk of trafficking to *provide individual support*
- *coordinate with local services* to support families or use the same *referral system* as in Axis 1
- develop *film and educational materials about internal trafficking*
- *provide technical support* to public schools
- *create alternative schools* in five very vulnerable villages for 200 children older than age 10 years who are former victims or at high risk of CT; *create preschools* for 150 children aged 4 to 6 years who are at high risk of trafficking
- issue *birth certificates*

Axis 3: Advocacy and Coordination

Axis 3, advocacy and coordination, was used to reduce the main risk factors of the macrosystem associated with CT in Bénin, with the participation of all actors at the central level. The expected results were the establishment of *national coordination* to fight CT and ensure that coordinated measures in the field of *judicial interventions* (protection of the child, prosecution of the trafficker, etc.) function until a new law against CT could be enacted and enforced. All institutions dealing with protection of children and trafficking issues were contacted and invited to participate in the creation of a national coordination group to combat CT. The judges of minors were contacted as well, and new judicial procedures were drafted. Some members of the team participated in drafting a new law to combat CT.

In 2001, a structured *monitoring and evaluation* system was implemented under the responsibility of a multidisciplinary team using the input–process–output–outcome–impact framework. Evaluations carried out at the end of 2001, 2002, and 2003 with the participation of the team and financial partners showed that annually an average of 415 children were protected at the Oasis Center (400 expected). Almost all children (95%) were safely reintegrated after 3 months (100% expected), and an increased number of children were reinserted

(25% in 2002 and 51% in 2003) after 1 year of intervention. Very few cases were considered to be failures or unresolved (in 2003 the recurrence of trafficking was only 5%). About 200 communities of origin were sensitized, and five villages were fully mobilized (10 expected). In addition, as expected, a national committee was created, and a law against CT was drafted, which was approved in 2006. This positive evaluation was the keystone for demonstrating the effectiveness of the system to national authorities and donors for the replication of the program.

COMMUNITY PARTICIPATION AND INTERSECTORAL COOPERATION

During the Axis 1 intervention, new organizations for referral were contacted, and the number of partners that referred victims of CT increased from three in 2001 to nine in 2004. At the end of the year, public institutions were informed about the results of the collaboration. Five health centers provided free vaccinations or low-cost hospitalization for very ill children. The private sector participated with donations of food, clothes, and other items. At the time of reintegration in each community of origin, the local authority, the director of the school, the health agent, and social services were contacted and invited to participate as members of a social network to protect the recovered child and avoid the recurrence of trafficking. The children's parents were considered to be partners as well. Employers were sensitized, and some of them paid the child a symbolic amount for his or her services.

To develop awareness materials (film, posters, and books) during the Axis 2 intervention, a communication project titled Anna, Bazil and the Trafficker[13] was developed and implemented with the participation of seven technical and financial partners (Tdh, Ministry of Health—MEPS, European Union, French Cooperation, UNICEF, Care International, Belgian cooperation). To create alternative schools in five villages for children older than 10 years of age, a new additional project was developed. Public local authorities were contacted, a technical partnership with two local NGOs was established, and the project was implemented with the financial support of the Swiss Development Cooperation and the Belgian cooperation. The communities participated by donating land and constructing the school.

Raising awareness of public institutions and actors involved in fighting CT during Axis 3 was one of the program's priorities. At least 30 institutions from all sectors (public, civil society, and journalists) were invited to participate in a national forum. The attorney and two judges of minors participated in the development of a procedure to protect children, and a lawyer's office defended children for free.

Five years after implementation of the program, a new strategic plan was developed that reinforced the mobilization of the communities at high risk for CT (Axis 2). For the sustainability of the program, there is a proposal to transfer the center to the government.

LESSONS LEARNED

- Baseline data should be obtained both through literature and directly in the field, including assessment of vulnerability. An adequate database containing the characteristics of the beneficiaries, follow-up activities, and results should be established. Instead of waiting for referrals from other institutions, actively identify beneficiaries through outreach. A good multisectoral two-way referral system should be established.

- There is a need for holistic services in complex problems. These should be based on the needs of the beneficiaries and human rights, with strategies to reduce the consequences of the problem, the risk factors, or the reinforcement of protective factors. Well-defined protocols, procedures, and approaches are necessary, considering tailored activities for each beneficiary. The infrastructure and materials need to be developed according to the special needs of the beneficiaries. The contribution of each Axis and its activities should be assessed and resources allocated accordingly.

- Team capacity building needs permanent reinforcement according to the team's needs and those of the project. The availability of a code of conduct for the team and beneficiaries should be ensured.

- In any case of biopsychosocial projects, a public health approach using a COPC model and principles is appropriate, with the active participation of a multidisciplinary team, multisectoral partners, and beneficiaries. There should be a good internal and external communication system and weekly planning of activities, and regular coordination meetings with the partners should be held.

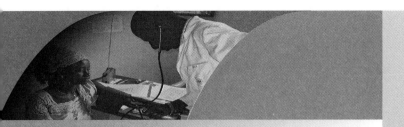

Discussion Questions

- Can an assessment about trafficking be based only on a literature review?

- How can trafficked children be identified in a community?

- How can child trafficking be prevented?

- Are children's rights respected in your community?

- Is there a need for an organization that advocates for children's rights in your community?

REFERENCES

1. Bénin Census. RGPH-3 3ème recensement général de la population et de l'habitation. Février; 2002.

2. Fourn L. Principaux enjeux de la santé publique au Bénin. Institut de Recherche Empirique en Economie Politique (IREEP). Document de travail préparé dans le cadre de la conférence: Échéance de 2006. Quels enjeux politiques et économiques. IREEP Bénin, 2005.

3. World Health Organization. Regional Office for Africa: Bénin country health system fact sheet 2006. http://www.afro.who.int/index.php?option=com_content&view=article&id=1016&Itemid=2040. Accessed April 2010.

4. UNICEF. The state of the world's children 2008: child survival. http://www.unicef.org/publications/index_42623.html. Accessed March 2009.

5. Dogbe C, Olowo J, Adegbidi FV, Degbo K, et al. Enquête sur les Enfants Travailleurs dans les Villes de Cotonou, Porto-Novo et Parakou, Vol. 1 et 2. UNICEF, Cotonou, Bénin, Décembre 1999. (Survey about child labour in the cities of Cotonou, Porto Novo and Parakou) UNICEF, Cotonou-Bénin. 1999.

6. Kielland, A, R Ouensavi. Child labor migration from Bénin. Magnitude and determinants: World Bank (WB), Carrefour d'Ecoute et d'Orientation (CEO), 2001.

7. United States Department of Labor. 2004 findings on the worst forms of child labor—Bénin. http://www.unhcr.org/refworld/docid/48c8ca453c.html. Published September 22, 2005. Accessed March 2009.

8. International Labour Organization. Convention No. 182. http://www.ilo.org/ipec/Campaignandadvocacy/Youthinaction/C182-Youth-orientated/C182Youth_Convention/lang—en/index.htm. Accessed August 2009.

9. United Nations. Protocol to prevent, suppress and punish trafficking in persons, especially women and children, supplementing the United Nations Convention Against Transnational Organized Crime. http://www.uncjin.org/Documents/Conventions/dcatoc/final_documents_2/convention_%20traff_eng.pdf. Published 2000. Accessed March 2009.

10. Australian Agency for International Development. AusGuideline activity design 3.3. The logical framework approach. http://www.ausaid.gov.au/ausguide/pdf/ausguideline3.3.pdf. Published October 2005. Accessed August 2009.

11. Ponce E, Houeto C, Gonzalez A. Internal evaluation of the "Child Errant" project 1999–2000. Terre des hommes, Oasis Center—Cotonou, Bénin [internal document]. 2000.

12. Kpadonou E. Report of the health situation of recovered children from the granite mines in Nigeria [Terre des hommes, Oasis Center—Cotonou, Bénin internal document]. 2003.

13. Matériels de Education pour la Santé (MEPS)-Ministère de la Santé Publique Bénin, Terre des hommes: Anna, Bazil et le trafiquant. www.youtube.com/watch?v=pWi5j8EOrU8. Accessed March 2009.

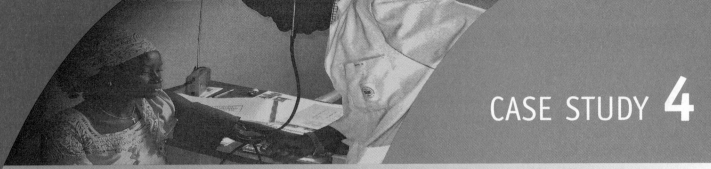

Averting Childhood Deaths in Resource-Constrained Settings Through Engagement with the Community: An Example from Cambodia

Henry Perry, Oun Sivan, Geof Bowman, Larry Casazza, Anbarasi Edward, Kay Hansen, and Melanie Morrow

BACKGROUND

Cambodia is a country of 14 million people surrounded by Vietnam, Thailand, and the Gulf of Thailand. In 1975, the Khmer Rouge took over the government, destroyed most of the country's infrastructure, and killed 3 million people—including most of the intellectuals and professionals in the country. Democracy arrived in Cambodia in 1995, and since that time there has been dramatic progress in getting the country back on its feet again. Nonetheless, Cambodia remains one of the poorest and least developed countries in Asia.

The United Nations Development Programme ranks Cambodia 131st out of the 177 countries of the world in its Human Development Index.[a] Indices of gender-related development and gender-related empowerment for Cambodia rank near the bottom of those countries for which data are available. Less than half of women older than age 15 years (46%) are literate. Thirty-eight percent of the population is younger than age 15 years, and one-third of the population is living on less than US$1 per day. Only 17% of the population has access to improved sanitation, and only 41% has access to improved water sources.[1]

World Relief is a Christian humanitarian relief and development organization established in 1944. It currently operates programs in 16 priority countries and participates in partnerships in many other countries.[b] It has been working in Cambodia for 14 years and has pioneered many innovative community-based maternal and child health programs around the world. This case study describes a community health project carried out by World Relief in Cambodia with financial support from the US Agency for International Development (USAID) and its Child Survival and Health Grants Program.[c]

The Community and Its People

The project was located in the east-central portion of Cambodia near the Vietnamese border, approximately 3 hours by road from Phnom Penh in the south-central portion of the country. Being part of the Mekong River Delta, the land is flat, and most of it is used for agricultural production and subsistence farming.

The great majority of people living in the project area are farmers, and rice is the main crop. However, there are small businesses in the area as well as scattered rubber plantations. The dominant religion is Buddhism, and there are numerous Buddhist temples located throughout the project area. In addition, about 11% of the project population is Muslim (Cham). According to the 1998 baseline survey, only half of the women of childbearing age in the project area had two or more years of schooling.

The project area was contiguous with that of Ponhea Kriek–Dombe Operational Health District of the Ministry of Health (MOH). Ponhea Kriek is one governmental administrative district, and Dombe is another. The two are combined into a single Operational Health District of the Ministry. The project began in five health areas (communes) of the Ponhea Kriek

[a]The Human Development Index is a composite of life expectancy, educational attainment, and adjusted real income.
[b]For more information about World Relief, see http://www.wr.org.
[c]For more information about this program, see http://www.usaid.gov/our_work/global_health/home/Funding/cs_grants/cs_index.html.

District in 1998. In 2003, USAID provided 4 additional years of funding, and the project expanded to include the entire Ponhea Kriek District and Dombe. The project began by serving a population of 78,000 people and then expanded to serve a total population of 185,000 people, with 20,000 children aged younger than 5 years and 26,000 women of reproductive age.

Health Services and Health Team

The ongoing health services in the project area are provided by the Ministry of Health, which operates a rudimentary hospital and a series of healthcare centers. During the latter period of the project's operation, the district health services of the MOH were managed by Save the Children Australia as part of a program financed by the Asian Development Bank.

The World Relief/Cambodia Light for Life Child Survival Project had a project director, four health field staff supervisors (referred to subsequently as supervisors), and 16 health field staff members (referred to subsequently as field staff members) who supervised community-based volunteers. In addition, there was one accountant and six behavior change communication specialists. The behavior change specialists focused primarily on puppet shows for the community, which conveyed key health education messages. They were the only men working on the project staff; all the rest were women. The project also had one four-wheel-drive vehicle and 23 motorcycles. All field staff members had two-way radios for communication via a central tower at the field office.

The most important members of the healthcare team were the community health volunteers called women health educators (referred to subsequently as educators), who were selected by the field staff members and community leaders. Each educator was responsible for the 10–15 households surrounding her own household, and 10 educators who lived nearby met monthly with a field staff member as a Care Group.[d] Each field staff member was responsible for 20–30 Care Groups. The educators worked 2–3 hours each week. At the time of expansion in 2003, the project recruited 49 of the best volunteer educators from the original project area to work 5 days a week in the expansion project area to provide support for newly formed Care Groups there.

THE HEALTH STATUS OF THE COMMUNITY'S CHILDREN

According to the 2006 Demographic and Health Survey in Cambodia, the overall under-five mortality rate is 83 deaths per 1000 live births (111 for rural Cambodia), and the overall ma-

ternal mortality ratio is 437 deaths per 100,000 live births, giving the country the highest rates of child and maternal mortality in Asia. Childhood malnutrition is common throughout the country, with 37% of children under-five moderately or severely stunted.[2] Pneumonia and diarrhea are the leading causes of death among children before they reach 5 years of age.[3]

The major health problems identified in the original baseline household survey in 1998 were low immunization coverage, malnutrition and micronutrient deficiencies, lack of hygiene, diarrhea, and low utilization of healthcare services for children with signs and symptoms of pneumonia.

THE INTERVENTION PROGRAM

Given the availability of funding to support these activities and the high levels of preventable mortality among children in the project area, the project focused its interventions on maternal and child health. The goals of the World Relief/Cambodia Light for Life Child Survival Project included the following:

- reduce the disease burden in children younger than 5 years of age and women aged 15–49 years
- strengthen the long-term sustainability of child survival interventions through an integrated, community-based approach in harmony with the MOH system

To achieve these goals, the project provided health education to mothers of young children. This education was about behaviors that would prevent disease, as well as the importance of healthcare services utilization for disease prevention and prompt treatment when warning signs occur in their children.

The volunteer educator visited the homes of the 10–15 women for whom she was responsible; occasionally these women met as a group as well. On average, she visited three houses per week. At that time she shared the most recent message she had learned. The educator also discussed with each woman the progress she had made in implementing the previous health messages she had received.

By the end of the project, there were 318 Care Groups and 2490 educators. At the midway point, the project also recruited 49 educator supervisors to work in the extension project area. The best educators from the original project area were paid to work 5 days per month with newly formed Care Groups in the extension project area.

During each Care Group meeting, the Care Group members learned a new message and practiced giving that message. During the same meeting, they also reported births and deaths that had occurred during the previous month. Finally, they discussed any problems encountered in their work during the previous month and any significant health problems encountered in the households.

---

[d]Further information about Care Groups is available at http://www.coregroup .org/storage/documents/Diffusion_of_Innovation/Care_Manual.pdf.

The project supported the functioning of a feedback committee for each area served by a health center. These committees were composed of Care Group leaders and one village leader from each village served by the health center. Once a month, this group met with the staff of the health center. At that time, the community representatives reported to the health center staff the number of births and deaths during the previous month, as well as any significant illnesses or other health problems in the communities. The health center staff shared any information that it thought would be valuable for the community to know. Together, they set the dates for the immunization outreach sessions in the communities during the upcoming month. The Care Group leaders, volunteer educators, and the village leaders informed the communities afterward. The project also worked to strengthen the quality of care provided to sick children at the health centers.

On a quarterly basis, the project measured the degree to which these objectives were being met, mainly by measuring the coverage of key child survival interventions. A few households selected at random were visited by each field staff member, and a brief questionnaire was administered. Only 100 of these interviews needed to be carried out each quarter to obtain representative information for the project area. Every 3 years or so, a full survey of a representative sample of households was carried out. Measures of nutritional status of children were obtained periodically, and the Care Groups kept monthly records of vital events. In addition, the project conducted qualitative assessments at several points.

Changes in Coverage of Key Child Survival Interventions

Indicators were measured separately in the original project area and in the extension project area. The level of childhood immunization coverage rose from 15% to 80%. Similar favorable changes were observed for coverage of pregnant women with tetanus toxoid immunization, use of iodized salt in the household, iron supplementation during pregnancy, initiation of breastfeeding within 1 hour of delivery, treatment of childhood diarrhea with oral rehydration therapy at home, and seeking early medical care for children with signs of pneumonia. Coverage levels for appropriate hand washing practices, treatment of the umbilical cord with a Betadine–alcohol solution, mothers' knowledge of danger signs of childhood illnesses, and provision of increased food and fluids during childhood illnesses were generally less than 20% when the project began, but by the end of the project coverage levels had increased in all cases to 80% or higher. A comparison of these changes with changes in coverage of the same or similar indicators in the Kampong Cham Province and Cambodia as a whole[2,4] indicated that, in all cases, progress was much stronger in the project area.

Changes in Nutritional Status

In 2002, 23% of the children in the original project area and the extension project area combined were moderately or severely malnourished.[e] In 2007, the level of malnutrition had declined to 13%. Levels of malnutrition in Kampong Cham Province and nationally in Cambodia declined as well,[2,4] but not to the same degree.

Changes in Mortality of Children During the First 5 Years of Life

An analysis of the data collected by the Care Groups indicated that in 2000, the under-five mortality rate in the project area (129 deaths per 1000 live births) was greater than in the Kampong Cham Province (111 deaths per 1000 live births) and the country as a whole (105 deaths per 1000 live births).[4] The analysis of the Care Group vital events data revealed that between 2000 and 2005 a dramatic mortality decline occurred in the project area, from 129 to 35 deaths per 1000 live births, a much greater decline than in the province or in the country as a whole during the same period (see Figure C4-1).[2] The achieved mortality rate of 39/1000 in the project area is what Cambodia will have to achieve nationally by 2015 if it is to achieve the Millennium Development Goals for children.[3]

Changes Observed Based on Qualitative Data

In 2004 and 2007, an external evaluation team held numerous structured discussions with staff members from the MOH, local authorities, community leaders, community members, and subsets of women. These reports confirmed that the project had been successful in working effectively with the MOH at the district level and that local authorities and community leaders were involved in the project and claimed ownership in it. Local community members perceived that their children were becoming healthier and fewer were dying. The local people also stated that they were saving money because they were spending less on health care. The volunteer educators indicated that their engagement had empowered them and that the community greatly appreciated their contribution. Community members also reported that their level of trust of MOH curative services had improved.

COMMUNITY PARTICIPATION AND INTERSECTORAL COOPERATION

Community participation and intersectoral cooperation were integral parts of the project from the outset and were important contributors to its success. Community leaders were

---

[e]A child with moderate or severe malnutrition is defined as a child whose weight for his or her age is less than 2 standard deviations below the international reference standard mean for children at that age.

FIGURE C4-1 Changes in Under-5 Mortality in Cambodia Nationally (1995–2005), in Kampong Cham Province (1995–2005), and in the Project Area (2000–2008)

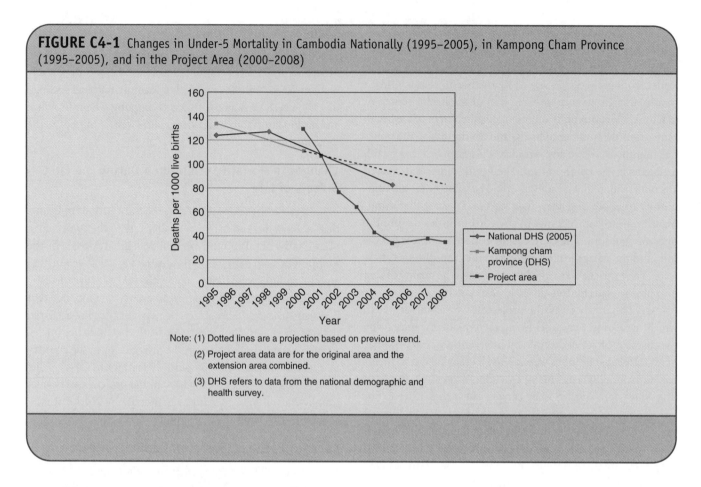

Note: (1) Dotted lines are a projection based on previous trend.

(2) Project area data are for the original area and the extension area combined.

(3) DHS refers to data from the national demographic and health survey.

engaged in the first steps of project planning. The formal community authorities helped to select the volunteer educators and promoted the full cooperation of the community in the project, ensuring that all households in the village were included in the project. A number of traditional midwives became volunteer educators. Community leaders volunteered their time to serve on feedback committees, which represented the communities in monthly meetings with the staffs of the health centers. The project worked with the salt vendors in the markets to promote the sale of iodized salt and the removal of noniodized salt from the marketplace.

LESSONS LEARNED

- The World Relief/Cambodia Light for Life Child Survival Project is a remarkable example of what communities can do to improve the health of their children if they have appropriate guidance and support. Changing health-related behaviors for the good has been a challenge for health programs for decades now. The Care Group approach is effective in improving child health, and it promotes women's health and community empowerment at the same time.[5,6] The total project cost was less than US$2 per capita per year.

- The project also demonstrated the power of community-based surveillance and the importance of reaching all homes with program interventions. Such approaches are inexpensive when volunteers are involved, and they engage the community as a partner in the effort to improve health.

- The achievements of the World Relief/Cambodia Light for Life Child Survival Project have been recognized by the donor community in Cambodia, and the project now serves as the foundation for the expansion of similar activities to a population of 1 million people covering 6 of 10 districts in Kampong Cham Province. The project served not only to mobilize the community, but it also acted as a catalyst to build a relationship of trust between the MOH and the people. Additionally, the project strengthened the capacity of each partner in the partnership. The effectiveness of the Care Group approach in Cambodia and other countries has led to its adoption by more than 15 other nongovernmental organizations (NGOs) working in more than 30 countries.

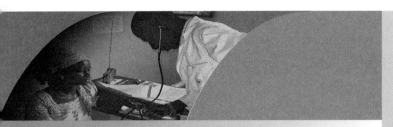

Discussion Questions

- How can this experience, and similar experiences, influence decision makers on the importance of involving communities and their representatives in all levels of planning, implementation, and evaluation of health programs?

- What clues does this case provide that might help us understand why only 16 of the 68 priority countries of the world (where 97% of the world's deaths among children occur) are on track to achieve Millennium Development Goal (MDG) 4 by 2015? (MDG 4 calls for a reduction by two-thirds in the under-five mortality rate compared to 1990 levels.)

- What was the catalytic role of World Relief that made it possible for the Ministry of Health and the communities to make such rapid progress in improving children's health? How can other organizations serve similar functions in other settings?

- What policies could international organizations, donors, and national governments adopt that could make the kinds of results demonstrated here more likely to occur?

- What can communities do to insist that they play a stronger role in planning, implementation, and evaluation of health programs that serve them?

REFERENCES

1. United Nations Development Programme. *Human Development Report 2007/2008. Fighting Climate Change: Human Solidarity in a Divided World.* New York, NY: Palgrave Macmillan; 2007. http://hdr.undp.org/en/media/HDR_20072008_EN_Complete.pdf. Accessed August 5, 2009.

2. National Institute of Public Health, National Institute of Statistics [Cambodia], ORC Macro. *Cambodia Demographic and Health Survey 2005.* Phnom Penh, Cambodia and Calverton, MD: National Institute of Public Health, National Institute of Statistics, ORC Macro; 2006. http://www.measuredhs.com/pubs/pdf/FR185/FR185%5BNov-11-2008%5D.pdf. Accessed February 2010.

3. Bryce J, Harris Requejo J, eds. *Countdown to 2015. Tracking Progress in Maternal, Newborn and Child Survival: The 2008 Report.* New York, NY: UNICEF; 2008. http://www.childinfo.org/files/Countdown2015Publication.pdf. Accessed August 5, 2009.

4. National Institute of Statistics, Directorate General for Health [Cambodia], and ORC Macro. 2001. *Cambodia Demographic and Health Survey 2000.* Phnom Penh, Cambodia, and Calverton, Maryland USA: National Institute of Statistics, Directorate General for Health, and ORC Macro. http://www.measuredhs.com/pubs/pub_details.cfm?ID=342&srchTp=type#dfiles. Accessed February 2010.

5. Laughlin M, World Relief Health Team. *The Care Group Difference: A Guide to Mobilizing Community-Based Volunteer Health Educators.* Baltimore, MD: World Relief; 2004.

6. Edward A, Ernst P, Taylor C, Becker S, Mazive E, Perry H. Examining the evidence of under-five mortality reduction in a community-based programme in Gaza, Mozambique. *Trans R Soc Trop Med Hyg.* 2007;101:814–822.

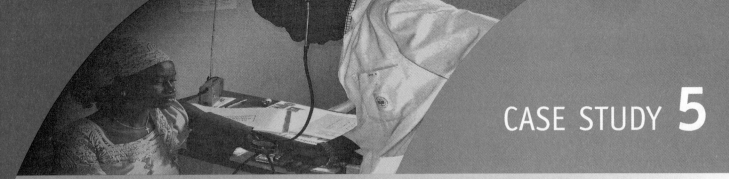

CASE STUDY **5**

Common Pathways: Worcester's Healthy Community Initiative

Suzanne B. Cashman and Clara Savage

BACKGROUND

Located in central Massachusetts and with a population of approximately 180,000 persons, Worcester covers a land area of 97.1 square kilometers (37.5 square miles). It is a largely blue-collar, working-class city with historic roots in the manufacturing industry. According to the 2000 census, whites make up 77.1% of the population, blacks 6.9%, Asians 4.9%, Native Americans 0.4%, and Native Hawaiians and other Pacific Islanders 0.1%. The remainder is of mixed heritage or unknown ethnicity. Hispanics, who may be of any race, and in Worcester are primarily from Puerto Rico and the Dominican Republic, make up 15.1% of the residents. The overall population has increased over the decades, from a total of 161,799 in 1980 to an estimated 175,454 in 2006.[1] The current overall socioeconomic and health status of the city is poorer than the state of Massachusetts.

Two Federally Qualified Health Centers in the community, Great Brook Valley and Family Health Center of Worcester,[a] have been serving the city's low-income population since the 1970s. In 1974, the University of Massachusetts Medical School, the then-new state medical school, graduated its first class of physicians. The university has grown over the decades and now houses a graduate school of nursing and a graduate school of biomedical sciences in addition to the medical school. Two large hospitals, at least nine others schools of

---

[a]A Federally Qualified Health Center (FQHC) is a type of provider defined by the Medicare and Medicaid statutes. FQHCs include all organizations receiving grants under Section 330 of the Public Health Service Act, which defines federal grant funding opportunities for organizations to provide care to underserved populations.

higher education, and many not-for-profit organizations also serve the city.

Although the university has a strong department of family medicine and community health, only intermittently has it taken a community-oriented primary care (COPC)[2] approach to identifying and addressing community health issues. Members of the department have, however, adopted a Healthy Communities approach to the health of city residents. As an ally to COPC, the Healthy Communities movement emphasizes a democratic approach to addressing community problems and includes nine principles: (1) broadly define *health*, (2) broadly define *community*, (3) share a vision based on community values, (4) address quality of life for everyone, (5) encourage diverse participation and widespread community ownership, (6) focus on *systems change*, (7) build capacity using local assets and resources, (8) benchmark and measure progress and outcomes, and (9) invest in youth leadership and development.[3] The approach is predicated on identifying a community's strengths and begins with lay and professional community members imagining what their neighborhoods and communities can become. This step of creating a shared vision, explicit in Healthy Communities but only implicit in COPC, is an important element of the process. It develops common bonds and identifies areas of shared concerns.

In 2003, leaders of two local health promotion initiatives, one of which had developed through a reorganization of State Department of Public Health regionalization, decided that merging the efforts of their small but passionate organizations could result in more effective approaches to improving the quality of life and health for the city's residents. Thus, the Worcester Healthy Community Task Force was born. With the help of an outside Healthy Communities leader–facilitator, the group began strategic planning and crafted draft vision and mission statements. Within several months, they had developed an outline of an organizational structure; a Leadership Council (LC) comprised of 18 to 22 members would meet quarterly and discuss and approve the organization's main goals and strategies. LC members represented leading public and private organizations in the city, as well as members of small not-for-profit agencies. In addition to the LC, a Leadership Support Team was formed, which consisted of members of the original two merging organizations and individuals from the State Department of Public Health, in particular the Office of Healthy Communities. People joined largely because of their commitment to a Healthy Communities approach to improving health and wellness. Because the organizers deemed it critical that the City of Worcester embrace this initiative, a city leader was included on the LC and the Leadership Support Team.

In January 2005, the LC decided to name this new organization Common Pathways (CP; www.commonpathways.org) and specified the two core functions that it would carry out: (1) create shared learning among diverse residents and key institutional stakeholders on current vital issues and (2) develop a consensus set of community indicators and benchmarks, thus broadening the base of decision makers and encouraging participants to set goals and track trends while supporting shared responsibility and performance compacts. Guided by Healthy Communities principles from the start, CP tried to make sure that people did not view it as another not-for-profit organization ready to dispense services; instead, leaders reiterated that the organization was focused on building civic infrastructure and promoting alignment of goals for work already under way. It would achieve this by promoting civic engagement and discourse concerning the community's values and methods for tracking progress toward reaching the community's goals. CP's vision is straightforward. It is to make "Greater Worcester a great place to be born, grow up, learn, live, work, raise a family, grow old and participate in community life." Its mission is "to promote shared learning, reflection and broad engagement that improve community decision-making and quality of life for residents of Greater Worcester." In 2005, with funds from a local health-promoting foundation, CP hired a full-time coordinator (CS).

From CP's inception, a medical school faculty member (SBC) with extensive experience in COPC and the clinical partner's vice president for community relations participated in developing and shaping CP; representatives from the community health centers contributed as members of a health promotion work group that developed as a result of a Boston-based initiative working in the Worcester community. These individuals served as a bridge between their institutions and this community-responsive and community-building initiative; their participation demonstrated clear institutional commitment.

THE HEALTH STATUS OF THE COMMUNITY

Like many similar-size communities with a high proportion of low-income households, Worcester faces significant health challenges, but it also offers numerous opportunities for progress. Compared with other communities in Massachusetts, the use of alcohol and illegal substances is high; a large percentage of Worcester adults are overweight or obese (35.2% and 20.9%, respectively) and get too little exercise; infant mortality, a key indicator of overall population health, is higher in Worcester than in any city in Massachusetts (in 2005, 13.9 versus 5.1 per 1000 live births); premature mortality rates, that is, death before age 75 years, were considerably higher in Worcester than in the state overall (410 versus 317 per 100,000, respectively); the teenage birth rate also continues to be higher in Worcester than in the state (37.2 versus 21.7 per 1000 girls 10–19 years old, respectively); and in some neighborhoods, 33% of residents smoke.[4] Compared to state averages, a considerably larger percentage of the population who are members of racial or ethnic minority groups speaks a language other than English at home and are foreign born. In part because the federal government designated Worcester as one of the refugee centers of entrance into the United States, there has been a dramatic increase in the number of immigrants from eastern Europe, Southeast Asia, Central America, South America, Africa, and lately from Iraq. Many of these individuals are victims of war and political persecution; a not insignificant proportion of them have spent time in refugee camps. In addition, it is believed that there is a significant group of immigrants without legalized status. In 2005, close to 20% of the people living in Worcester were below the federal poverty level.[1]

THE INTERVENTION PROGRAM

At one level, the entire process of developing CP has been an ongoing intervention; it has been about building capacity and ensuring that, to the extent possible, activities of existing organizations are aligned. Fundamentally, it is about synergy and collaboration. Developing shared aims brings people together to identify areas of common interest. Although these are often people who know or at least know about one another, like everyone else they work within their own silos and do not often have the opportunity to come together around common ground. This collaborative effort provides that common ground while offering valuable learning opportunities.

The work has not been without conflict and misunderstanding, however. For example, after approximately 4 years spent functioning in a very loosely structured, organic manner, it became clear that CP needed defined structure and operating principles. It wasn't clear to people how they could take a leadership role, what the LC members' terms were, how responsibility was assumed or shared, and so forth. Consequently, a subgroup comprising members of the Leadership Support Team and LC began meeting to draft operating principles that would spell out clearly how CP is governed and how residents could participate. This process was cumbersome, stirred up underlying conflict, and consumed approximately 6 months. Although participants reminded themselves and one another that conflict meant they were being honest and were experiencing an inevitable stage of development, this process included painful discussions and hurt feelings. Working through this step successfully is a testament to participants' shared commitment to CP's goals and to the Healthy Communities processes.

On the basis of the work that developed through CP's extensive and intensive community involvement processes (see the next section), CP's coordinator convened work groups comprising 15 to 20 individuals for each of the six priority themes. The Public Health and Medical Services group is promoting healthy weight among residents of Worcester. They are doing this by taking a multipronged approach aimed at promoting physical activity, wellness, and healthy nutrition for children, youth, families, employees, and the community at large. The Education work group has laid out a plan of activity that focuses on working with the city schools to implement the Youth Risk Behavior Surveillance System (YRBSS) and then sharing anonymous results with organizations promoting healthy youth development. Their focus is on youth academic success and healthy emotional development. The work group addressing the improvement of Mental Health and Social Services has developed a plan to improve the current capacity of the 2-1-1 information and referral service[b] so that it is better known, accessible, and accurate for use by members of diverse communities. The work group coalesced around housing issues has partnered with local housing organizations and is working to prevent foreclosure and receivership. More specifically, the group is updating information about initiatives such as a receivership effort to rehabilitate foreclosure buildings and return them to the rental market to serve low-income and minority residents. The group looking at transportation issues initiated an intervention with the Worcester Regional Transit Authority to boost ridership and promote use of public transportation. Focused on economic

development, the sixth group has elected to tackle the issue of jobs for youth and is working with several other local organizations to promote development of these jobs.

Each work group meets monthly to plan, implement, and evaluate its activity aimed at supporting initiatives. One participating organization in each group has agreed to function as its convening organization. This means that the organization assigns an individual to assume the responsibility of convening group members, facilitating meeting logistics, and ensuring that meeting minutes are developed and distributed. Each work group has included an evaluation outline in its work plan. With the work groups beginning to implement their activities, an independent evaluator has been contracted to track the work groups' progress toward reaching their stated objectives.

COMMUNITY PARTICIPATION AND INTERSECTORAL COOPERATION

Developed according to Healthy Communities principles, CP used several approaches to ensure that community voices and priorities were included and that meaningful community involvement and intersectoral participation guided all decision making. Gathering community input occurred initially through asking people three questions at several venues and events: (1) What do you like about Worcester? (2) What don't you like about Worcester? and (3) How can we improve as a city? The questions and responses formed the basis of community discussions and information gathering.

In the fall of 2005, CP held a well-publicized community forum at a local not-for-profit agency. Approximately 150 participants attended to learn about this newly developing organization and to discuss the three questions. Simultaneously, during several summer months, the city residents' responses to these same questions were solicited through a series of small group discussions with community members at nearly 100 one-on-one interviews, many ethnic festivals, and more than 70 surveys of people who live or work in Worcester. From these community conversations, the CP Leadership Support Team and LC identified 11 themes that undergirded the residents' comments and responses. These themes—Civic Engagement, Culture and Recreation, Economic Development, Education, Environment, Diversity and Multiculturalism, Housing, Public Health and Medical Services, Public Safety, Social and Mental Health Services, and Transportation—captured residents' priorities and concerns for their city. In the spring of 2006, at a second community forum held at a local university, approximately 75 participants again gathered. Through discussion and voting, they prioritized the 11 themes. The top six themes selected for initial attention and action were Economic Development, Education, Housing, Public Health and Medical

---

[b]In Massachusetts, 2-1-1 is a phone number used to provide information and referrals for health and human services providers. There is no charge for the service; it is available 24 hours a day every day, and it can provide assistance in more than 30 languages via an interpreter service.

Services, Social and Mental Health Services, and Transportation. CP LC members concurred that these six themes represented challenges and opportunities for the city.

With the six priority themes identified, CP commissioned a professional researcher to gather data about each one and convened a Community Indicators Work Group to identify key indicators for each of the six priority areas. Co-led by the clinical system's CEO and a local university president, the work group did this through reviewing data availability (current and longer term), understandability of the indicator, and relevance of the indicator for measuring achievement toward either short-term or long-term goals. In addition, work group members consulted other city indicators reports to obtain ideas of specific indicators used for similar themes and obtained valuable help from the state's public health department. Throughout the process, the work group shared progress on developing specific indicators with members of the Leadership Support Team and LC. The indicator development process was lengthy and drawn out, taking about 2 years to complete.

At a third community forum held in the spring of 2008, approximately 150 individuals, among them several community-based primary care physicians, met to review the Community Indicator Report for the six priority themes. Participants divided themselves into small groups, each focused on one of the themes. After selecting a facilitator–leader, they agreed on an indicator of focus and then identified those agencies and organizations that could take specific actions needed to address it. Each group has continued to meet and has developed a detailed action plan, complete with time lines, short-term measurable objectives, and long-term goals. Each work group has committed to move forward the selected indicators by focusing on actions that are achievable in a short period of time, that will foster participation, and that are linked to long-term goals.

LESSONS LEARNED

As in any major endeavor, we learned many lessons through the process of developing CP and no doubt would do many things differently if we were to do this again. Our suggestions for anyone engaging in a similar activity are the following:

- Resist remaining with an organic type of loose structure too long; develop clear guidelines and operating principles relatively early in the process.
- Even though you may want to be sure that the public sees the endeavor as representing a broad definition of health, include local medical leaders from the start.
- Build diverse leadership and resident participation and ownership from the beginning.
- Have a core group of strong and positive supporters who are committed to the long-term goals while continually identifying and embracing new community input. Committed charismatic and recognized leaders can stimulate community engagement and pride at critical phases of the intervention.
- Expect criticism and skepticism along the way, increase your capacity for listening and processing what you hear, and welcome conflict as a reflection of diverse views and beliefs while staying true to the principles of community well-being.
- Engage skilled individuals to develop specific, measurable indicators that are appropriate, are relevant, and have data sources for measurement.
- Hire a coordinator and staff person. Although coalitions can accomplish a great deal with dedicated people who volunteer their time, a paid staff is key to advancing goals and aims. These individuals leverage the energy and commitment of the participants.
- Carve out dedicated time to observe and reflect on the relationships and social networks developed among the members of participating groups. This can deepen the understanding of organizational development.
- Recognize that new organizations are often ignored until they begin to gain traction. Then they attract notice and the political jockeying for resources begins. It helps to be prepared for this change.
- Acknowledge mistakes and celebrate success. This honors candor and retains commitment.

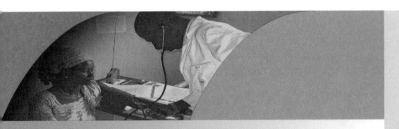

Discussion Questions

- If we think about health as a result of multiple factors, including where we live, the jobs we have, and the relationships we enjoy, what implications does this hold for medical and other healthcare professional training?

- How well do you know the different sectors and neighborhoods of the community where you are working? What are the sources of your information?

- How do the COPC and Healthy Communities processes and approaches complement and differ from each other? (See Chapters 3 and 4 for a full explanation of COPC.)

- How might the medical community leaders have played a more prominent role?

- What should be the role of the state and local health departments in a Healthy Communities initiative?

REFERENCES

1. Worcester Police Department 2008 Annual Report http://www.ci
.worcester.ma.us/uploads/4d/c2/4dc235b05ee35f7e6dc31f85210f6d20/wpd-
annual-report-2008.pdf

2. Mullan F, Epstein L. Community-oriented primary care: new relevance in a changing world. *Am J Public Health*. 2002;92:1748–1755.

3. Cashman SB, Stenger J. Healthy communities: a natural ally for
community-oriented primary care. *Am J Public Health*. 2003;93:1379–1380;
author reply 1380.

4. Massachusetts Office of Health and Human Services. MassCHIP.
http://masschip.state.ma.us. Accessed April 2009.

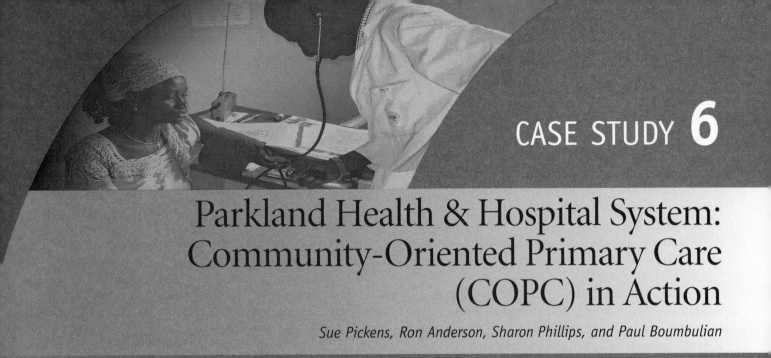

Parkland Health & Hospital System: Community-Oriented Primary Care (COPC) in Action

Sue Pickens, Ron Anderson, Sharon Phillips, and Paul Boumbulian

BACKGROUND

Parkland Health & Hospital System is one of the nation's largest and busiest public hospital and health systems. It has been serving the citizens of Dallas County for more than 115 years and evolving to meet changing community needs. It is a regional Level I trauma facility and burn center and a Level III neonatal intensive care unit and provides several other highly sophisticated services that are critical to the broader north Texas community.

Parkland is a quaternary care health system that, in 2008, provided more than 43,000 inpatient discharges, 16,000 births (nearly 35% of all births among Dallas County residents), more than 70% of the county's major trauma care, and more than 60% of the county's AIDS-related services. In 2008, Parkland's total outpatient visits numbered more than 1 million.[1] In recognition of its outstanding performance in terms of service provision, *U.S. News & World Report* has listed Parkland among the nation's top hospitals for 15 consecutive years.[2]

Parkland Health & Hospital System is owned and operated by a special taxing jurisdiction of the State of Texas that is coterminous with the Dallas County geographic boundaries. This special taxing jurisdiction is called the Dallas County Hospital District. Hospital district jurisdictions are separate from the public health funding structures of the state, city, and county. The Texas statute that created this hospital district requires the district to provide or purchase medical care for the indigent and needy residents of the county. Parkland is governed by an independent board of managers, appointed by local elected officials, the county judge, and four county commissioners. The commissioners also set county property tax rates for the hospital district.

Sociodemographics of the Population

The north Texas region is home to more than 6.3 million people. The 12-county Dallas–Fort Worth Consolidated Metropolitan Statistical Area (CMSA) was the fastest-growing metropolitan area in 2007.[3] Dallas County is home to 2.3 million people, and there has been a dramatic demographic shift, with the region becoming much more Hispanic. Dallas County, the primary service area for Parkland, has become a minority majority county, with the following demographics: 39.1% Hispanic, 20.4% African American, 34.4% white, and 6.1% other.[4] More than 18% of the population is non-US citizens. The primary growth for Dallas County came from natural increase and international migration.[5] An estimated 40% of the total Dallas County population is twice the federal poverty level, representing over 930,000 people who are uninsured or medically indigent. However, the median household income in Dallas County is $46,372, indicating a bimodal population of very wealthy and very poor groups, with a limited middle class.[6]

Development of Parkland's COPC Program

Parkland began its transformation in 1980 when Dallas County residents, in support of the new governance and leadership at Parkland, passed a bond referendum to renovate Parkland's teaching hospital and campus specialty outpatient clinics. The renovations were completed in the mid-1980s. As soon as these facilities opened, they were filled to capacity. At this point, Parkland began to examine different options for decentralizing primary care.[7]

In 1986, Parkland undertook a community planning effort to meet the challenges of the growing outpatient volume. The results of this community planning effort were Parkland's plan for decentralization, *Community Oriented Primary Care: A Plan for Dallas County*. This plan included an increase in the tax allocation for the incremental implementation of the community-oriented primary care (COPC) program. The COPC program envisioned a series of outpatient primary care facilities to provide primary and preventive care on six key elements: (1) assessment of community needs and assets, (2) community prioritization through community conversations, (3) collaboration with community organizations, (4) provision of primary health care, (5) evaluation, and (6) financing.[8]

Outside of the Parkland hospital COPC system, there are an additional 26 voluntary clinics, many of which are church affiliated. Some of these facilities operate one or two days a week, but others, including three independent Federally Qualified Health Centers,[a] operate full time but are not part of the Parkland COPC health center system. There is also a program called Project Access that supports health care access for the underserved. Operated by the Dallas County Medical Society, Project Access works with Parkland, the voluntary clinics, local nonprofit hospitals, and private physicians to assist in the provision of primary and specialty care for the poor and uninsured population that is not eligible for the Parkland system. Parkland coordinates and cooperates with these clinics to help navigate patients through the available services within Dallas County.

Community Health Care System: Parkland's COPC Program

Parkland's COPC program provides care in both traditional and nontraditional settings. Services are offered through a system of 11 large health centers and 11 youth and family centers located on the grounds of the Dallas Independent Public School District and the Carrollton, Addison, Farmers Branch Public School District; four mobile clinic vans to more than 25 homeless shelters; a geriatric program that includes a separate geriatric assessment center and a senior house calls program; and the Dallas County Adult and Juvenile Jail System. The Parkland COPC services are therefore provided in 23 separate fixed sites, four mobile vans, and five jail locations. Services are provided via multidisciplinary teams composed of a mix of midlevel practitioners and primary care physicians, nurses, social workers, language assistants, psychologists, psychiatrists, and business staff. Innovations in healthcare delivery models,

such as shared medical visits and integration of mental health services into primary care, have been steadily developed to mold health care to the changing landscape of population needs. COPC physicians are board certified and also have clinical faculty status at the University of Texas Southwestern Medical School (UTSW). In addition, special efforts are made to match physicians and COPC employees to the communities they serve; more than 20% of the COPC providers are bilingual, 55% are minorities, and more than 60% are women. Four of the centers are practice sites for approximately a third of UTSW pediatric residents, with COPC pediatricians serving as their supervising physicians.

Partnerships and Community Collaborations

Parkland has established a partnership with community organizations to provide other health and social services, creating a one-stop shopping network covering all primary care disciplines and dental health. Parkland's Women's and Infant's Specialty Health service is responsible for women's health services at the majority of COPC sites and at two stand-alone sites. Community Dental Health, a private not-for-profit organization providing dental services to low-income adults and children of Dallas County, are also colocated in several of the COPC sites. Parkland Youth and Family program is a collaborative with the Dallas Independent Public School District and Dallas Mental Health Authority to provide services to students at the public school campuses. Parkland also partners with the Dallas Housing Authority to provide services in the communities of subsidized housing.

Parkland's COPC program provided primary health care to nearly 139,000 unique patients in 2008, which resulted in more than 449,562 visits. The women's health and family planning program provided another 249,378 visits to women in Dallas County. The jail health program sees more than 3500 patients a month in the Dallas County Adult and Juvenile Jail System and distributes medicine to between 2300 and 2500 inmates daily. Parkland is the principal provider of prenatal care to uninsured women in Dallas County. Roughly 97% of the patients who delivered a baby at Parkland received such care. These services are offered in COPC health centers and freestanding health centers throughout the community.

THE HEALTH STATUS OF THE COMMUNITY

Parkland developed its COPC system around a detailed community health assessment. Since the mid-1990s, this assessment has been conducted on an annual basis. The assessment is epidemiologically based and is used as a management tool to position community health centers and focus public health outreach activities. The assessment (the most recent edition

---

[a]A Federally Qualified Health Center (FQHC) is a type of provider defined by the Medicare and Medicaid statutes. FQHCs include all organizations receiving grants under Section 330 of the Public Health Service Act, which defines federal grant funding opportunities for organizations to provide care to underserved populations.

of which is *The Community Health Checkup, 2008*) is produced in conjunction with the Dallas–Fort Worth Hospital Council Needs Assessment Committee. The checkup is made available to the community at large by posting it on the Parkland Health & Hospital System's and council's Web sites.[9] Local data are used in the assessment, including information on population variables such as age, ethnicity, and income; birth outcomes and birth-related variables; death rate variables; morbidity data, such as infectious diseases, chronic disease prevalence, and health risk survey data; access to primary care; preventable hospitalizations; and hospital utilization.

The results from this assessment are different for each defined service area within Dallas County; however, the health outcomes of significant concern include the following:

- increasing infant mortality since 2001 throughout the county, but particularly in south Dallas County
- high diabetes and heart disease rates in south Dallas County
- significantly higher rates of people without health insurance
- lack of mental health and substance abuse services, as well as high rates of poor mental health as evidenced in south and west Dallas County
- significant trauma volume at the hospitals, and high fatality rates due to automobile crashes, falls, and other injuries throughout Dallas County

This community assessment is provided to the COPC outreach program. A series of Community Conversations were held in which community leaders, residents, and political representatives were invited to participate. Focus groups were conducted in English with instant Spanish translation via headphones. Approximately 8 to 10 community members attended each of these sessions. Five Community Conversations were held in 2007. Priorities were established for each group, with follow-up continuing toward implementation. The priorities established by these groups target the issues that have direct bearing on health status but have little to do with the medical care system. The issues chosen as priorities by the groups included safety, education, and employment. COPC outreach services are supporting these Community Conversations and the action plans that are developed from them as one means of improving the health of their communities. Specific health assessment data supplied to the Community Conversations groups included the following:

- There are significant rates of asthma in southeast Dallas.
- The mortality and morbidity indicators for birth outcomes, cancer, heart disease, and diabetes are worsening for east Dallas.

- West Dallas fares better than the rest of Dallas County on only 2 of the 12 health indicators.
- More people are being diagnosed with chronic diseases, such as diabetes, high blood pressure, or asthma, within selected service areas such as west Dallas.
- Mortality rates in selected service areas indicate no change in chronic disease rates after implementation of COPC in those areas. This suggests a lack of access to care, necessitating more services than are currently available through the existing COPC system. This lack of access may be allowing chronic diseases to go undetected longer than in service areas that have better access to care.

In addition to the Community Conversations, each health center has established a community advisory board to provide input into clinic operations and community health needs. The advisory boards have sponsored projects that have an impact on community health, such as interventions aimed at reducing teenage pregnancies.

Additionally, an analysis of community needs was conducted in 2008 to indicate where to expand COPC health centers. Using data from the census, patient origin data, a community needs index,[10] preventable hospitalizations, and avoidable emergency department visits, each zip code was evaluated and organized into communities of need. Five geographic areas were identified where the conditions indicated a significant lack of access to primary care.

THE INTERVENTION PROGRAM

An important part of the COPC program is assessment of health outcomes and data on the cost of healthcare services.[11] Parkland has conducted numerous assessments since 1995. Most recently, the analysis of community needs within Dallas County showed that areas where COPC health centers are located have fewer inpatient admissions for potentially avoidable hospitalizations and lower rates of inappropriate emergency department use.

In 1998 to 2002, the rate of stillbirths per 1000 live births among mothers with at least one prenatal care visit was 5.6, compared to 13.0 among mothers who received no prenatal care. Corresponding neonatal death rates per 1000 live births were 3.7 and 11.4. Also, Parkland's neonatal mortality outcomes by ethnicity were significantly better than those for the United States overall and for African Americans and Hispanics residing in Texas.[12] Parkland preterm births in minority women from 1988 to 2006 significantly decreased, coinciding with increased prenatal care.[13] These outcomes are a result of the establishment of the women's and infants' health centers located within the COPC health centers. These health centers provide over 120,000 prenatal care visits a year, and more than 97% of women who gave birth had prenatal care at Parkland. Additionally, Parkland has a complications prenatal service for high-risk pregnant women within its system, as well as an antenatal inpatient unit for women who need inpatient hospitalization prior to delivery.

Healthy Living with Diabetes, a COPC program approved by the American Diabetes Association, consists of five classes. For those who completed the program, their hemoglobin A1C tests dropped by 1.34 points. The overall medical costs by program participants versus nonparticipants were statistically significantly lower.[14]

COMMUNITY PARTICIPATION AND INTERSECTORAL COOPERATION

Parkland has entered into numerous partnerships and collaborations. The COPC health center outreach services sponsors community coalitions representing the communities served by the major health centers. Parkland also supports the Perinatal Periods of Risk collaborative that is identifying the root causes of fetal and infant deaths. This collaborative includes several health organizations. Examples of other collaboratives that Parkland COPC participates in include the Cancer Disparities Coalition in south Dallas, Dallas County Children's Obesity Collaborative, and the south Dallas pediatric education collaborative.

Parkland also gives community residents a key role in defining the services they provide as well as deciding on priorities for their communities. As described earlier, each COPC clinic has a community advisory board made up of community members and users of the system. These boards meet monthly and work to improve the services of the clinic as well as identify and work on health improvement projects within the community. Also as described earlier, the Community Conversations continue to meet with members of the community, advisory board members, and other interested parties in implementing the priorities established by each of these conversations. Parkland uses a community-based participatory research (CBPR) model when doing research or interventions in the community, and community members are asked to participate in the design and implementation of these projects. Additionally, town hall meetings are scheduled for projects that are high profile or impact a large component of the community.

Parkland has also instituted a systemwide program to monitor patient satisfaction and identify patient clinical and safety issues as seen from the patient perspective. In 2008, more than 15,000 patient satisfaction surveys were completed using a telephone survey methodology in both English and Spanish. The telephone methodology is used to help overcome low literacy levels, especially in a medically indigent population. The results of these surveys, patients' comments, and any "hot comments" are provided to health center managers, the community advisory board, senior leadership, and the systemwide quality improvement committee. This process helps improve the quality and services at each of the health centers.

LESSONS LEARNED

- Under current funding mechanisms that are based on employee-sponsored health insurance, improvements to community health status often do not accrue to the bottom line of healthcare institutions, but they are realized in other social and economic sectors. An evaluative mechanism is needed to determine outcomes and benefits when institutions such as Parkland invest in community health status improvements.

- Parkland is in the process of establishing a Community Health Improvement Measurement and Evaluation System (CHIMES), which could act as such an evaluation system to help document areas in which community health investment has produced savings for the community, whether in the form of fewer hospitalizations, fewer days lost from work, or less school absenteeism. A Center for Health Innovation has also been established. It is designed to be a quality improvement organization for inpatient care. Although the current work targets readmission rates, future work will concentrate on the relationship between social determinants of health and community health status.

- Additional issues arise when funding becomes difficult. When this occurs, eliminating the COPC system is seen as one option. It is important to maintain outcome information that shows the value of COPC to the community and the overall health system. When the value of primary and preventive healthcare services are communicated, the citizens of the county often support the system with additional tax revenue, as they did in 2000 when Parkland was facing an $83 million budget deficit; again in 2008, more than 82% of Dallas County voters approved a bond package to replace the current Parkland main campus and expand the current COPC system. This package includes an additional 2.5¢ per $100 valuation of property taxes for the citizens of Dallas County.

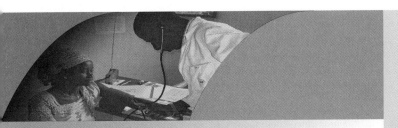

Discussion Questions

- How can facilities be aligned to meet growing demand?

- How does the dispersion of poverty populations away from the city center and into the suburbs affect the current service providers, and what new locations need to be established to support this change?

- How can a tax-based system be funded at the appropriate level with decreasing tax revenue and increasing unemployment?

- How can the funding structure of a program that serves patients of a multicounty region (such as trauma or burn services) be changed to reflect the regional nature of its service structure without depending on a single county tax base?

- How does COPC continue to be relevant to our communities and meet their ever-changing needs?

- How does COPC develop and design services that will affordably treat, promote, and maintain communities' and residents' wellness?

REFERENCES

1. Parkland Health & Hospital Decision Support Services, TII database proprietary data, Parkland Decision Support System, 2008. http://www.parklandhospital.com/whoweare/at_a_glance/index.html. Accessed April 2010

2. *U.S. News & World Report.* Parkland Memorial Hospital, Dallas. http://www.usnews.com/listings/hospitals/6740950. Accessed February 25, 2009.

3. US Census Bureau. Dallas–Fort Worth leads metro areas in numerical growth. http://www.census.gov/Press-Release/www/releases/archives/population/011671.html. Published March 27, 2008. Accessed February 2009.

4. Neilson Claritas Propietary Population data base. 2008. http://en-us.nielsen.com/tab/expertise/segmentation_and_targeting/demographics

5. US Census Bureau Population Division. *Table 5: Estimates of the Components of Population Change for Counties of Texas: July 1, 2006 to July 1, 2007.* Washington, DC: US Census Bureau; 2008. CO-EST2007-05-48.

6. US Census Bureau. American Community Survey, 2007. http://factfinder.census.gov/servlet/DTTable?_bm=y&-context=dt&-ds_name=ACS_2007_1YR_G00_&-CONTEXT=dt&-mt_name=ACS_2007_1YR_G2000_B05001&-mt_name=ACS_2007_1YR_G2000_B19001&-mt_name=ACS_2007_1YR_G2000_B19013&-mt_name=ACS_2007_1YR_G2000_B17002&-tree_id=307&-geo_id=05000US48113&-search_results=01000US&-format=&-_lang=en. Accessed February 2009.

7. Pickens S, Boumbulian PJ, Anderson RJ, Ross S, Phillips S. Community oriented primary care in action: a Dallas story. *Am J Public Health.* 2002;92:1728–1732.

8. Anderson RJ, Boumbulian PJ. Comprehensive community health programs: a new look at an old approach. In: Korn D, McLaughlin CJ, Osters M, eds. *Academic Health Centers in the Managed Care Environments.* Washington, DC: Association of Academic Health Centers; 1995:119–135.

9. Strategic Planning Department, Parkland Health & Hospital System. *The Community Health Checkup.* Dallas, TX: Dallas–Fort Worth Hospital Council; 2008.

10. *Community Need Index database.* Thomson/Reuters; Propietary data. http://thomsonreuters.com/products_services/healthcare/?view=Standard 2007. Accessed April 2010.

11. Rhyne R, Boque R, Kululka G, Fulmer H, eds. *Community Oriented Primary Care: Health Care for the 21st Century.* Washington, DC: American Public Health Association; 1998.

12. *Parkland Community Benefit Plan and Report,* 2008/2009. Dallas, TX: Planning and Population Medicine Department, Parkland Health & Hospital System, 2008.

13. Levino KJ, McIntire DD, Bloom SL, Sibley MR, Anderson RJ. Decreased preterm births in an inner-city public hospital. *Obstet Gynecol.* 2009;113:578–584.

14. Parkland Health & Hospital System. Parkland Community Health Plan and Dallas County Hospital District meetings schedule. http://www.parklandhospital.com/media/pdf/BOM_022409.pdf. Published February 24, 2009. Accessed February 2009.

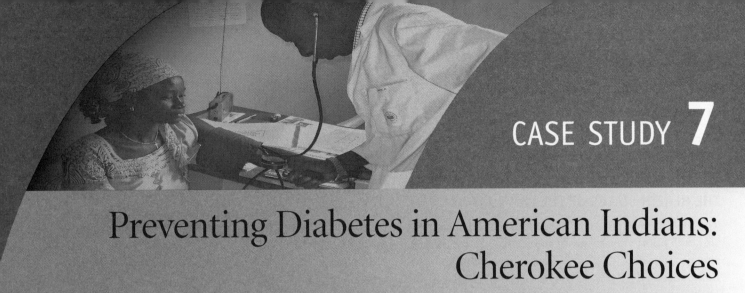

CASE STUDY 7

Preventing Diabetes in American Indians: Cherokee Choices

Patrik Johansson and Jeffrey J. Bachar

BACKGROUND

The majority of the 13,400 Eastern Band of Cherokee Nation (EBCN) tribal members live on the Qualla Boundary, a 56,000 acre Indian reservation in western North Carolina held in trust by the US federal government specifically for the EBCN.[1] The EBCN is a federally acknowledged tribe, and as such is a sovereign nation that maintains government-to-government relations with the United States. The Honorable Michel Hicks, Chief of the EBCN, describes the unique history and political status of the Cherokee Nation in the following statement: "In 1762, the Cherokee Nation was a world power. We were viewed by the British as an important military ally, valued trading partner. We were making treaties with Great Britain and with the colonies of Virginia and South Carolina for years before we began a nation-to-nation relationship with the United States government."[2] In 1838, the US government forcefully removed many Cherokees living in the East to Indian Territory in Oklahoma. One-fourth to one-half of the 16,000 Cherokees died before reaching Oklahoma. The EBCN citizens of today descend from individuals who hid in the Appalachian Mountains to avoid removal and others who returned to their homeland following removal. Gradually, and with great effort, tribal members have created the present-day vibrant, sovereign nation.[3] Today, as a result of federal acknowledgement, EBCN tribal members are eligible for services funded through the Indian Health Service (IHS) of the US Department of Health and Human Services. The median household income of EBCN tribal members, $31,884, falls below the state median income of $46,335,[1,4] and tribal members are less likely to have completed college and attended graduate school than other residents of North Carolina.[5]

The EBCN provides health services to tribal members through the Cherokee Indian Hospital Authority and the Eastern Band of Cherokee Indian Health and Medical Division. The Cherokee Indian Hospital is a 20-bed hospital with an average census of eight patients. The outpatient clinic and the emergency room have approximately 22,000 and 1500 visits per year, respectively. The Eastern Band of Cherokee Indian Health and Medical Division is a community-focused health system that provides an array of health services that include public health nursing services, diabetes services, home health services, women's health services, and youth health services. Through the Cherokee Choices Program, the Health and Medical Division also conducts health promotion activities aimed at increasing physical activity and promoting well-being and healthy choices, which can reduce the risk for obesity and diabetes among tribal members.[6,7]

The Centers for Disease Control and Prevention (CDC) of the US Department of Health and Human Services funded the Cherokee Choices Program in 1999 through Racial and Ethnic Approaches to Community Health (REACH) 2010, the cornerstone of CDC's efforts to eliminate racial and ethnic disparities in health. The fundamental objective of REACH is to address the Healthy People 2010 goal to eliminate health disparities among different segments of the population, such as by race, ethnicity, education, income, or geographic location.[8]

The Cherokee Choices Program received REACH 2010 funds to develop a community-based intervention to improve the health and prevent the rise in diabetes among tribal members. The mission of Cherokee Choices is to delay the onset of Type II diabetes and related complications by working with community and other organizations to develop and deliver community-based behavior change interventions.[9] The Cherokee Choices Team includes a principal investigator, research coordinators, focus group facilitators, and community-outreach workers.

THE HEALTH STATUS OF THE COMMUNITY

The REACH 2010 program funded interventions addressing six health priority areas—breast and cervical cancer screening and management, cardiovascular disease, diabetes mellitus, immunizations, HIV/AIDS, and infant mortality—in at least one of the following racial and ethnic minority groups: African Americans, American Indians, Alaska Natives, Asian Americans, Pacific Islanders, or Hispanics/Latinos. In consultation with community members through key informant interviews and focus groups, the Cherokee Choices Team underwent a prioritization process to identify the most pressing health concern among the six health priority areas. They reviewed existing data on the prevalence and impact of the health conditions and chose to address Type II diabetes because this condition has reached epidemic proportions among tribal members. According to the National Opinion Research Center (NORC), among EBCN tribal members, the prevalence of Type II diabetes was 26.6% for men and 30.2% for women, versus 8.1% and 8.8% among all races of North Carolina men and women aged 18 years and older.[5] In addition, an even larger proportion of tribal members are at risk for Type II diabetes because of a high prevalence of obesity. According to NORC, 50.9% of EBCN males and 52.3% of EBCN women were obese, compared to 24.0% and 24.4% of all North Carolina men and women, respectively.[5]

Furthermore, of great concern with regards to the future potential deterioration of quality of life from chronic diseases, the high obesity prevalence is also reflected among tribal children. Analyses of the EBCN Resource Patient Management System (RPMS), the IHS Electronic Health Record, indicated that 53% of tribal members between the ages of 2 and 18 years were categorized as either obese or overweight, and this problem seems to worsen with age.[10] A diet high in fats and sugars from an increased consumption of fast foods, coupled with a sedentary lifestyle, may be contributing to the alarming increase in childhood obesity and ensuing risk factors for complications from chronic disease among tribal members.[11] More than 19 fast-food restaurants are available within 3 miles of the primary district in the town of Cherokee.[9] A survey of 85 tribal children revealed that 18% eat at fast food restaurants five or more times per week, and 52% reported eating out at least twice per week.[12] There is one grocery store and a seasonal farmers' market (May to September) in Cherokee that provides limited fresh produce, and some individuals maintain personal gardens. In comparison to the surrounding towns, fresh produce is more expensive in Cherokee.[13] According to Frederick Bradley, tribal elder, former hospital administrator, and a former teacher in the local public school system, many people opt for fast food because fresh produce is less available and more expensive.[13]

Initial research by the Cherokee Choices Team and a professional marketing agency indicated an interest in the prevention of Type II diabetes, particularly among children. As a way to incorporate parents in the interventions, the team identified the elementary school, work sites, and local churches as locations for intervention components. In consultation with tribal agencies and community groups, the team developed a community action plan that encouraged strategies to (1) engage individuals interested in a school intervention for children, (2) target tribal employees interested in losing weight and improving health, and (3) create opportunities for increased physical activity and nutritional information among church members.[9]

The marketing agency identified an attitude of indifference toward diabetes among tribal members: "Because diabetes has touched so many Cherokee families, there is a broad awareness of diabetes throughout the Cherokee community, accompanied by a general apathy. Because diabetes is so rife, it has unfortunately created an almost fatalistic acceptance of diabetes as an 'inevitable fact of Cherokee life' and a widespread belief that the disease is not preventable."[14] To reverse this perception of fatalism, the team decided that any intervention would have to include visual messages, mechanisms of educational and emotional support, and an overarching approach that would create community coalitions with the single vision of making people healthier.[9]

THE INTERVENTION PROGRAM

The Cherokee Choices Program includes three main programs: (1) elementary school mentoring, (2) work-site wellness for adults, and (3) church-based health promotion. Moreover we will outline the work-site wellness for adults program. In addition, a social marketing component, television advertisements, and a television documentary series support the Cherokee Choices Program (Bachar, 2006).

Moreover we will examine the program which challenged teams of employees from different tribal agencies to participate in weekly educational and support activities and to increase time spent in physical activity. Fitness workers, nutritionists, and dietitians (wellness staff) conducted activities where teams competed for prizes by attending exercise classes, nutritional assessments, healthy cooking demonstrations, and stress management workshops, in addition to meeting physical activity and dietary goals. Participants supported one another through communal exercise activities and by attending the monthly Lunch and Learn in-service education program where a healthy catered lunch was served. Participants also received personal support and encouragement each week from the wellness staff and learned ways to exercise and form healthy shopping habits.[9]

In addition, the wellness staff maintained an open-door policy that encouraged people to drop in for talks and one-on-one support. Over the course of the program, more than 100 employees formed nine teams. Each team selected a team leader whose role included keeping track of team members' weekly exercise habits, as well as their participation in support and educational activities. Each leader served as a liaison with Cherokee Choices, sent out regular e-mails encouraging members to continue the program, and solicited volunteers to attend wellness activities. Cherokee Choices visited each tribal agency at least weekly for encouragement and support.

The teams engaged in a 16-week competition-based program where participants received weekly to biweekly support from the Cherokee Choices Program staff, who based the winning team's performance on change in weight, change in body fat, participation in activity, and overall behavior change. To increase physical activity, each tribal agency formed teams that challenged one another to volleyball, racquetball, and basketball games. Team members accrued points through self-reported minutes of exercise per week, through the number of Cherokee Choices events attended, and for participation in and winning of scheduled athletic events. Furthermore, a social marketing component, television advertisements and a television documentary series, supported the Cherokee Choices Program.[9]

The Cherokee Choices Team collected baseline and follow-up data on participants through personal interviews and clinical measurements. In the interviews, participants described their eating and physical activity habits. In collaboration with Cherokee Choices, a local diabetes clinic conducted clinical measurements for fasting blood glucose, blood pressure, fasting lipid panel, height, weight, and body fat percentage. The Cherokee Choices Team conducted interviews on goal attainment and follow-up measures every 6 months over the project's three-year period.

Evaluation

The proportion of individuals who lost weight and decreased body fat increased among those who met physical activity recommendations. Almost two-thirds of participants lost weight and maintained weight loss. One-third of participants lost one or more points in body mass index. Additional program milestones included the following:

- Participants increased their physical activity and healthy eating behaviors.
- Eighty-eight percent of individuals completed the program.
- Fifty-six percent of participants met goals.
- Ninety-four percent of participants would participate again.
- Following completion of the program, some participants have been able to decrease or eliminate the use of diabetes and antihypertensive medications.[9]

In qualitative assessments, participants identified the following factors as incentives to participate in the program: to feel better, to look better, to improve health, to support coworkers, and to be a positive role model for their families and community. Participants also perceived the program as a start down a healthier path in life.

Furthermore, participants listed the following reasons as incentives to sustain their involvement in the program: obtain information about how to eat and improve health; receive support for change; and receive assistance with exercising, losing weight, and feeling better. Program participants also reported satisfaction with the delivery of weekly health baskets by fitness and nutrition specialists that encouraged healthy snacking, in addition to wellness-related prizes for accumulated exercise time (gift certificates to a local sports store, hand weights, basketballs, stress balls, yoga mats, and jump ropes).[15]

COMMUNITY PARTICIPATION AND INTERSECTORAL COOPERATION

In designing a culturally competent intervention, the Cherokee Choices Team employed principles of community-based participatory research and sought continuous community consultation on the development of the health promotion program through focus groups and interviews with key informants. The focus groups sought community perceptions and opinions on diabetes and diabetes-related health issues, as well as intervention design and implementation. In addition, meetings between the Cherokee Choices Team and community groups and tribal agencies enhanced capacity building and planning activities that culminated in the development of a community action plan. The community action plan adopted strategies to "engage individuals interested in a school intervention for children; target tribal employees interested in losing weight and improving health; and create opportunities for increased physical activity and nutritional information among church members."[9] With support from program managers, supervisors, and tribal leadership who attended many of the Cherokee Choices activities, employers have given employees time off to exercise. The Cherokee Choices Team gives biannual program and evaluation updates to a community coalition composed of a cross section of individuals from the three main programs in addition to other community members and elected officials from the tribal council. Furthermore, the Cherokee Choices Team consults with coalition subgroups and conducts discussion groups with them to assess the progress of the program.

LESSONS LEARNED

Over the course of the program, Cherokee Choices Program Principal Investigator Jeff Bachar has identified the following important lessons:[16]

- Funding sources must be diversified. The precarious nature of federal funding makes it unreliable as the sole source; local resources are essential to ensure sustainability and to promote investment in the intervention.
- Regular feedback from community members is essential. Establishing a system to obtain input from those involved in the intervention is crucial. This system provides a means to allow the intervention to be sensitive to cultural needs, it can mitigate problems at the earliest possible point, and it can be an incubator for new ideas and solutions to problems. Listening to community members in the design phase is essential. This takes time—more time than one might expect, especially in communities where input has not been sought regularly. People may not be accustomed to being truly involved in designing an intervention; thus, initial input may be hard to obtain, and the quality may not be at a useful level. Establishing a system to show people that their input will actually be used is crucial. Trust must be established in this regard, and patience is required. Persistence is needed to dig deeper for more feedback and to obtain information that may not come right away.
- Integrating and collaborating with other programs is a key to success. Although Cherokee Choices is a health program, we have to think of our partners (transit, city planners, and businesses) as being relevant outside of the health system. Wellness as an economic issue resonates with the business community.
- At times, you have to be fearless and willing to be seen as a rule breaker. You have to be willing to try things that have never been tried. Overcoming the mentality of "that's the way we've always done it" is a challenge that the program must be ready to meet.
- Establishing trust over years will enable the program to take more risks later. It may be prudent to hold back initially while being watchful for opportunities to act on more assertively later. Being politically astute is an essential skill.

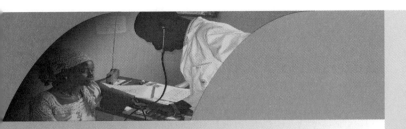

Discussion Questions

- Why might the diabetes prevalence be higher among EBCN tribal members than other residents of North Carolina?

- Why is community involvement and intersectoral participation important in a program such as Cherokee Choices?

- Why is it important to delve below the surface of health issues in the community?

- Why did building community trust take time, and why was it important in this project?

- What do you think was the most important lesson learned by the principal investigator, and why?

REFERENCES

1. Eastern Band of Cherokee. Official web site. http://www.nc-cherokee.com/. Accessed March 2009.

2. Museum of the Cherokee Indian. Emissaries of peace. *The 1762 Cherokee and British Delegations Exhibit Catalogue.* 2006:v.

3. Cherokee, North Carolina. History and culture. http://www.cherokee-nc.com/index.php?page=56. Accessed April 2009.

4. Martin E. Reservations: gambling has changed life for the Cherokee. *Business North Carolina.* 2004;March; p.49.

5. National Opinion Research Center. *REACH 2010 Risk Factor Survey Year 4 Data Report for Eastern Band of Cherokee Indians.* Chicago, IL: National Opinion Research Center. 2006.

6. Cherokee Indian Hospital Authority, http://www.ihs.gov/jobscareer develop/CareerCenter/Vacancy/pdf/27703-06172008030407.pdf. Accessed April 2010.

7. Eastern Band of the Cherokee Nation. Health and medical division: Eastern Band of Cherokee Indians. http://www.cherokee-hmd.com/. Accessed March 2009.

8. Centers for Disease Control and Prevention. Racial and ethnic approaches to community health: about REACH 2010 (1999–2007). http://www.cdc.gov/reach/reach_2010/index.htm. Accessed March 2009.

9. Bachar JJ, Lefler LJ, Reed L, McCoy T, Bailey R, Bell R. Cherokee Choices: a diabetes prevention program for American Indians. *Prev Chronic Dis.* 2006;3:A103.

10. Tribal Epidemiology Center, Tribal Health Program Support, United South and Eastern Tribes Inc. Nashville, TN, *Obesity in Cherokee Children.* [Internal document]. 2009.

11. Sturm R. Childhood obesity—what we can learn from existing data on societal trends, part 2. *Prev Chronic Dis.* 2005;2:A20.

12. Cherokee Choices. *Daily Eating Habits Questionnaire (Modified)* [internal document]. 2004.

13. Johansson P. Interview with Mr. Frederick Bradley, Eastern Band of Cherokee tribal elder. April 11, 2009.

14. The Goss Agency. *Marketing Strategy Report* [internal document]. 2004.

15. Cherokee Choices. *Internal Evaluation Report* [internal document]. 2005.

16. Johansson P. Interview with Mr. Jeff Bachar, principal investigator, Cherokee Choices Program. April 8, 2009.

The Health Commons: An Expansion of the Community Health Center Concept in New Mexico

Saverio Sava and Arthur Kaufman

BACKGROUND

Today we are witnessing a historic unity among US primary care specialties in their joint call for universal access to a primary care medical home.[a] This call is emerging at a time of economic crisis in the country and in the world and amidst a growing realization that the US healthcare system is broken, too expensive, too short on access, and too low in value. The heavy investment in fragmented, specialized care and the unbridled use of technology for some, instead of for prevention and primary care for all, has placed the United States 37th in the WHO's international ranking of healthcare systems.[1]

The concept of the primary care medical home has been used for many years. This has recently been refocused by the major primary care organizations and the Centers for Medicare & Medicaid Services as the more elaborately defined concept of the primary care patient-centered medical home. One of the origins of the current refocusing on a primary care patient-centered medical home is the community health center movement in the United States, which is largely credited to the work of Drs. Jack Geiger and Count Gibson, who proposed how to provide community-based health care to people of disenfranchised neighborhoods that lacked basic health care in 1964.[2] Although these health centers have served as a safety net for the uninsured, they have also progressed as breeding grounds for innovation in delivering health care to communities and are an integral factor in the work of alleviating the health disparities that exist in the United States.

The Health Commons described in this case study is one such innovation and is really a broader concept of the patient-centered medical home, recognizing the essential link between clinic and community.[3] This case study will outline the evolution of community-based primary care in an underserved community in New Mexico from storefront community health centers, to multiservice community health networks, to Health Commons.

The Southeast Heights Experience

The University of New Mexico (UNM) Department of Family and Community Medicine has worked with several communities, community health centers, and the New Mexico Department of Health in developing the concept of the Health Commons.[4] The Health Commons was built upon and extended beyond the community health center model. Its concept grew out of a recognition that intractable health problems in our society, such as health disparities between economic and ethnic groups, poor access to care, and alarming increases in uninsured populations, have social determinants as their root cause. These problems cannot be addressed by the healthcare system alone; they require an unprecedented integration and collaboration among many community stakeholders, pooling resources to address community-prioritized health needs. In the process, the healthcare system must become transformed and serve a broader purpose in its community.

[a]An approach to providing comprehensive primary care for children, youth, and adults. The PC-MH is a healthcare setting that facilitates partnerships between individual patients, their personal physicians, and when appropriate, the patient's family. http://www.medicalhomeinfo.org/Joint%20Statement.pdf Accessed April 1, 2010.

One component of the Health Commons is one-stop shopping, where in one site patients can obtain services of primary care, behavioral health, oral health, social services and case management, health education, and public health. Another component is the relationship between the clinic and community, in which the priority needs of the community drive the services and programs of the health center. This is accomplished through community boards and a prominent role for community health workers or promotoras who serve as links between the community and the clinic. And finally, Health Commons has community-based components linked to, but based outside of, the clinic to broaden access to services and to address social determinants of disease. These components can reside in school health centers, work sites, or more marginal communities within the catchment area of the clinic and address such issues as high school dropout rate, access to a clean water supply, reliance on commodity foods, access to services for undocumented immigrants, or local economic development.

This concept of the Health Commons truly has been a work in progress influenced by the interplay of community, providers of care, and public health in urban and rural areas of New Mexico. We will trace the emergence of this model in an urban site that is fostered by an academic health center.

THE HEALTH STATUS OF THE COMMUNITY

The east central neighborhood of Albuquerque, New Mexico, is characterized by a young population, high mobility, ethnic diversity, poverty, and social stresses, including inadequate housing, social isolation, and violence. It is the entry point for poor immigrants to the city, predominantly from Mexico, Central America, and Vietnam, and has the highest concentration of urban American Indians and under-five children in Bernalillo County. Health problems include a heavy burden of diabetes and cardiovascular disease, teen pregnancy, and a high rate of behavioral health disorders, including depression and substance abuse.

THE INTERVENTION PROGRAM

The intervention program developed throughout the years includes the involvement of academic departments, health clinics, social services, and other providers that were organized in the framework of a healthcare mall.

The Storefront

Recognizing the lack of access to healthcare services in this community, the UNM Health Sciences Center began outreach into this community in the early 1980s. In 1981, the Young

Children's Health Center (YCHC) was established as an outreach of the UNM School of Medicine Department of Pediatrics. The first YCHC clinic was located in a storefront complex of offices.

During the first year of operation, the State Department of Health office was located in this same shared space. Next, the City of Albuquerque's Department of Family and Community Services, recognizing the extraordinary health and human service needs in the neighborhood, created the East Central Multi-Service Center (ECMSC) in 1984, which then housed these clinical programs in addition to senior services and the Women, Infants, and Children (WIC) program.

To meet the growing health care needs of the community, the University Hospital, together with the UNM School of Medicine Department of Family and Community Medicine, created the Southeast Heights Center for Family Health in 1992 in a storefront adjacent to the YCHC. The concept of a healthcare mall was thus initiated, and collaboration was created at many levels. The mall had evolved to provide families with a range of services in close geographic proximity. With primary healthcare services as the foundation, families could also receive support services (such as WIC) and participate in personal enrichment activities (such as classes in English as a second language) in the ECMSC. The center was also used for a senior lunch program and a community meeting room.

A successful collaborative effort was the initiation of a monthly meeting between YCHC, the Family and Community Medicine Department, and agencies that provided health or social services in the community. This group grew to include many of the other service providers, such as the local child care agency, the schools, Catholic Family Services, and the Department of Health. This meeting was not only an effective means to share information about services, but it also helped build relationships and broaden the spirit of collaboration.

As the mall concept grew over the ensuing years, there emerged a realization that to achieve the next level of collaboration, structure needed to follow function. From the community perspective, the mall concept allowed easy shopping for services in close proximity to one another but often without coordination between those services.

Emergence of the Health Commons

These efforts led to the renovation of the shared space to create a structure more conducive to the Health Commons model. The renovation brought all of the clinical services together in a building with a large shared entrance and an adjacent child outreach area. An attempt was made to locate as many of the wrap-around services as possible in this shared space. This includes eligibility workers, case managers, social workers, diabetic educators, smoking cessation counselors, promotoras, and mental health workers.

With the creation of this Health Commons, patients truly have one place to go for multiple services. A technique called *warm handoff* is frequently practiced. When a provider has a patient with an identified need, the appropriate resource person is frequently brought right to the exam room to establish contact with that patient. This saves the patient multiple visits and allows increased interaction and mutual learning among different service providers.

Meeting space is creatively used to provide group visits and learning sessions. This ranges from a group Centering Pregnancy Class coordinated and taught by a team that includes a doula, a social worker, and one of the resident physicians; to a group diabetes education class in Vietnamese; to a meal preparation class coordinated by the child life resource worker.

In its early stages, this collaborative model of care has not only been found to be more effective but also has been, in general, well received by the community and by the providers of care. However, attempting to integrate three separate services that report to three separate administrators and institutions (Department of Pediatrics, Department of Family and Community Medicine, and Department of Health) has been challenging. Not only had three separate cultures and ways of working been established long before the merger into the Health Commons, but there was fear in some quarters that the benefits of collaboration could be outweighed by a potential loss of jobs. Public health nurses, for example, worried that if the family physicians absorbed all immunizations into their well-child clinics, then fewer public health nurses would be needed to provide immunization services.

The Southeast Heights Center for Family Health has already outgrown the present structure, and a new Health Commons facility, three times the size, has just opened in the same neighborhood to accommodate this function.

COMMUNITY PARTICIPATION AND INTERSECTORAL COOPERATION

As the service entities continued to grow and collaborate, efforts shifted to better involve the community. Grant funding helped support the development of a community-based agency called Community Health Partnerships. Its purpose was to form a more effective bridge between the community and the health and social service agencies that served them. Community Block Leaders became an essential link among them. These community workers were able to directly bring the community voice to meetings and planning sessions.

Future of the Health Commons: Expanding the Capabilities of the Patient-Centered Medical Home

Four national primary care associations—the American Academy of Family Physicians, the American College of Physicians, the American Academy of Pediatrics, and the American Osteopathic Association—have jointly called for the creation and support of a new model of care based on the patient-centered medical home.[3] Its potential and pitfalls are being debated nationally. This model characterizes the practice as having a personal physician, being physician directed, and having a whole-person orientation with coordinated and integrated care. There are quality and safety measures, including evidence-based medicine, health information technology, and continuous quality improvement, with payment structured to reflect quality. The home embodies the core features of primary care (first contact, patient-focused over time, comprehensive, coordinated, family oriented, culturally competent, and community oriented). However, community orientation appears to be a small component of the model and may suffer the same fate as it did with weak support in the current community health center arrangements. Neither the present medical home model nor the community health center model ensure integration with the communities in which they operate or serve.

LESSONS LEARNED

- The development of the Health Commons, from an isolated storefront with scattered outpost activities to a coordinated system of services, provided a framework to overcome professional isolation and space division and contributed to developing a culture of service among the different Health Commons components.
- The process of creating a shared work space encourages collaboration and overcomes traditional, professional divisions. The first major progression was the creation of a healthcare mall, which colocated and coordinated the diverse types of services that clients and patients would utilize. The Health Commons concept moves beyond location to the coordination of services for the patient.
- A well-constructed Health Commons includes both structural and functional components. The structural components are provider commons, meeting rooms, teaching spaces, resource desk, telehealth facility, and space for eligibility workers, counselors, promotoras, and other nontraditional components of health care. The functional components are the warm handoff, regular team meetings, eligibility workers, community interface, and the community extension programs.

- Although the Health Commons was conceptually embraced by the participating partners, there have been very real barriers to overcome in translating the concepts into practice. These barriers included fear of job loss, fear of identity loss, different components of the Health Commons reporting to different authorities, ignorance of the training and abilities of other healthcare professionals, limited funding, historic suspicions, misunderstandings, and turf issues.
- The Health Commons reaches beyond individual health to look at community factors and social determinants of poor health that lead to health disparities. It offers a service model without walls in which community input guides the priorities and programs of the clinic, with community stakeholders helping to identify and address those factors. Thus the Health Commons should be held up as a comparative model to enrich planning and discussion of the patient-centered medical home.

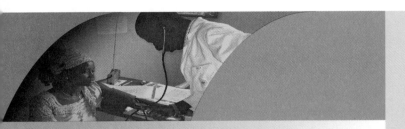

Discussion Questions

- How does a Health Commons differ from a community health center?

- How does a health service mall differ from a Health Commons?

- How does a Health Commons address the social determinants of health and disease?

- What barriers must be overcome to create a Health Commons?

REFERENCES

1. World Health Organization. *World Health Report 2000—Health Systems: Improving Performance.* Geneva, Switzerland: World Health Organization; 2000.

2. Mullan F, Epstein L. Community oriented primary care: new relevance in a changing world. *Am J of Public Health.* 2002;92:1748–1755.

3. Rosenthal T. The medical home: growing evidence to support a new approach to primary care. *J Am Board of Fam Med.* 2008;21:427–440.

4. Kaufman A, Derksen D, Alfero C, et al. The health commons and care of New Mexico's uninsured. *Ann Fam Med.* 2006;4(suppl 1):S22–S27.

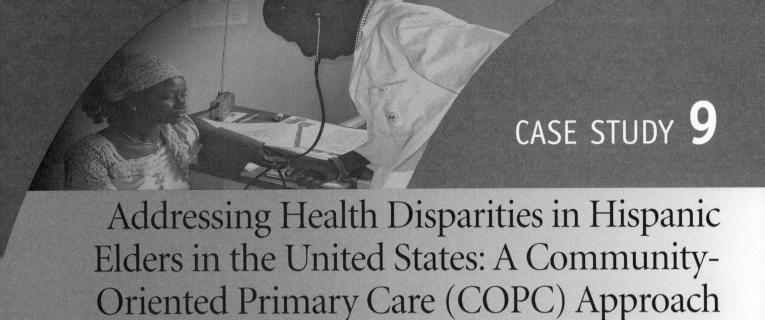

Addressing Health Disparities in Hispanic Elders in the United States: A Community-Oriented Primary Care (COPC) Approach

Patrik Johansson, Jennifer Tsai, Melissa Klein, and Jaime Gofin

BACKGROUND

The Office of Management and Budget's (OMB) *Classification of Federal Data on Race and Ethnicity* defines Hispanic/Latino as "a person of Cuban, Mexican, Puerto Rican, South or Central American, or other Spanish culture or origin, regardless of race."[1] Because race and Hispanic origin are viewed as separate concepts by OMB, Hispanics may be of any race. According to the US Census Bureau, in 2004, the majority of Hispanics (58.5%) indicated that their race was white alone, and 35.2% indicated that they were "Some Other Race."[2]

With 46.7 million self-identified individuals who represent 15% of the total US population, Hispanics are the largest minority group in the United States.[3] Furthermore, demographers project that the Hispanic population will triple to 132.8 million during the 2008 to 2050 time period and that the proportion of Hispanics in comparison to the nation's total population will double from 15% to 30%.[3] In 2004, the US Census Bureau indicated that the three largest Hispanic subgroups in the United States included Mexican Americans (28.3 million), Puerto Rican Americans (4 million), and individuals of Central American origin (3.4 million). [4]

In addition to the great diversity that exists among Hispanic communities through multiple national backgrounds, the length of residence in the territory that has become the United States adds to the heterogeneity in this population. There are Hispanic communities in the United States whose origins predate the founding of the country; however, their neighbors may include recently arrived Hispanic immigrants. According to the US Census Bureau, in 2004, close to three-quarters of Hispanics were US citizens, either through birth (about 61%) or naturalization (about 11%), and 28% of

Hispanics were foreign born and had not become US citizens. English language fluency varies among new arrivals and long-term residents of the United States.[2,5] Educational attainment and income vary significantly among Hispanic subpopulations; however, on average a smaller proportion of Hispanics complete college than non-Hispanic whites. In 2004, 12.7% of Hispanics had a bachelors or more advanced degree, in comparison to 29.7% of non-Hispanic whites.[2] In 2007, the median income for Hispanic households was $38,679, in comparison to the median income of $54,920 for non-Hispanic white households.[6] Furthermore, it is significant to note that overall, Hispanics have the highest uninsured rates of any racial or ethnic group in the United States. Between 2005 and 2007, Hispanics had an average uninsurance rate of 32.8% in comparison to non-Hispanic whites, who had an uninsurance rate of 14.5%.[6]

Different Hispanic subpopulations reside in different states. For example, in California and Texas, the largest subgroup is Mexican Americans, and in Florida and New York, the largest subpopulations include Cuban Americans and Puerto Rican or Dominican Americans, respectively. The Hispanic population is young in comparison to the total US population. In 2007, the Hispanic population had a median age of 27.6 years, and that of the total population was 36.6 years. Nearly 34% of the Hispanic population was younger than 18 years old, compared with 25% of the total population.[7] By 2050, demographers predict that Hispanics will be the fastest-growing population in the 65 years and older age cohort, reaching 15 million.[8]

Healthcare disparities refer to differences in the access, use, quality, or outcomes of healthcare services received by racial or ethnic minority groups.[9] According to the *National Healthcare Disparities Report*—an annual report to the US Congress published by the Agency for Healthcare Research and Quality, part of the US Department of Health and Human Services (HHS)—Hispanic elders experience significant healthcare disparities in comparison to the non-Hispanic white elderly population in forms ranging from poorer access to health care to poorer diabetes control.[10]

In 2007, in response to the findings from the report, five agencies[a] of HHS announced the creation of the HHS Improving Hispanic Elders' Health: Community Partnerships for Evidence-Based Solutions Initiative (the Hispanic Elders Project). The project involved eight coalitions across the United States participating in a pilot initiative aimed at bringing together coalitions of local leaders from communities with large numbers of Hispanic elders. The coalitions reviewed the latest research findings and promising practices to create and implement their own local plans to address one or more health disparities facing their respective communities.[10]

THE HEALTH STATUS OF THE COMMUNITY

The National Institutes of Health defines health disparities as "differences in the incidence, prevalence, mortality, and burden of diseases and other health conditions that exist among spe-

---

aThe five agencies included the Administration on Aging, the Agency for Healthcare Research and Quality, the Health Resources and Services Administration, the Centers for Disease Control and Prevention, and the Centers for Medicare & Medicaid Services.

cific population groups in the United States."[11] Different populations affected by disparities include racial and ethnic minorities, the elderly, individuals with disabilities, and residents in rural areas.

Type II diabetes disproportionately affects the elderly and racial and ethnic minority groups, including Hispanic subpopulations.[12] Estimates by the Office of Minority Health (part of HHS) observe the following:[13]

- In a national survey conducted from 2003 to 2006, Mexican Americans were almost two times more likely than non-Hispanic white adults to have been diagnosed with diabetes by a physician.[12,14]
- In 2002, Hispanics were 1.7 times as likely to start treatment for end-stage renal disease related to diabetes, compared to non-Hispanic whites.[15]
- In 2005, Hispanics were 1.6 times as likely as non-Hispanic whites to die from diabetes.[16]

Healthcare disparities in quality of care exist between Hispanics and non-Hispanic whites. Studies indicate that Hispanics are less likely than non-Hispanic whites to receive recommended services for diabetes care, such as hemoglobin A1C (HbA1c) testing, eye examinations, and foot examinations.[2,17,18] HbA1c is glycosylated hemoglobin; it provides information about blood sugar levels over a 3-month period and indicates how well one is controlling his or her diabetes. Eye and foot examinations are recommended because diabetics are more prone to retinopathy, which predisposes to blindness, and nonhealing foot sores that can lead to amputations.

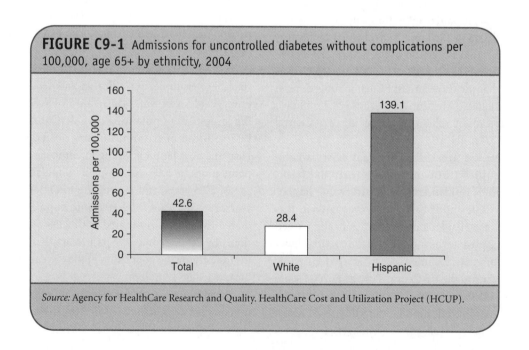

FIGURE C9-1 Admissions for uncontrolled diabetes without complications per 100,000, age 65+ by ethnicity, 2004

Source: Agency for HealthCare Research and Quality. HealthCare Cost and Utilization Project (HCUP).

Disparities between Hispanics and non-Hispanic whites persist for receipt of HbA1c tests and foot exams, even after controlling for socioeconomic status.[17]

Diabetes requires constant monitoring by both the provider and the patient. Loss of control of the condition can lead to hospitalizations. Figure C9-1 shows the number of admissions per 100,000 for the elderly and indicates that Hispanics are more than three times as likely to be hospitalized for diabetes as whites.

Hispanic elders represent the fastest-growing segment of the US elder population and experience health disparities in the form of a disproportionate burden of diabetes. In addition, they experience healthcare disparities by means of poorer diabetes control and access to care. Hispanic elders face many obstacles to health care, including linguistic and cultural barriers that may contribute to these disparities. For example, although Hispanic community organizations may provide medical care, nutrition counseling, exercise classes, or other programs, very few maintain sufficient resources or expertise to meet the needs of the growing elderly population. Culturally and linguistically appropriate services for elderly Hispanics are not always available across the country, and social services organizations that have long-standing histories of serving English-speaking populations often do not employ a sufficient number of bilingual staff members or translators.[2,19]

THE INTERVENTION PROGRAM

To address health and healthcare disparities facing Hispanic elders, the Administration on Aging, the Agency for Healthcare Research and Quality, the Centers for Disease Control and Prevention, the Centers for Medicare & Medicaid Services, and the Health Resources and Services Administration convened community coalitions tasked with creating and implementing their own local plans to address one or more health disparities affecting Hispanic elders. On the basis of a competitive selection process that took into account the presence of large Hispanic populations, HHS selected sites in Chicago, Illinois; Houston, Texas; Los Angeles, California; Lower Rio Grande Valley, Texas; Miami, Florida; New York City, New York; San Antonio, Texas; and San Diego, California.[19] Each site engaged in a coalition-building process with relevant community organizations, including at least one representative from a local Hispanic community organization, aging services provider, healthcare provider, public health agency, health services research organization, and Area Agency on Aging.

Employing principles of community-oriented primary care (COPC) with technical assistance from the George Washington University School of Public Health and Health Services Department of Prevention and Community Health, community coalitions undertook the following steps:

1. Defining and characterizing a target community of Hispanic elders experiencing health disparities within their area.
2. Prioritizing a health disparity issue to address through an intervention in the target community.
3. Conducting a detailed assessment of the health disparity issue.
4. Planning an intervention to address the health disparity issue.
5. Implementing the intervention.
6. Evaluating and reassessing the intervention.

The availability of resources, existing data on the target population, and coalition composition drove the proposed interventions for each site participating in the initiative. All eight community coalitions prioritized diabetes as one of the highest-ranking health problems facing the community. Because of the high prevalence of Hispanic elders who had already been diagnosed and were treated for diabetes, coalitions did not focus on primary prevention, which seeks to delay or halt the development of diabetes. In conducting detailed assessments, community coalitions prioritized secondary prevention (the prevention of complications of diabetes in individuals already diagnosed with the disease) and tertiary prevention (the controlling of complications of diabetes).[20]

Interventions varied by site; common elements included implementing new or expanding existing diabetes or other chronic disease self-management programs, increasing coordination or linkages among provider services and aging or social services, improving physician adherence to diabetes standards of care to reduce complications and improve quality of care, and implementing other evidence-based programs for prevention of complications from diabetes.

Evaluation

An evaluation of the Hispanic Elders Project revealed that all community coalitions created an intervention plan that addressed diabetes disparities in the target population. In addressing diabetes, the eight coalitions focused primarily on secondary and tertiary prevention. Six of the eight coalitions based their interventions on the Stanford Chronic Disease Self-Management and Diabetes Self Management Programs (CDSMP/DSMP).[21,22] The programs are workshop-based initiatives given in community settings, such as senior centers, where at least one trained non-health-professional leader with a chronic disease him- or herself facilitates the program. The programs designed to enhance regular treatment and chronic disease-specific education, such as diabetes instruction.[21] In employing the CDSMP, one site conducted 10 workshops that reached more than 110 participants. Other evaluation efforts focused on coalition-building aspects of the project. Telephone interviews were conducted by the designated coalition coordinators and consultants from the Department of Prevention and Community Health of the George Washington University School of Public Health and Health Services. The interviews revealed that perceived successes of the coalition included raising awareness of the healthcare disparities affecting Hispanic elders at local, county, and state levels; bringing together new and diverse partners who shared resources and built ongoing relationships to create an intervention program; putting together a plan to address healthcare disparities affecting Hispanic elders; engaging in interdisciplinary efforts; and getting much done with no direct funding.

COMMUNITY INVOLVEMENT AND INTERSECTORAL COOPERATION

From its inception, the Hispanic Elders Project underscored the importance of interdisciplinary work across organizational boundaries to link aging services providers, medical care providers, Hispanic community organizations, health services research organizations, and public agencies to promote the use of evidence-based prevention programs, new Medicare benefits, and other initiatives that could reduce health disparities among Hispanic elders. Each community coalition included representation from the local Area Agency on Aging, community-based organizations with a focus on Hispanic elders, the local public health agency, healthcare providers, other senior services providers, and health services research organizations. Staff from each of the five federal agencies, consultants from Academy-Health, and experts from the National Council on Aging and the Department of Prevention and Community Health of the George Washington University School of Public Health and Health Services provided technical assistance in the form of community-level data on health indicators; tailored site visits; facilitation of learning and the exchange of information and best practices among teams through conference calls and confer-

ences; and guidance on COPC implementation with particular emphasis on prioritization, detailed problem assessment, and intervention planning. HHS agencies provided national leadership and key technical assistance in the following forms:

- data tools to help communities target interventions to populations and geographic areas with the greatest need
- resource guides to help communities design effective, sustainable, culturally appropriate services
- a virtual office for electronic housing and sharing of resources

LESSONS LEARNED

- Preventing and managing complications of diabetes (secondary and tertiary prevention, respectively) in the elderly was a priority in the communities participating in the HHS Hispanic Elders Project.
- In addressing diabetes, the coalitions favored a community-based approach, primarily in the form of the CDSMP.
- Ongoing technical assistance based on the COPC approach constituted a relevant component in the systematic process focused in the community setting, with the goal of creating an intervention plan addressing one or more disparities among Hispanic elders.
- The coalitions succeeded in implementing interventions aimed at addressing health disparities in Hispanic elders.
- The formation of community coalitions allowed for new professional relationships and partnerships to form, sharing of resources, networking opportunities, and interdisciplinary work to take place that would not have otherwise.
- Both long-distance learning via electronic communication and close attention to personal individual needs appear to have facilitated the implementation of evidence-based interventions by the coalitions in the communities.

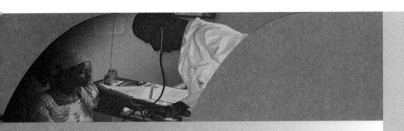

Discussion Questions

- How does the US Office of Management and Budget define *Hispanic*?

- What are the challenges with grouping Hispanic subgroups into one category when developing healthcare interventions for members of this community?

- What are health disparities versus healthcare disparities? Please give examples of each within the context of Hispanic elders.

- Why did the US Department of Health and Human Services choose to address health disparities through a focused effort on Hispanic elders?

- How did the HHS Hispanic Elders Project employ principles of COPC in the project's development?

REFERENCES

1. Office of Management and Budget. Office of Management and Budget revisions to the standards for the classification of federal data on race and ethnicity. http://www.whitehouse.gov/omb/fedreg_1997standards/. Accessed July 2009.

2. US Department of Commerce Economics and Statistics Administration, US Census Bureau. *The American Community—Hispanics: 2004.* 2007. Available at http://www.census.gov/prod/2007pubs/acs-03.pdf. Accessed April 10, 2010.

3. US Census Bureau. An older and more diverse nation by midcentury. http://www.census.gov/Press-Release/www/releases/archives/population/012496.html. Accessed July 2009.

4. US Census Bureau. Hispanics in the United States. http://www.census.gov/population/www/socdemo/hispanic/files/Internet_Hispanic_in_U.S._2006.ppt#504,15,Top "Top Five States by Hispanic Population Size: 2006." Accessed July, 2009.

5. Pew Hispanic Center. English usage among Hispanics in the United States. http://pewhispanic.org/files/reports/82.pdf. Published November 29, 2007. Accessed November 2009.

6. Denavas-Walt C, Proctor BD, Smith JC. *US Census Bureau, Current Population Reports, P60-235, Income, Poverty, and Health Insurance in the United States: 2007.* Washington DC: U.S. Government Printing Office.

7. US Census Bureau. US Hispanic population surpasses 45 million; now 15 percent of total. http://www.census.gov/Press-Release/www/releases/archives/population/011910.html. Accessed July 2009.

8. Federal Interagency Forum on Aging-Related Health Statistics. *Older Americans 2008 Key Indicators of Well-Being.* Federal Interagency Forum on Aging-Related Statistics. Washington, DC: U.S. Government Printing Office, March 2008,

9. LaVeist T. *Minority Populations and Health: An Introduction to Health Disparities in the United States.* San Francisco, CA: Jossey-Bass; 2005.

10. AcademyHealth. Improving Hispanic elders' health: community partnerships for evidence-based solutions. http://www.academyhealth.org/ahrq/elders/#growth. Accessed July 2009.

11. National Cancer Institute. Defining health disparities. http://crchd.cancer.gov/disparities/defined.html. Accessed July 2009.

12. Agency for Healthcare Research and Quality. *2008 National Healthcare Disparities Report.* 2008. AHRQ Publication No. 09-0002.

13. Office of Minority Health. Diabetes and Hispanic Americans. http://www.omhrc.gov/templates/content.aspx?lvl=2&lvlID=54&ID=3324. Accessed July 2009.

14. National Center for Health Statistics. *Health, United States, 2008 with Chartbook.* Hyattsville, MD: National Center for Health Statistics; 2009:276.

15. Centers for Disease Control and Prevention. Data & trends national diabetes surveillance system end stage renal disease. http://www.cdc.gov/diabetes/statistics/esrd/mRatePerDiab.htm. Accessed April 2010.

16. Centers for Disease Control. *National Vital Statistics Report.* 2008. Vol. 56. No. 10. Table 17.

17. Mainous AG III, Diaz VA, Koopman RJ, Everett CJ. Quality of care for Hispanic adults with diabetes. *Fam Med.* 2007;39:351–356.

18. Varma R, Torres M, Peña F, Klein R, Azen SP, and Los Angeles Latino Eye Study Group. Prevalence of diabetic retinopathy in adult Latinos: the Los Angeles Latino Eye Study. *Ophthalmology.* 2004;111:1298–1306.

19. Medical News Today. Eight communities selected to participate in HHS Hispanic elders initiative, USA. http://www.medicalnewstoday.com/articles/80773.php. Accessed July 2009.

20. US Department of Health and Human Services. Diabetes prevention and control: a public health imperative. http://www.healthierus.gov/STEPS/summit/prevportfolio/strategies/reducing/diabetes/prevention.htm. Accessed November 2009.

21. Stanford School of Medicine, Department of Education. Chronic disease self-management program. http://patienteducation.stanford.edu/programs/cdsmp.html. Accessed July 2009.

22. University of Illinois at Chicago, Midwest Latino Health Research, Training and Policy Center, Jane Addams College of Social Work. Diabetes empowerment education program (DEEP). http://www.uic.edu/jaddams/mlhrc/Programs/DEEP.htm. Accessed November 2009.

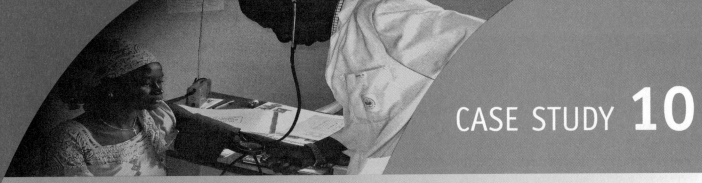

A Community-Oriented Multisector Intervention to Improve Sexual and Reproductive Health and Reduce Violence in Moldova, Eastern Europe

Elizabeth Ponce, Emma Garcia, and Elena Mereacre

BACKGROUND

Moldova is a small country (33,843.5 square kilometers) situated in southeastern Europe between Romania to the west and Ukraine to the north, east, and south. In 2008, the population was 3.57 million. Moldova became independent in 1991 following the disintegration of the Soviet Union, and the capital is Chisinau. The ethnic composition is Moldovans (75.8%), Ukrainians (8.4%), Russians (5.8%), and others (10.0%). Eastern Orthodox Christians make up more than 90% of the population, and Moldovan is the official language. About 59% of the people live in rural areas.[1] The economy depends on agriculture, featuring fruits, vegetables, tobacco, and a wine industry. In 2005, 48.5% of the population was under the national poverty line. Moldova is classified as medium in human development (ranked 111th out of 182 countries)[2] and remains, after Montenegro, the poorest country in Europe in terms of GDP.[3] Since 1994, after the main economic crisis, about 800,000 Moldovans have migrated to other European countries in search of work.[4] In 2006, 36% of the gross domestic product (GDP) depended on work remittances.[5]

Health Services

During the Soviet times, the healthcare system in Moldova promoted hospital-based care, creating a surplus of hospitals and specialists and a shortage of primary healthcare services. The primary care sector has seen significant reform since 1996 and is now based on a model of family doctors. Secondary care is provided through general hospitals at the rayon (municipal) level.[6] The healthcare services are emergency health care, primary health care, hospital and specialized outpatient health care, mother and child health care, and family planning. There are state sanitary epidemiologic services and a national program for combating tuberculosis and HIV/AIDS, as well as a national immunization program.

In 2008, the infant mortality rate in Moldova was 12.2/1000 live births, and life expectancy was 69 years. Almost 100% of young people and adults are literate. For the last 10 years, Moldova has faced a declining population growth rate as a result of a declining birth rate and increased death rate (10.9/1000 and 11.8/1000, respectively, in 2008).[7] For several decades, abortion was a means of preventing births and has been a prominent aspect of reproductive health in other countries in the former Soviet Union.[8] In 2006, the fertility rate was estimated at 1.4 children per woman; the percentage of pregnant adolescents was 13%. HIV/AIDS continues to be a major public health problem, with an increasing number of cases every year (254 in 2003 and 731 in 2007), especially in young people aged 15–29 years (49.5% of the cases in 2007). The prevalence of syphilis is very high at more than 250/100,000 per year.[9] High rates of illegal emigration could explain the increased cases of trafficking in persons (TIP) for sexual or labor exploitation, with very serious consequences to the victims. Most of the victims of TIP have been victims of physical or sexual abuse before departure.[4]

THE HEALTH STATUS OF THE COMMUNITY

This program deals with three rural communities in the Ialoveni District of Moldova: Costesti, Molesti, and Hansca villages, located 14 to 20 kilometers from Chisinau. The population in 2004 was about 18,000 people. The three villages are among the poorest in Moldova, despite multiple local and international actions addressing poverty and recent progress from its small economic base (agriculture, fishing, vegetables, and wine). The communities are characterized by very high rates of unemployment and migration. In the last 10 years, there were 56 identified cases of TIP in Costesi.

The number of HIV cases and sexually transmitted infections (STI) in 2002 and 2004 were 64 and 73, respectively; adolescent pregnancies accounted for 37% of all pregnancies in Hansca. In 2006, the baseline Knowledge, Attitudes, and Practices assessment among schoolchildren aged 13–19 years showed high rates of risk behaviors related to pregnancy and STI/HIV—7.1% had a sexual experience before the age of 18 years; 32% had unprotected sex; 46% consumed alcohol very often; and 24% reported domestic violence and sexual violence on the streets and discotheques.[10]

The main determinants associated with the risk behaviors were lack of information; communication problems with parents and friends about sexual issues; lack of life skills; lack of access to condoms; lack of adolescent supervision as a consequence of parents' migration (about 37.4% of young people aged 10–14 years has at least one parent abroad); lack of access to healthcare services; and lack of educational and leisure facilities. Gender inequality and poverty were probably associated with the spread of violence and the high rate of migration and TIP, especially among young people.

THE INTERVENTION PROGRAM

The target population for the intervention program was aged 13 to 30 years (about 5000 people in the three communities). In 2005, given the situation of this population, the local NGO Compasiune[a] and the Swiss association Vivere[b] created a comprehensive, community-based program in Costesti, Molesti, and Hansca, applying the community-oriented primary care (COPC) approach. The program was developed as follows.

Identification of Main Needs

Two meetings were organized for identifying the main needs with representatives of the target population, local authorities, and leaders to share the findings of Compasiune and Vivere.

Setting Priorities

It was evident that there was a community syndrome with strong and complex relationships among sexual and reproductive health (SRH), HIV/AIDS, violence, and TIP. Young

people with STIs and the victims of sexual violence and TIP, with the purpose of sexual exploitation, are more vulnerable to HIV or high-risk behaviors. Thus STIs, HIV, unwanted pregnancies, violence, and trafficking were selected as priorities for intervention.

Planning

Using a logical framework approach (LFA),[11] a program for youth on SRH, violence, and trafficking was drafted. The objective was to create a community-based comprehensive model to prevent unwanted pregnancies, STIs, HIV, gender-based violence, and TIP and to rehabilitate TIP victims. The activities included the following:

Services: Provide comprehensive, free, and confidential services that are coherent and integrated with national youth policies, and develop a multisectoral intervention.

Community interventions: Protect human rights and address gender issues, resilience, risk, and protective factors among vulnerable populations; develop relevant skills among youth and implement peer-to-peer education; strengthen the community response and support local youth initiatives; and carry out capacity-building activities.

Procuring financial resources: Three proposals were written and approved.

Capacity building: Hire and train a multidisciplinary team consisting of an educator, psychologist, family doctor, gynecologist, nurse, and social assistant. The training would include survey methodology, health promotion and education, counseling, outreach, integrated communications for behavioral change, and other relevant issues for the program.

Program Implementation

Five axes (alternatives of interventions) were developed:

- Axis 1, health promotion and prevention: This axis was aimed at increasing young people's access to an integrated communication program (ICP) to promote a healthy lifestyle. The activities included training of volunteers; a communication program through mass media; seminars about SRH, HIV, STIs, unwanted pregnancy (**A**bstinence, **B**e faithful, and **C**ondom approach), violence, and TIP; counseling and hotline services; and condom distribution.
- Axis 2, creation of a youth-friendly health center (YFHC): A fully equipped Avante YFHC was created in the building of the local health center. Holistic, confidential, and free services were provided 5 days a week for 4 hours in

the afternoon. The services provided were care, information, and counseling on general health, SRH, HIV, STIs, nutrition, and hygiene; management techniques for violence and trafficking; mental health and social support; support for very poor victims of violence or TIP; and a multisectoral two-way referral system (MSRS). Local and regional institutions (health, social, legal, and education institutions from the public, private, and civil society sectors) were contacted to create the MSRS. Outreach activities were developed to identify vulnerable people. Avante was included in the YFHC network, and records and a database were developed and shared with 11 YFHC centers that were created by the government in Moldova.

- Axis 3, vocational training: Axis 3 was aimed at improving the socioeconomic status of women and reduce gender inequalities. Four vocational courses (sewing, hairdressing, cooking, and computer courses) for very poor women or victims of violence and TIP were organized in 2008.
- Axis 4, community mobilization: A key strategy for community mobilization included influencing decision makers to change or implement SRH and violence policies and increase resource allocation for youth. The program developed the partnership approach where local authorities and youth themselves become partners in the action. This axis integrated participatory advocacy tools to reach policy makers and local authorities and provided opportunities for learning and sharing information about SRH, violence, and TIP and to increase awareness about the youth situation.
- Axis 5, creation of a youth-friendly sports center (YFSC): Axis 5 was aimed at increasing young people's access to appropriate leisure facilities for better supervision. The activities included the creation of a sports center (Avante YFSC) and the support of young people in arts and crafts.

Evaluation

In 2006, the Vivere and Compasiune team applied the input–process–output–outcome–impact framework for monitoring and evaluating the program. Knowledge, attitudes, and behavior changes were assessed before and after the implementation of the ICP among young people, volunteers, parents, teachers, and local leaders. Monthly monitoring and biannual process and outcomes evaluations were organized with the participation of formal partners, local leaders, and youth representatives.

A process and outputs evaluation on December 31, 2008, showed the following:

- Axis 1, health promotion and prevention: One hundred volunteers received diplomas as peer-to-peer educators; young people, parents, authorities, and local leaders (1598 in total) were reached through seminars; 551 calls were registered at the hotline service; and more than 4000 condoms were distributed. The constraints were a great migration of young people aged 19 to 29 years or difficulties in reaching them.
- Axis 2, creation of a youth-friendly health center (YFHC): The YFHC provided consultations to 935 young people, and 26 vulnerable people received comprehensive assistance. The constraints were a lack of specialists at the local level and team turnover, and the lack of a heating system reduced the demand in winter.
- Axis 3, vocational training: A total of 68 young people received professional training.
- Axis 4, community mobilization: As a result of individual meetings, roundtables, seminars, lobbying activities, negotiations, and project visits, three formal partnerships were established and more resources were allocated. In addition, 23 local leaders were mobilized to create local committees that discussed and resolved individual cases. The local police was sensitized to identify and refer more victims of violence. Representatives of three local churches participated actively in the project roundtables.
- Axis 5, creation of a youth-friendly sports center (YFSC): A total of 204 young people frequented the YFSC; 10 dance performances were performed by youths, with at least 1200 spectators; and the youths also contributed to the decoration of the center.

An evaluation of the effects and impact of the program in December 2008 showed the following:

Knowledge and behavior: The participants' knowledge improved for contraception, HIV, and STIs; the youths felt more comfortable talking with friends about sex and condoms; there was an increased demand for condoms (from 0 to more than 4000); and the youths were better informed or searched for more information about HIV and TIP.

Life skills: There were reported improvements in refusing sex without a condom and saying no to migration (however, there was an increased percentage of people who desired to go abroad to search for work); and there was better communication with parents, friends, and boy- or girlfriends.

Community involvement: Community leaders were mobilized in multisectoral and multidisciplinary committees; volunteers with improved life skills created a local youth council and two local NGOs for youths; and church representatives no longer impeded activities, and their messages were complementary.

Health situation: There was an increase in the frequency of disclosing violence and TIP and seeking consultations to get information about STIs, HIV, and pregnancies; there was a marked decrease in the incidence of HIV and STIs; and denunciation and prosecution of violence and TIP increased, with several TIP and violence victims rehabilitated.

Reassessment: The situation was reassessed by the team and volunteers, and new problems were identified, such as increased alcohol and cigarette consumption among very young people. New actions and continuous capacity building will be implemented by the team, stakeholders, beneficiaries, and volunteers to respond to these new challenges.

COMMUNITY PARTICIPATION AND INTERSECTORAL COOPERATION

The involvement of community members and different stakeholders was embedded in the program, as seen in Axes 1–4. The youths were key actors in the program. The concerted actions of different sectors of the community were crucial for the implementation of activities and the success of the program.

After 3 years of implementation, in January 2008, the Avante YFHC was transferred to the Ministry of Health, and it continues developing the same activities that are now financed by the National Health Insurance. In 2009, Vivere was still providing technical and complementary financial support.

LESSONS LEARNED

- A COPC approach is appropriate for biopsychosocial interventions.
- A comprehensive community-based program is possible with the commitment of all members of the team, partners, stakeholders, beneficiaries, and volunteers. Formal agreements with partners ensure long-term commitment. Volunteers and peer-to-peer educators stimulate the quality of the results. They increase the coverage and ensure the continuity of activities.
- Human resources availability at the local level should be secured before starting the action. They should be trained and involved in all decisions. Good salaries could reduce turnover. Participation in a national network could ensure financial and training opportunities.
- Holistic, friendly, and free services with well-defined protocols, procedures, and approaches that consider tailored activities for each beneficiary could increase access for young people. Outreach activities are very effective in identifying vulnerable people.
- Cultural sensitivity should be considered when making key messages.
- Assessing the frequency of migration of the target populations ensures coverage.

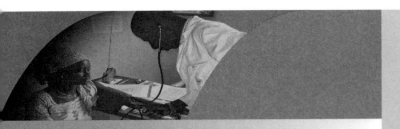

Discussion Questions

- What is the role of primary care in reproductive health, violence, and trafficking?

- What is the role of foreign NGOs and Ministries of Health in developing a trafficking prevention and reha-bilitation program?

- Is there a need for a control group to study changes in knowledge, attitudes, and practices in this intervention?

- How can sustainability be assured in this type of program?

- Is there enough evidence to spread the project's activities to other regions in Moldova? To other countries?

REFERENCES

1. National Bureau of Statistics of the Republic of Moldova. 2004 population census. http://www.statistica.md/pageview.php?l=en&idc=350&id=2208. Accessed August 2009.

2. United Nations Development Programme. Human development report, 2009. http://hdrstats.undp.org/en/countries/country_fact_sheets/cty_fs_MDA.html. Accessed July 2009.

3. World Bank. Gross domestic product 2008. http://siteresources.world bank.org/DATASTATISTICS/Resources/GDP.pdf. Accessed July 2009.

4. International Organization for Migration. Moldova. Trafficking as it is: a statistical profile. 2005-2006 update. http://www.iom.md/materials/brochures/3_ct_traff_eng.pdf. Accessed February 2010.

5. Ratha D, Zhimei X. *Migration and Remittances Factbook 2008.* Washington, DC: World Bank Group; 2008. http://publications.worldbank.org/ecommerce/catalog/product?item_id=8084331. Accessed July 2009.

6. Atun R, Richardson E, Shishkin S, et al. Moldova: Health system review. *Health Systems in Transition.* 2008; 10(5): 1–138:p 17. http://www.euro.who.int/observatory/CtryInfo/CtryInfoRes?COUNTRY=MDA&CtryInput Submit=

7. National Bureau of Statistics of the Republic of Moldova. Statistical data. http://www.statistica.md/index.php?l=en#idc=34&. Accessed February 2010.

8. Ashford L. *Reproductive Health Trends in Eastern Europe and Eurasia.* Washington, DC: Population Reference Bureau; 2005. http://www.prb.org/Publications/PolicyBriefs/ReproductiveHealthTrendsinEasternEuropeand Eurasia.aspx. Accessed July 2009.

9. National Scientific and Applied Center for Preventive Medicine, *Information Bulletin About the Epidemiological Situation of HIV, Ministry of Health and Social Protection, Moldova, 2007.*

10. Ponce E, Mereacre E, Garcia E, Dunai L, Spino E, Bivol E. *Sexual and reproductive health and violence: Effectiveness of training courses in changing knowledge, attitudes and behaviours of young people and parents in the villages of Costesti and Hansca.* Vivere- Chisinau, 2006–2008. In press.

11. Australian Agency for International Development. AusGuideline activity design 3.3. The logical framework approach. http://www.ausaid.gov.au/ausguide/pdf/ausguideline3.3.pdf. Published October 2005. Accessed August 2009.

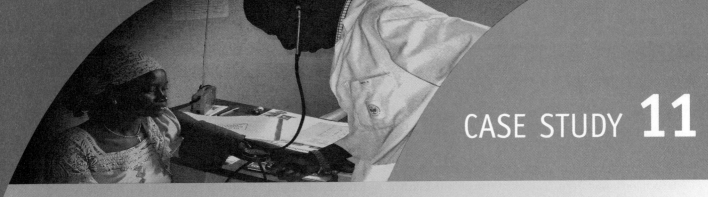

Community-Oriented Public Health (COPH): The Case of Catalonia, Spain

Josep Lluís de Peray and Angelina González

BACKGROUND

Catalonia is a region in the northeast of Spain with a wide political and administrative autonomy, which includes the Catalan Health System. The Catalan Health System governance is divided into eight health regions, each of them divided into a number of health zone authorities (Govern Territorial de Salut, or GTS). The GTS is the decision-making entity in which healthcare decisions are made and performed by the healthcare providers with the participation of the community. The GTS is the smallest public health entity run by a public health team (PHT). There are 36 GTS in Catalonia.

Public health is understood as the responsibility of the public administrations and the organized community, which takes into consideration the healthcare needs and determinants of health of the population and acts through performing its functions (see Chapter 5). This is done through activities of health protection, health promotion and disease prevention, and public health surveillance.

The reform of the Catalonian public health system is being developed in different directions: (1) legal actions, with the creation of a public health law; (2) organizational activities, with the creation of a new public health agency across the eight health zones and 36 GTS that include change management; and (3) demonstrative activities to test the feasibility of the model. Seven survey areas are testing the feasibility of the model, and they are developing team work in public health within the public health agency in coordination with primary health care and other agents to address the most important health needs of the population. The activities that are being supported by the agency are availability and management of demographic and epidemiologic data; criteria and methods for health needs assessment; tools and experiences of participative prioritization; and design and evaluation of health programs, as well as the performance of good practices in the coordination of services to improve overall system efficiency.

The new public health agency is a shared framework between public health and primary health care, thus providing an opportunity to describe and analyze some community-oriented experiences. Two key elements of public health reform are (1) improving the value of public health actions when they are addressed to social health determinants through intersectoral actions and (2) orienting the public health services to the main community needs in specific territories, such as districts or neighborhoods.

In addition, this process is concurrent with the progressive consolidation of a model of community-oriented primary health care, which covers 10% of the 400 primary healthcare teams of Catalonia. These centers are part of the AUPA (Actuant Units per a la Salut—Towards Unity for Health) network (see Case Study 12) that gathers both the experience of community-oriented primary care (COPC) and The Network: Towards Unity for Health (TUFH).[1] Other centers have been included in AUPA through a plan of community development led by the municipality.

The Catalan Healthcare System

In Spain, the total amount of public investment in health care is €1.250 per inhabitant per year (US$1.700), which is 6% of the GDP. This investment is financed by taxes and is administered across the health departments of each of the 17 autonomous communities into which Spain is divided.[2] The

Spanish system is universal, free in the provision of healthcare services, geographically based, multidisciplinary, equitable, and efficient.

In Catalonia, of the total of resources dedicated to health, 61% is spent on hospital care, 22% on primary health, and 5% on social health care. In Catalonia, there are 400 primary health centers, 61 hospitals, 37 mental health centers, 65 drug addiction centers, 200 social health centers, and 36 public health offices. Regarding human resources, there are 2.2 physicians, 2.7 nurses, and 1.9 auxiliary nurses per 1000 inhabitants.

Primary health centers are open 24 hours a day, 7 days a week through the whole year. There is a referral system to the next level of care (i.e., for specialists and mental health). Primary health centers have diagnostic and treatment capacity to solve more than 85% of the health problems. The rate of visits is high, with more than seven consultations per inhabitant per year.[3]

The healthcare system in Catalonia, like the rest of Spain, is based on primary care teams. Teams are formed by family doctors, pediatricians, nurses, midwives (in some teams), social workers, and administrative professionals. Every team attends to an assigned population that is geographically delimited, ranging from 7500 to 30,000 people. The teams provide continuous care through the life course.

The professionals and workers of the primary health teams receive a salary with benefits, depending on the job conditions, characteristics of the place where the team is based, and for performing management and teaching tasks. For the users, there is not direct payment for the service, but there are copayments for some pharmaceutical products.

THE HEALTH STATUS OF THE COMMUNITY

The Catalan region, which covers 32,000 square kilometers, has a population of 7.5 million (14% are immigrants). In Catalonia, there are 11.7 births per 1000 inhabitants, and the standardized mortality rate is 6.8 deaths per 1000 inhabitants. There are 105 persons older than 65 years for each 1000 persons who are younger than 15 years. The life expectancy is 77 years for men and 84 years for women. The infant mortality rate is 2.87 per 1000 live births. Fifty percent of the population older than 75 years needs help with the basic activities of daily living.[4]

Regarding lifestyle, 25% of people aged 15 years and older are sedentary. There is an increased prevalence of overweight and obesity, especially among the population younger than 15 years old. The percentage of smokers among the age group 15 to 75 years is 29%. The most common chronic diseases are chronic back pain, arthritis and degenerative osteoarthritis, problems of the circulatory system, hypertension, varicose veins, migraine and headache, and depression and anxiety.[5]

The main infectious diseases according to compulsory reports are tuberculosis, legionellosis, hepatitis A and B, HIV/AIDS, and sexually transmitted diseases. The main causes of death for all age groups are problems of the circulatory system, cancer, respiratory diseases, gastric system diseases, mental problems, neurological diseases, and external causes, in this order. The causes of premature death are traffic accidents, AIDS, suicides and self-injury, lymphoma, pneumonia, and leukemia.[2]

THE INTERVENTION PROGRAM

The new public health agency, through the public health team in the various GTS, is involved in different community health programs, one of them being Health in the Neighborhoods.[6] This program shows many elements of public health action working together with primary care services to address the main health needs of the community.

Health in the Neighborhoods was born after the law for the improvement of neighborhoods, urban areas, and villages with special needs was passed (Law 2/2004, June 4). This law was promulgated by the Catalan government to promote an intensive improvement of infrastructures and resources of neighborhoods with urban problems and at risk of social exclusion. The process is initiated when the municipalities present a project in a yearly competitive call. Selected projects receive funding from both the municipality and the central government. The funding is spent in neighborhood gentrification to stop urban regression processes, improve residents' life conditions, and facilitate social cohesion. In each of the selected neighborhoods, a follow-up commission is created to evaluate the process. Citizens are part of that commission. During the 5 years since the approval of the law, €1000 million have been invested in 92 neighborhoods where 700,000 people live (10% of the total Catalonian population).

The urban project has been joined by other departments of the Catalonia government, among them the Department of Health (DOH) with the program Health in the Neighborhoods. The DOH realizes that urban gentrification offers not only an opportunity to identify places, sectors, and collectives that are especially vulnerable with respect to health, but it also provides an opportunity to make changes in the health determinants of the community from different perspectives.

Health in the Neighborhoods started with an analysis of determinants and mechanisms of inequalities to determine and promote the implementation of concrete actions (from the healthcare system and from the municipality) to minimize their effects. The public health agency was appointed to develop and administer this program. The strategy is based on the following premises:

1. Analysis of social and cultural determinants that produce inequalities in health
2. Cooperative work with municipalities in planning, action, and evaluation
3. Promotion of community health by working on disease prevention and health promotion together with primary healthcare teams
4. Prioritization in the development and improvement of healthcare services for specific areas with higher social and health needs

In each neighborhood a Local Leader Team (LLT) for the program is formed. LLT members are regional health authorities who are responsible for health and social services in the municipality. The LLT forms a nominal group (NG), which is an interdisciplinary group of all healthcare professionals working in the neighborhood, as well as the social workers or other local workers and nongovernmental organizations (NGOs). The NG follows a working process, using qualitative methods, guided by a team of experts. The NG is responsible for defining needs and possible actions to be carried out to reduce inequalities. The level, as well as the timing, in which population participation is included in the process varies with the history and characteristics of the place.

When the NG has diagnosed the health needs in the neighborhood and has proposed some actions, the LLT prioritizes actions that will become the specific health program for that neighborhood. The LLT establishes the distribution of responsibilities among the local health agents.

To complement local actions, the DOH offers a specific catalog of health promotion services in these neighborhoods. Some examples of the services funded by the DOH are free pills to help people stop smoking, workshops addressed to primary health teams or municipalities (healthy life education for elderly people; food advice for different cultural groups; and identification and prevention of violence in elderly people, women, and children), and workshops addressed to schools (promotion of vegetables and fruits and review of food menus). Moreover, those selected neighborhoods are high-priority action zones for all initiatives of the DOH.

The assessment helped identify five groups with specific characteristics—children, youth, women, elderly people, and immigrants. Neighborhoods were assessed for similar health problems, like higher burden of disease than in the general population and early exposure to risky environments.

Prioritized actions by the different LLTs are classified in three ways: (1) actions related to the most prevalent health problems in vulnerable groups; (2) actions that address the reorganization of services and training of professionals; and (3) actions

to develop specific interventions or a catalog of specifically designed actions for neighborhoods with special needs.

In 2009, 40 out of 92 selected neighborhoods have completed the needs assessment. Actions and improvement programs have been started in eight of those areas. Each of the actions contains its own follow-up and evaluation process. Parallel to the needs assessment and prioritization of actions in each of the selected neighborhoods, the process has generated a shared work space where social workers and healthcare professionals meet. This has happened at the primary health and health administration levels. In some places these dynamics were already in place, but for others it has been one of the benefits of the program.

COMMUNITY PARTICIPATION AND INTERSECTORAL COOPERATION

Community organizations of different kinds and backgrounds are basic elements for the effective development of community activities. These organizations act as process facilitators, perform key activities, and mediate with health services, thus allowing community participation. The increased presence of these organizations has become the third sector of social and health services activity as seen from a broad perspective.

LESSONS LEARNED

- The articulation of public health services through primary health services with a community orientation is an opportunity to develop effective community health care.
- There is a need for networking among the different agents—public health, municipalities, and primary health agents. It is important to know who these agents are, what they do, and which programs are being implemented. Moreover, agents need to have the ability and flexibility to work together.
- Intersectoral cooperation and working, starting from the local level and including the managers, is needed to have more effective health policies.
- For the success of these projects, it is essential that decision makers in the neighborhood's health structure (the ones forming the LLT) perceive the process (the methodology and assessment) as an opportunity to improve the health of the vulnerable groups in their area.
- The assessment process for the 40 neighborhoods provided rich information about health-related problems. In most cases it is not possible to solve them within the local level; answers are needed at a regional level. There is a need to find new answers to the problems that arise, like undesired pregnancies, drug consumption by youths, and lack of social networks among elderly people.

- The assessment results may question the need to repeat all phases of the program in each neighborhood. But the fact that the process itself creates a shared identification of health needs and reinforces a common interest among different agents to act together indicates the importance of implementing all phases in each neighborhood.
- Gender, poverty, and other living conditions give birth to a specific pattern of vulnerability that is constant in Catalonia, thus creating inequalities in health. The need for specific actions or resources in these neighborhoods is evident. The process generated by the law has helped to open one path toward reducing health inequalities in Catalonia. Public health services facilitate and extend the actions of the healthcare system beyond the walls of the health centers. This is one of the values of the public health reform.

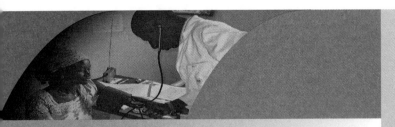

Discussion Questions

- With the available information, can you characterize the healthcare system in Catalonia, Spain?

- With the available information, can you characterize the main health problems in the present context?

- In your opinion, should neighborhoods be an object of special actions?

- Which are the methodological elements that you identify in the program Health in the Neighborhoods?

- Where can you identify the community's participation and the responsibilities of the healthcare system in the presented program?

REFERENCES

1. The Network: Towards Unity For Health. What is The Network: Towards Unity for Health? http://www.the-networktufh.org/home/index.asp. Accessed June 2009.

2. Departament de Salut. Salut en Xifres. Generalitat de Catalunya. Barcelona, 2008. http://www.gencat.cat/salut/depsalut/html/ca/xifres/salutxifres_2008.pdf. Accessed June 2009.

3. Navarro V, Martin Zurro A. La Atención Primaria de Salud en España y sus comunidades autónomas. IDIAP Jordi Gol, 2009. http://www.actasanitaria.com/fileset/doc_49401_FICHERO_NOTICIA_31035.pdf. Accessed June 2009.

4. Departament de Salut. Salut en Xifres. Generalitat de Catalunya. Barcelona, 2008. http://www.gencat.cat/salut/depsalut/html/ca/xifres/salutxifres_2008.pdf. Accessed June 2009.

5. Generalitat de Catalunya. Department de Salut. Salut en Xifres. Direcció general de Planificació i Avaluació. Barcelona 2009. http://www.gencat.cat/salut/depsalut/html/ca/dir1935/salutxifres2009.pdf.

6. Sierra I, Cabezas C, Brugulat P, Mompart A. Estrategia «Salud en los barrios»: actuaciones focalizadas en territorios de especial necesidad social y de salud. *Med Clin (Barc)*. 2008;131(suppl 4):60–64.

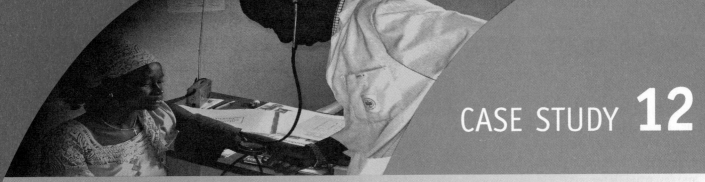

Community-Oriented Primary Care (COPC)—Atención Primaria Orientada a la Comunidad (APOC)—and the Development of a Network of Community-Oriented Health Services: The Case of Catalonia, Spain

Gonçal Foz

BACKGROUND

Community-oriented primary care (COPC) is being implemented in Spain, most significantly in Catalonia. The development of that experience will be presented in this case study.

Historical Framework

In 1983 a group of young family doctors in Catalonia were exposed to a recently published book by Sidney L. Kark, *The Practice of Community-Oriented Primary Health Care.*[1] By 1986, the Catalan Society of Family and Community Medicine (CAMFIC) organized a course, inspired by Kark's book, for family doctors and residents (Primer curs d'Atenció Primària Orientada a la Comunitat, Barcelona, February 1986). In the same year, this group of young doctors met Dr. Jaime Gofin, a member of Kark's team, who was invited by the Catalan government to a seminar for the development of primary health care.

At that time, the Catalan government was starting a process of primary healthcare reform. This was the origin of a fruitful collaboration between Dr. Gofin and the COPC working group of CAMFIC (which he helped to create); the group continues to be active today. Throughout the years, the working group developed and carried out, among other activities, capacity-building courses and workshops on COPC, which has trained more than 500 primary care professionals to date. Community-oriented primary care was then translated into Catalan (and Spanish) as Atención Primaria Orientada a la Comunidad (APOC). Additionally, the COPC working group was involved in promoting the publication of a new book on COPC by Sidney L. Kark, Emily Kark, J. H. Abramson, and Jaime Gofin,[2] which was originally written in English and

translated into Spanish for the extensive readership in Spain and Latin American countries. The working group also developed a guide on how to carry out a preliminary examination of the community, later published by CAMFIC.[3] Members of the group have also presented papers at conferences, produced other publications,[4–7] and developed a Web site.[8]

For many years, COPC was mainly a teaching experience in Spain, but presently (perhaps after a needed time to produce effects) many primary care teams in Catalonia are COPC oriented. As explained later, the development of a network of community-oriented primary care teams, Actuant Units per a la Salut (AUPA), inspired by The Network: Towards Unity for Health WHO program[9] from which it takes its name, has led to a significant increase in the community orientation of primary health care in the region.

Contextual Framework

Catalonia is one of the 17 autonomous communities in which Spain is politically organized. This political system is similar, in fact, to a federal state. The national health system of Spain is also federally constituted; every autonomous community has a specific health service, so the national health system of Spain is organized in 17 autonomous health services coordinated in a federal council.

The Spanish health system is a public system with universal coverage, and primary health care is organized in health areas of 10 to 40,000 inhabitants covered by a primary care team that works in a health center that is accessible to all the population of the area. The primary care team is composed of family physicians (1:2000 inhabitants), pediatricians (1:1200 children), nurses (1:1800 inhabitants), and a social worker.[10] The organization of health services and primary care in Spain is appropriate for the development of COPC because of its territorial base and universal coverage.

In the last census, the population of Catalonia was 7.5 million inhabitants. The Catalan health service is organized into seven health regions (Lleida, Tarragona, Terres de l'Ebre, Girona, Central, Alt Pirineu-Aran, and Barcelona) that cover between 200,000 and 700,000 inhabitants each, except the Barcelona metropolitan region, which covers more than 5 million inhabitants, and the Pyrenees region (Alt Pirineu-Aran), which covers 70,000 inhabitants.[11] The Catalan population is a typical population of a developed country—aging with a low birth rate. Since the year 2000, Catalonia has experienced the highest percentage of immigrants among all Spanish regions. Immigrants come mainly from South America, north and central Africa, eastern Europe, China, and Pakistan. These immigrants are contributing to population growth and to an increase in fertility and birth rates.

The health status is similar to other developed countries, with a low infant mortality rate and high life expectancy, and cardiovascular diseases and cancer are the main causes of death. Concomitantly, there is a high incidence of other health problems, like AIDS and unwanted pregnancies, and deleterious behaviors, such as drug abuse, smoking, alcoholism, and gender violence.

THE ORIGIN AND DEVELOPMENT OF THE AUPA NETWORK

The AUPA network was created in 2003 by the Department of Health of the Catalan Autonomous Government, co-led by the Institut d'Estudis de la Salut (Institute of Health Studies, the Catalan public institution for the training of healthcare professionals) and the Catalan Society of Family and Community Medicine (through its COPC working group), as a network to provide mutual support and training to primary care teams involved in community health activities. After the AUPA network was formed, other institutions were incorporated and support the network, including the Department of Social Psychology of the Autonomous University of Barcelona, the Association of Family and Community Nurses (AIFICC), and the Agency of Public Health of Barcelona (ASPB).

AUPA AND COPC IN THE CATALAN HEALTH SERVICE

In July 2009, 43 health teams were already incorporated in AUPA, representing more than 10% of the total Catalan primary health teams. Of these 43 teams, 15 are COPC practices, and 9 are at the preliminary stages of developing a COPC process; the rest are doing other types of community activities. Table C12-1 presents the geographic distribution and stage of COPC development.

A sizeable number of health teams are in the preliminary steps of development and became members of the network in the last 2 years. This growth expresses the current attraction of AUPA and the interest of many Catalonian health teams in extending the individual focus of their practices to beginning a community healthcare process. It is expected that most of the teams will progress to the implementation of intervention programs.[12] In some of the primary care practices, health teams are involved in community development, a process to improve the neighborhood living conditions that addresses all the pop-

TABLE C12-1 Geographic Distribution and Stage of COPC Development of Primary Care Teams in the AUPA Network

Catalan health region	Incorporation to AUPA	AUPA network		
		COPC practice	COPC preliminary steps	Community activities
Girona	2004 to 2007	3	-	1
Lleida	2009	-	2	-
Central	Since 2003	-	-	2
Barcelona	Since 2003	10	7	15
Tarragona	2003 to 2007	2	-	1
Total	Since 2003	15	9	19

ulation's identified needs in a participative way. Some of the teams are part of a Catalan government program that adresses deprived neighborhoods (see Case Study 11).

SPECIFIC FEATURES OF THE COPC PROCESS IN CATALONIA

Primary care practices in Catalonia that are involved in COPC have adapted the COPC steps to their practices, considering their local realities and resources.

Preliminary Examination

As a result of teaching COPC from 1986 to 2000 and the publication of a guide on preliminary examination of the community, many health teams in Catalonia collected data about their communities. This began soon after their exposure to COPC in the 1990s. They applied the methodology proposed in the COPC workshops, that is, a preliminary examination that includes the definition and characterization of the community and identification of health needs. Health data were gathered by the primary care teams in collaboration with public health services and with the participation of the community. The detection of health needs included the use of quantitative and qualitative methodologies. The term *preliminary examination* is frequently heard in the jargon of primary care teams in Catalonia, along with *community health diagnosis*, which describes the same concept.

Prioritization

All the teams involved in COPC practice, as well as community health processes that do not follow the COPC methodology, do prioritization analysis, frequently with community participation and intersectoral collaboration. The most frequently used process is a Nominal Group with members of the health team and representatives of other services and community institutions that consider the magnitude of the health problems as well as the effectiveness and the feasibility of the interventions. This is remarkable because in Spain, prioritization is not a usual feature in primary care practices without community intervention. Examples of prioritized groups and conditions in those practices are frail elderly; promotion of healthy habits at all ages; children, schools, teenagers, and immigrants; substance abuse in adolescents; childhood obesity; mental health; promotion of physical activity and nutritional habits; and prevention of falls in the elderly.

Community Diagnosis–Detailed Assessment

Four of the COPC teams are involved in or have completed a process of community diagnosis–detailed assessment of the prioritized health condition as proposed by the COPC approach. The diagnosis was done for the following health issues: falls in the elderly, mental health, health of immigrants, obesity, nutrition, and physical activity in children.

Evaluation

Only 1 of the 15 teams developed a complete evaluation process, reflecting the relatively short time of our experience and the need to strengthen evaluations of community health interventions.

THE FUTURE OF COPC IN CATALONIA

The historic evolution of AUPA has been an exciting process of growing and learning. As mentioned, 24 primary care teams presently practice COPC at various stages of development. It is expected that nine practices that are in the preliminary stages will further develop to become COPC practices. The experience of AUPA might provide evidence and insights about the feasibility of the process and subsequently about its effectiveness. To assist the primary care teams in their development of COPC, there is a need for follow-up and support in the early stages of their community orientation. This might be possible through the AUPA network and institutional support.

LESSONS LEARNED

- The development of COPC is a lengthy process.
- The network has allowed the teams to learn and get support from teams that already developed COPC practices. Follow-up on the development of the primary care teams' community health processes, which was not possible before creation of the network, was facilitated by the creation of AUPA.
- During the first years after a significant number of professionals were trained in COPC, some started COPC practices. Since its creation, AUPA has taken an inclusive approach to considering community-oriented activities, at any level and using any method, as candidates to be in the network. This flexibility has been key to the growth of the network, from eight health teams in 2004 to 43 teams in 2009.

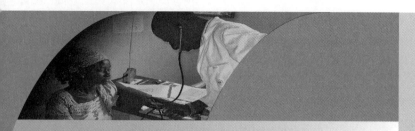

Discussion Questions

- Why is the development of a COPC practice a lengthy process?

- What are the factors that influenced the growing experience of primary care teams' community orientation in Catalonia?

- What are the benefits of a network of primary care practices?

REFERENCES

1. Kark SL. The practice of community-oriented primary health care. New York, NY: Appleton-Century-Crofts; 1981.

2. Kark SL, Kark E, Abramson JH, Gofin J, eds. Atención Primaria Orientada a la Comunidad (Community-Oriented Primary Care—COPC). Barcelona, Spain: DOYMA; 1994.

3. Grup de treball en APOC de la Societat Catalana de Medicina Familiar i Comunitària. *Aproximació al coneixement de la comunitat en Atenció Primària. Guia de recollida de dades per a l'examen preliminar de la situació de salut d'una comunitat.* 2nd ed. Barcelona, Spain: EDIDE; 2003.

4. Foz G, Martin C, Gofin J. The training in community medicine of family physicians. Presented at: Wonca European Regional Conference; 1990; Barcelona, Spain.

5. Foz G, Pañella H, Martin C, Pou R, Montaner I, Peray JL. Atención Primaria Orientada a la Comunidad. Fundamentos conceptuales y metodológicos. *Atención Primaria.* 1991;8:252–254.

6. Foz G, Gofin J, Montaner I. Atención Primaria Orientada a la Comunidad (APOC): una visión actual. In: Martin Zurro A, Cano Pérez J, eds. *Atención Primaria. Conceptos, organización y práctica clínica.* 6th ed. Madrid, Spain: Elsevier; 2008:345–366.

7. Gofin J, Foz G. Training and application of community-oriented primary care (COPC) through family medicine in Catalonia, Spain. *Fam Med.* 2008;40:196–202.

8. Societat Catalana de Medicina Familiar i Comunitària. Grup de Treball en Atenció Primària Orientada a la Comunitat—APOC. http://www.apoc-copc.org/home.htm. Accessed August 2009.

9. Gofin J. The community oriented primary care (COPC) approach and Towards Unity for Health: unity of action and purpose. *WHO Newsletter Towards Unity for Health (TUFH).* April 2000; 1: 9–11.

10. Larizgoitia I, Starfield B. Reform of primary care: the case of Spain. *Health Policy.* 1997;41:121–137.

11. Catsalut. Servei Català de la Salut. Oficina Central de la Targeta Sanitària Individual. Dades de població de referència 2009. Barcelona, Spain. Generalitat de Catalunya, Departament de Salut; 2009.

12. López E, Forcada C, Miller FA, Pasarin M, Foz G. Factors involved in the development of the community projects. Observational study of the Catalonian primary care centers AUPA network. Atención Primaria 2010;42: 218–225.

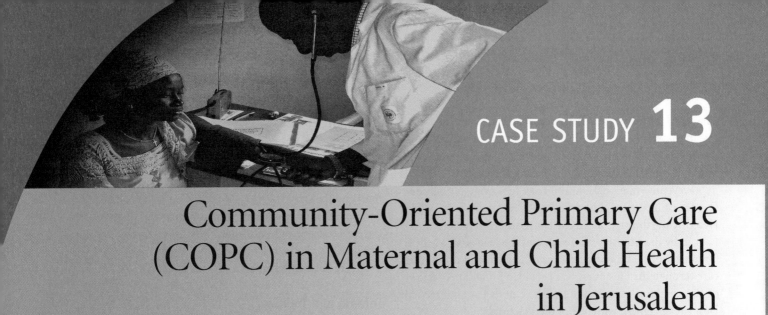

CASE STUDY **13**

Community-Oriented Primary Care (COPC) in Maternal and Child Health in Jerusalem

Rosa Gofin

BACKGROUND

The Kiryat Hayovel neighborhood was founded in 1951 in southern Jerusalem, Israel. Located about 7 kilometers from the city center, it was then in the outskirts of the city in a sparsely populated area. Housing was mostly government owned, built of concrete, with a size of about 40 square meters. Some of the housing was small units built with asbestos. There was electricity, water, and a sewage system, but houses were inhabited even before these facilities were in place or roads were finished. Public transportation was scarce, and private cars were scant. Shops covering the essential needs of the population were available, and there were educational facilities.

The original inhabitants of the neighborhood came from various regions of the world; there were recent immigrants from 25 different countries, mainly of Middle Eastern and north African origin, and from central and eastern Europe, mostly Holocaust survivors. There were also a few Israeli-born inhabitants and some early immigrants to the country who were government employees or veteran trade union members.

In many cases this population mix, with varied cultural backgrounds, languages, behaviors, food habits, and dressing patterns, cohabited the same building, or alternatively, lived in distinctive sections of the neighborhood. The differences among the different groups of the population or different sections of the neighborhood were striking and posed a challenge for the health services, or any services, provided to the population.

With the passing of time, the neighborhood reached about 25,000 inhabitants, and the standard of living improved. Public transportation linked the neighborhood with all other neighborhoods in the city. Houses were enlarged, and new ones were

built; dormitories for university students were erected in the area; shopping and recreation facilities were added. Because rent in the neighborhood was, and still is, relatively low compared to other parts of the city, young families populate the neighborhood but move out when they can afford the ownership of a home or a larger home. At some point, the poor and unhealthy asbestos housing was dismantled, and their inhabitants moved to other regions in the city. Overall, the neighborhood has retained its middle-to-low socioeconomic status.

Regarding the mother and child population, with time the proportion of immigrants decreased, and Israeli-born mothers were the majority. There was an increase in educational level and socioeconomic status.[1]

Health Services

The curative health services of Israel are provided by four sick funds. Until 1994 they were financed through voluntary insurance and covered about 95% of the population. Since 1995 there has been a National Insurance Law that entitles all citizens to basic basket of services. Preventive services for mothers and children are provided by Mother and Child (MCH) clinics known as *Tipat Halav* or *Drop of Milk*. MCH clinics were started by the Hadassah Medical Organization in 1916, and today they encompass about 1200 clinics, mostly belonging to the Ministry of Health, two local governments, and in some cases the sick funds. These MCH clinics serve the whole country, including all citizens in rural and urban areas. They required a small out of pocket fee.

Health care for the population of Kiryat Hayovel was provided through the Hadassah Community Health Center, which was founded by the Hadassah Medical Organization (see

Chapter 3 for history and development). Hadassah also owns two of the four hospitals in the city of Jerusalem (a third-level, 800-bed hospital in the vicinity of the health center and a community hospital in the northern part of the city).

Preventive maternal and child care to a geographically defined area in the neighborhood was provided by the MCH Health Unit through an MCH clinic (in agreement and financed by the Ministry of Health and the Hadassah Medical Organization), and comprehensive curative and preventive care through the life course was provided for another section of the neighborhood by the health center's Family Practice Unit (in agreement with one of the sick funds).

The health teams in the MCH clinics were nurse centered. Immunizations, growth and development surveillance, and health promotion activities are typically provided by the nurses, and doctors (generalists, pediatricians, family physicians, and gynecologists) attended mostly to the medical needs of the expectant mothers and children. The ratio of nurses to number of births varied during the years but was around 1:180. Other members of the teams include social workers (from the Municipality Welfare Department local office), and when the budget allows, a psychologist.

The services provided by the MCH clinics (both of the MCH and Family Medicine Units) were as follows:

For prenatal care: Early detection (congenital and pregnancy-related conditions), counseling, and health education and promotion were provided to pregnant women. High-risk pregnant women received care according to their needs, and they were referred accordingly. The coverage of pregnant women in the 1970s was about 85% in the preventive-care-only clinic and 100% in the comprehensive clinic of the family practice area. With time and the availability of new technologies offered by specialized clinics (which were not available at the health center), the coverage of prenatal care in the MCH clinics decreased markedly. Women opted for services that could offer the most advanced, specialized care that could be afforded by their insurance or privately. All deliveries take place in the hospital and are covered by the insurance.

For children aged 0–5 years: Immunizations (according to the Ministry of Health recommendations), growth and development surveillance, screening, counseling, health promotion, and referrals were provided. The population coverage in these clinics was close to 100% (according to a review of birth certificates and surveillance activities by the nurses).

THE HEALTH STATUS OF THE COMMUNITY

The health status will be described for pregnant women and infants and toddlers.

Pregnant Women

Health surveillance carried out during pregnancy pointed to the presence of anemia, bacteriuria, and deleterious behaviors, such as smoking. This prompted a detailed assessment of anemia[2] and the smoking status[3] of pregnant women. The prevalence of anemia was higher among women with high parities, low social class, and poor diets. The prevalence of smoking reached 27% in the mid-1970s. Smoking was associated with the degree of acculturation to the society.

Infants and Toddlers

Infant mortality and infectious diseases were relatively high and comparable to the rest of the country when the neighborhood was founded. Improvements in the physical environment and socioeconomic conditions of the population were also translated into the improvement of infant mortality and morbidity.[2] However, other types of problems in this multiethnic and multicultural population were evident. Studies indicated gaps in the educational achievements of children according to ethnic origin and socioeconomic background.[4,5] Findings also indicated a different growth pattern according to ethnic origin and social class.[6,7]

It was therefore decided to carry out a more in-depth analysis to quantify the problems under study and their determinants. The target population was children aged 0–2 years. Information about births was routinely obtained through the Jerusalem District Health Office of the Ministry of Health, which gets information about births from the hospitals and then transmits it to the respective MCH clinic. Nurses carried out an active demographic surveillance covering children who enter the area after birth and those who leave the area before their second birthday. In the 1970s, when the program was started, there were about 400 births in the area per year.

The development assessment showed that at age 24 months there were lower development quotient (DQ) scores (measured by the Brunet Lèzine test[8]) among children whose mothers had less education and in large families,[9] showing a need for verbal stimulation. Growth studies revealed that there were no gross growth delays or poor general nutritional status[10]; however, there was a high prevalence of nutritional anemia, and breastfeeding was low for infants at age 6 months.[11] Following these initial assessments, additional health problems were addressed, such as injuries (at home and in traffic, which showed a relatively high incidence in children aged 0–2 years), needs for home safety improvement, and use of car restraints.[12] Oral health was assessed regarding the incidence of early childhood caries, which was shown to be high among 3 year olds.[13]

THE INTERVENTION PROGRAM

On the basis of the previously mentioned assessments and with evidence emerging about effective interventions starting at an early age, the health team decided that the MCH clinics could offer an appropriate framework for the implementation of an Early Stimulation program to decrease the gaps among population groups and through the possible determinants of these gaps—mother's educational background, family size, short intervals between births, nutritional habits, and rearing practices. Thus the Promotion of Development (PROD) Program was started. Other programs followed, and all were integrated into the routine of the MCH clinic. Nurses provided counseling and guidance in routine encounters with the parents. To guide and structure the advice, checklists were designed for the early stimulation program, family spacing, injury prevention, breast feeding, and oral health.

The intervention programs included the population as a whole (pregnant women and children), and although high-risk groups were identified, the activities were all-inclusive to avoid stigmatization of selected groups of the population.

Pregnant Women

The anemia prevention program included advice on nutrition and iron supplementation,[14] and it showed the benefits of iron supplementation over the treatment of anemia. The early diagnosis of asymptomatic bacteriuria showed a positive outcome in the offspring.[15] The family spacing program addressed issues such as couples' decision making and appropriate contraceptives, which were provided or subsidized by the clinic, and advice on stopping smoking was given to the pregnant women.[16]

Infants and Toddlers

The program related to the growth and nutrition of the children was mostly of a surveillance nature, and parents were given advice when there were deviations from expected growth (mostly overweight).

A program was implemented to increase the initiation and duration of breastfeeding. The program started during the last trimester of pregnancy for those who received care at the MCH clinic.[11] It included education and advice regarding the benefits of breastfeeding, the usual problems encountered and how to cope with and solve them, and support to breastfeeding mothers. Other recommendations on feeding habits were related to appropriate weaning practices and foods for infants and toddlers. Iron supplementation was recommended in the form of medicines, and when formula became affordable to the population, the nurses ensured that babies received the recommended amount of iron.

The Early Stimulation program was started from birth, and was mainly based on verbal stimulation and parent–child interaction. Emphasis was placed on using the routine home activities of the caretaker, mainly the mother, as a vehicle for appropriate language exchange, use of age-appropriate toys, and developmentally tailored play interaction.[9] Workshops were organized for parents in which toys were prepared with home materials (bottles, cups, etc.), but they were discontinued when educational toys became more affordable and the mothers were no longer interested in this activity. In addition, group meetings were organized to discuss issues regarding child rearing. These groups had an uneven history because participants who would have benefited the most from this participation (i.e., parents with low education levels) attended the least.

The injury prevention program was geared to the promotion of safety behavior and injury prevention at home, as well as the use of car restraints.[12] The program used a developmental approach and repetitive messages on injury prevention and safety through the first 2 years of life. For the oral health program, advice was given to the parents regarding the use of bottles and sugary beverages.[13]

Immunizations were integrated into the routine of the MCH service according to the schedule of the Ministry of Health. Coverage was consistently high (more than 95% for most vaccines), according to the periodic reviews at the clinics.

Evaluation

A controlled evaluation of the breastfeeding program showed an increase in breastfeeding and longer durations,[11] and anemia prevalence decreased over the years.[17]

The time trend evaluation of the Early Stimulation program showed that after 2 years of implementation there was a decrease in the 24 months DQ gap between children whose mothers had 0–8 years of education and those with more education.[9] The continuous surveillance of the population showed that this gain was not maintained over the years.[1] Mothers who had low education in the 1980s and 1990s were a special group. Because most of those mothers were born in the country, they enjoyed free education for at least nine years. Those who were early dropouts may have had specific limitations that precluded them from continuing school, and the intervention in the clinic may not have been enough to promote the development of their children. However, another at-risk group benefited from the program—the mothers who were late high school dropouts whose children's DQ was maintained over the years.

A process evaluation of the injury prevention program showed the feasibility of introducing it into the routines of the clinics, and the oral health program demonstrated an increase in knowledge about early childhood caries and improved practices regarding tooth brushing.[13]

One of the programs was discontinued because of changes in the health system. Family planning maneuvers, like insertion of IUDs, could be performed only by gynecologists or after certification, which at the time was not feasible. The family planning program was transformed into a counseling-only service.

COMMUNITY PARTICIPATION AND INTERSECTORAL COOPERATION

Mothers were involved in the organization of toy-making workshops and taking over some of the group educational activities by opening their homes for meetings. When there was a threat to close the health center, the community mobilized to protest.

Because the MCH service was mainly preventive, there was a referral mechanism with the sick funds for cases that needed additional care. Welfare and social services were, as mentioned, provided by the local Welfare office.

LESSONS LEARNED

- The inclusion of the *whole population* was possible through an organized system of birth reporting.

- It was *feasible to integrate the programs* through the routines of the clinic by providing in-service training and prioritizing activities within the clinic.
- The programs were *sustainable*; some lasted about 3 decades. The *adaptation* of the programs to the *changing characteristics of the population* was possible because of the intimate knowledge of the population by the health team and the new knowledge that was being accumulated regarding interventions. Some of the programs were later adopted as *national policies* by the Ministry of Health (anemia prevention) or adapted by other providers of care.

The end of the service in 1999 resulted from a change in policy of the Hadassah Medical Organization (mainly a tertiary care provider), which stopped its support of the health center. As a consequence, the service as offered until then was discontinued.

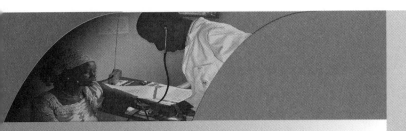

Discussion Questions

- Were COPC steps followed in the development of the programs?

- How feasible is it to adapt the MCH programs to a population elsewhere?

- How feasible is it to obtain information on the births in a community that you know about or work in?

- Is community participation an essential component for the success of a program?

REFERENCES

1. Gofin R, Adler B, Palti H. Time trends of child development in a Jerusalem community. *Paediatr and Perinat Epidemiol.* 1996;10:197–206.

2. Kark SL. *The Practice of Community-Oriented Primary Health Care.* New York, NY: Appleton-Century-Crofts; 1981.

3. Gofin J. Smoking in pregnancy. A community survey. *Harefuah.* 1979;96:278–281.

4. Lieblich A, Ninio A, Kugelmass S. Effect of ethnic origin and parental SES on WPPSI performance of pre-school children in Israel. *J Cross Cultural Psychology.* 1972;3:159–168.

5. Ortar G. Educational achievements of primary school graduates in Israel as related to their socioeconomic background. *Comp Educ.* 1967;4:23–35.

6. Flug D. Height and weight growth of children in two different neighborhoods. Cited by: Kark SL. *The Practice of Community-Oriented Primary Health Care.* New York, NY: Apple-Century-Crofts; 1981.

7. Epstein LM. Growth in weight of infants in the western region of Jerusalem, Israel. *J Trop Pediatrics.* 1968;14:139–148.

8. Brunet O, Lèzine I. *Le dévelopment psychologique de la première enfance.* Paris, France: Presses Universitaires de France; 1951.

9. Palti H, Zilber N, Kark SL. A community-oriented early intervention programme integrated in a primary preventive child health service. Evaluation of activities and effectiveness. *Community Med.* 1982;4:302–314.

10. Palti H, Adler B, Reshef A. A semilongitudinal study of food intake, anemia rate and body measurements of 6–24 month old children in a Jerusalem community. *Am J Clin Nutr.* 1977; 30:268–274.

11. Palti H, Valderrama C, Pogrund R, Jarkoni J, Kurtzman C. Evaluation of the effectiveness of a structured breast-feeding program integrated into a maternal and child health service in Jerusalem. *Isr J Med Sci.* 1988;41:731–735.

12. Gofin R, De Leon D, Knishkowy B, Palti H. Injury prevention program in primary care: process evaluation and surveillance. *Inj Prev.* 1995;1:35–39.

13. Sgan-Cohen H, Mansbach IK, Haver D, Gofin R. Community-oriented oral health promotion for infants in Jerusalem: evaluation of a program trial. *J Public Health Dentistry.* 2001;61:107–113.

14. Gofin R, Adler B, Palti H. Effectiveness of iron supplementation compared to iron treatment during pregnancy. *Public Health.* 1989;103:139–145.

15. Gofin R, Palti H, Adler B. Bacteriuria in pregnancy and growth and development of the infants. *Early Human Dev.* 1984;9:341–346.

16. Gofin J, Fox C. A smoking cessation program for pregnant women: minimal input intervention. *Harefuah.* 1990;118:525–527.

17. Gofin R, Palti H, Adler B. Time trends of hemoglobin levels and anemia prevalence in infancy in a total community. *Public Health.* 1992;106:11–18.

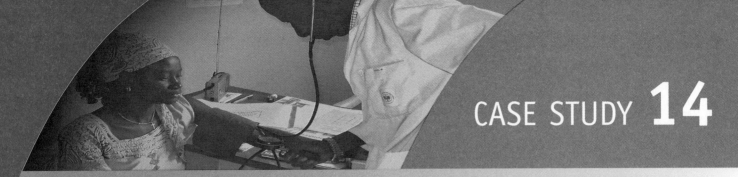

A Community-Oriented Primary Care (COPC) Program for the Control of Cardiovascular Risk Factors: The CHAD Program in Jerusalem

Jaime Gofin

BACKGROUND

In 1953, the Hadassah Community Health Center was founded in Kiryat Hayovel, a western Jerusalem neighborhood. The center provided integrated curative and preventive care for individuals through the life course through its family practice unit. This care was financed by an agreement with the larger sick fund (one of the four sick funds in Israel) through which nearly all the population was insured.[1] The center also provided maternal and child care and additional services to the larger neighborhood area (see Case Study 13).

The population served by the family practice unit consisted of about 2700 residents, composed mostly of Holocaust survivors from central and eastern Europe, immigrants from Middle Eastern countries, and Israeli-born civil servants. Doctors and nurses comprised the family practice team that provided care in the clinic and through outreach activities. Additionally, a support team consisting of a health educator–community organizer, health recorder, epidemiologists, and a social psychiatrist provided support and services. All team members were trained in public health (see Chapter 3 for details). The team that provided primary care was also responsible for implementing community programs. These programs were based on three related components: (1) consultations at the clinical practice, (2) periodic reviews of special groups at risk, and (3) planned community health surveys.[2,3]

THE HEALTH STATUS OF THE COMMUNITY

Because of the multiethnic population the health center served, it was important to seek information about the differences in risk factors and atherosclerotic morbidity and mortality among the different groups. Striking differences in myocardial infarction were already evident among the different ethnic groups that composed the Israeli population in the 1950s. Ashkenazi Jews of European origin presented higher rates than Jews of Oriental origin. These differences decreased with time as the population assimilated to the country. Moreover, among the immigrants from Yemen, for example, those who recently arrived in the country had lower cholesterol levels compared to those with longer residence. Deaths due to atherosclerotic conditions and diabetes were much higher among the latter than among recent immigrants. This was primarily associated with differences in dietary patterns, mainly the consumption of fats and sugar. North Africans, particularly women, had an increasing death rate associated with atherosclerotic heart disease. Death rates from cerebrovascular diseases were also increasing in this population, while for those of European origin, it was decreasing.[4] Given this evidence, information gathered at the health center was analyzed.

In the late 1960s, more than half of the deaths in the defined population were due to cardiovascular diseases (CVD). A review of records provided information about risk factors. However, the review revealed that records of blood pressure and cholesterol measurements or smoking habits were missing for about half the population. Thus, information was obtained on CVD, diabetes, and their risk factors through a comprehensive health survey, the Community Health Study (see Chapter 3). This study also included a comprehensive appraisal of health status and sociocultural determinants.[5,6] The survey included not only the population that was targeted for intervention, but also the remaining neighborhood, which afterward became a comparison group. The findings from the

Community Health Study were part of the community diagnosis of CVD and diabetes and were the basis for the intervention program for the control and prevention of these conditions.

THE INTERVENTION PROGRAM

On the basis of this baseline community diagnosis, the CHAD (Community syndrome of Hypertension, Atherosclerosis, and Diabetes) program was initiated in 1969 for all people aged 25 years and older, approximately 1000 people.[1,7,8] The program objectives included (1) to improve behaviors regarding diet, smoking, and exercise; (2) to shift the distribution of blood pressure, weight–height indexes, and serum glucose and lipid levels at the community level; (3) to decrease the incidence of hypertension, hypercholesterolemia, diabetes, and obesity; and (4) to encourage community response regarding prevention of CVD.

On the basis of the findings of the clinical records and the survey, the program team developed a plan of action at the individual and family levels. The intervention program included activities for healthy people (to promote their health and prevent the development of risk factors or the targeted diseases) and for those with risk factors (according to a tailored program in accordance with their individual risk profile) and treatment and rehabilitation for those who had hypertension, diabetes, or CVD. A central feature of the program included an individual record for each person that was updated at regular intervals in accordance with the risk profile (which determined the frequency of visits to the clinic). The record contained demographic information, risk status, specific planned and performed intervention activities, and examination results. Intervention activities were performed at each clinic visit or at home (by physicians or nurses), and special CHAD clinics were organized by appointment. Most of the program activities were carried out through face-to-face encounters with individuals or families.

In 1978, 8 years after the inception of the program, 34% of participants were receiving active treatment for established CVD, 51% were in the at-risk group, and 15% required only surveillance.[2] Surveillance of health and monitoring of program activities enabled the early detection of changes in health status and quality of care.

Evaluation

The program trial design (an intervention and comparison group) allowed for the evaluation of program effectiveness. At the end of the first 5 years of the intervention, a controlled evaluation was carried out by examining the intervention population (regardless of degree of individual participation and compliance) and comparing it with the adjacent population in the neighborhood that received its usual care from another clinic. The comparison population was almost three times larger than the intervention population. The results from more than 2500 people aged 35 years and older at the beginning of the program who were examined in 1975 and 1976 showed in the intervention group a decrease in the prevalence of hypertension (33%), cigarette smoking (23% in men), hypercholesterolemia (31%), and overweight (13%).[9–11] There were also decreases in the comparison population, although to a lesser degree.

Ten years after the program, an evaluation of risk factor status in the intervention community was implemented on the basis of the program's records. All people who were in the program since its inception were included in this evaluation. The analysis suggested further decreases in mean systolic and diastolic blood pressure and in the prevalence of hypertension.[12] The proportion of hypertensive patients whose condition was under control had risen from 65% to 78%. There was also a decrease in cigarette smoking, but national surveys showed no decline. No changes in weight and cholesterol levels were evident.

A third evaluation took place 15 years after the program; this time it also examined the control population aged 50 years and older (response rate of 84%). The results suggested decreases in the prevalence of risk factors in both the intervention and control populations, although the mean blood pressure was lower in the CHAD population as compared to the rest of the community. Additionally, the prevalence of hypertension (based on current measurements) was considerably lower in the CHAD population.[9] The results also showed improvement in the recording of activities and results, with high rates of risk factor measurements. This was present in both populations, although measurement rates were higher in the CHAD population. This explains the impact of the CHAD program in the surrounding area, along with increased-risk factor control.

The CHAD program was a pioneer experience of a *multifactorial program integrated in primary care*. The multifactorial approach was recommended by the World Health Organization for noncommunicable diseases in 1983.[13] On the basis of the CHAD experience, the major sick fund in Israel adopted the program for hypertension in their 1300 clinics.[14] The program was sustained for approximately 30 years. In 1999, the health center closed as a result of a change in ownership.

COMMUNITY PARTICIPATION AND INTERSECTORAL COOPERATION

In the preparation and implementation of the Community Health Study from 1969 to 1971, community members were actively promoting the participation of the residents. This was initiated and developed with the assistance of the health educator and the health team. Together with members of other community agencies, they created a community group. This group participated in recruitment and practical support during the surveys and provided feedback and information to the rest of the community. Additionally, they participated in the publication of a neighborhood newspaper and in educational activities at primary schools in the neighborhood. Although this participation became more sporadic, relations between the community and the health center were maintained throughout the entire implementation of the program.

LESSONS LEARNED

- The program evaluation provided evidence for the feasibility and effectiveness of a comprehensive (prevention, promotion, and treatment) and multifactorial (addressing several risk factors) program integrated into primary care.
- The work of the clinical team was benefited by the support of epidemiological and health behavior disciplines. This was facilitated by an academic environment.
- A control community that is adjacent to the intervention population may be influenced by the intervention program activities.
- The program could be adapted to other primary care clinics.
- The integration of a community program in the regular clinic strengthened the relationship between the community and the health center.
- The program constituted an essential component of the teaching of COPC and research in the Jerusalem School of Public Health and Community Medicine.

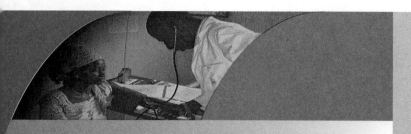

Discussion Questions

- What COPC principles were adopted by the CHAD program?

- What are the differences between a community-oriented primary care service and a regular primary care service?

- What are examples of constraints in comparing an intervention population with an adjacent control population?

- What is the role of community surveys in the development of a community health program?

REFERENCES

1. Epstein L, Gofin J, Gofin R, Neumark Y. The Jerusalem experience: three decades of service, research, and training in community-oriented primary care. *Am J Public Health.* 2002;92:1717–1721.

2. Kark SL. *The Practice of Community-Oriented Primary Health Care.* New York, NY: Appleton-Century-Crofts; 1981.

3. Kark SL, Abramson JH, Gofin J. A community oriented multifactorial cardiovascular program in a family practice. In: Kark SL, Kark E, Abramson JH, Gofin J, eds. *Atencion primaria Orientada a la Comunidad (APOC).* Barcelona, Spain: DOYMA; 1994:chap 13;pp121–133.

4. Kark SL. *Epidemiology and Community Medicine.* New York, NY: Appleton-Century-Crofts; 1974.

5. Kark SL, Gofin J, Abramson JH, et al. Prevalence of selected health characteristics of men: a community health survey in Jerusalem. *Isr J Med Sci.* 1979;15:732–741.

6. Gofin J, Kark SL, Mainemer N, Abramson JH, Hopp C, Epstein LM. Prevalence of selected health characteristics of women and comparison with men: a community health survey in Jerusalem. *Isr J Med Sci.* 1981;17:145–159.

7. Kark SL, Kark E, Hopp C, Abramson JH, Epstein LM, Ronen I. The control of hypertension, atherosclerotic diseases, and diabetes in a family practice. *J R Coll Gen Pract.* 1976;26:157–169.

8. Abramson JH. Community-oriented primary care—strategy, approaches, and practice: a review. *Public Health Rev.* 1988;16:35–98.

9. Abramson JH, Gofin J, Hopp C, Schein M, Naveh P. The CHAD program for the control of cardiovascular risk factors in a Jerusalem community: a 24-year retrospect. *Isr J Med Sci.* 1994;30:108–119.

10. Abramson JH, Hopp C, Gofin J, et al. A community program for the control of cardiovascular risk factors: a preliminary evaluation of the CHAD program in Jerusalem. *J Comm Health.* 1979;5:3–21.

11. Abramson JH, Gofin R, Hopp C, Gofin J, Donchin M, Habib J. Evaluation of a community program for the control of cardiovascular risk factors: the CHAD program in Jerusalem. *Isr J Med Sci.* 1981;17:201–212.

12. Gofin J, Gofin R, Abramson JH, Ban R. Ten-year evaluation of hypertension, overweight, cholesterol and smoking control: the CHAD program in Jerusalem. *Prev Med.* 1986;15:304–312.

13. Glasunov IS, Grabauskas V, Holland WW, Epstein FH. An integrated programme for the prevention and control of non-communicable diseases: Kaunas report. *J Chron Dis.* 1983;36:419–426.

14. Silberberg DS, Baltuch L, Hermoni Y, Viskoper R, Paran E. The role of the doctor–nurse team in control of hypertension in family practice in Israel. *Isr J Med Sci.* 1983;19:752–755.

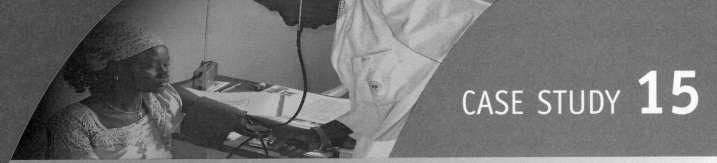

CASE STUDY 15

The Healthy Municipalities Movement in Nocaima, Cundinamarca, Colombia: Academia–Community Partnership in Action

Ricardo Alvarado

ACKNOWLEDGMENTS

To the people and municipality authorities of Nocaima and to X Semester medical students for their participation in the Healthy Municipalities Movement in Nocaima.

BACKGROUND

Colombia is a country that had a population of 46,741,000 in 2008,[1] 31% of whom were children younger than age 15 years; only 25% of the population lived in the provinces. People move to the cities because of job scarcity, the influence of the armed conflict, drug trafficking, terrorism, common delinquency, and media influence. Colombia is ranked second in worldwide population displacement.[2] In 1994, the death rate from violent causes was 129/100,000 population,[3] and from 2005 to 2008 the rate decreased to 41.5/100,000.[4] Still, an average of 41 homicides per day were recorded in 2008.[5] The infant mortality rate was 15/1000 in 2008.[4] The GNP is US$105 billion,[6] of which 7.7% is dedicated to health.[7] The main products are coffee, sugar cane, nickel, and livestock. Grain and other basic food products are both produced locally and imported.

Nocaima is one of 1102 municipalities in Colombia, located 66 kilometers west of Bogotá. It has an urban nucleus surrounded by land plots. The population is mainly composed of families that were displaced from rural areas because of local violence in 1996. Of the 7734 habitants, 34% live in the urban area. Regarding the socioeconomic status, 90% of the population is in levels 1 and 2 (lowest), and 28% are under the poverty level. Unmet basic needs decreased from 59% in 2001 to 32% in 2007. The homes are constructed with brick, concrete, or adobe materials. In rural areas 48% had a mud floor in 2001,

and in 2007 this proportion decreased to 25%. In the urban area the proportions were 36% and 3%, respectively. During the same years, in the urban area, the availability of toilet systems increased from 54% to 75%, and the availability of tap water increased from 80% to 93%, while in the rural areas the availability remained at 35%. The sewage system availability in the urban area increased from 70% to 85%, but there is still no sewage system in the rural areas. Wood was used for cooking in 53% of the households in rural areas in 2001, and this has not improved.[8–10]

The major economic activity in the area is the growth of sugar cane to produce *panela*, a nationally consumed beverage that is mixed with milk to provide a basic caloric intake for Colombian babies.[8]

The majority of the population (80%) receives financed or subsidized health care from the government. Those who are in socioeconomic levels 3 to 6 contribute to their health care in a proportional manner, and 13% of the population has a prepaid plan that is deducted from their salary. An additional 8% are not registered in the healthcare system but attend the health center through an enhanced plan. Care is provided by a health center in Nocaima, and referrals are sent to the closest hospital, which is located in the municipality of La Vega and is 20 minutes away by car. The health center has two physicians, one dentist, three auxiliary nurses, one microbiologist, and 13 health promoters.

Healthy Municipalities Movement

The Healthy Municipalities Movement (HMM) is a development strategy that promotes the commitment of citizens to individual and community health. It also includes social well-being components, such as employment, education, food, housing, clothing, security, roads, communication, justice, ecosystem, basic services (water, sanitation, garbage disposal, and electricity), and sports and recreation.[8] Nocaima started its process to become a Healthy Municipality on March 15, 2001.[8] It used an action framework based on an adaptation of the community-oriented primary care (COPC) approach[11,12] for the development of its programs as follows:

> Planning: Form a work team; characterize the population; identify the health status of the community and its determinants; monitor trends in health and socioeconomic conditions; develop the Health-Promoting Schools Initiative; develop intersectoral participation and establish agreements among sectors; develop a strategic and operational plan (determining what will be done, who will do it, and how it will be done)

> Doing: Establish a Joint Task Force to bring together local authorities and community leaders that will carry out the activities identified in the planning stage; conduct a community diagnosis; implement activities to promote healthy environments and lifestyles

> Verifying: Carry out surveillance monitoring and evaluation

> Action: Reexamine actions and strategies for decision making about the continuation and modification of the program

The process started with a formal agreement among local organizations, citizens, and elected municipal authorities.[8] This was followed by the development and implementation of an action plan to continuously improve the environmental and social conditions that will promote and sustain the health and well-being of all citizens. This HMM process used qualitative and quantitative methods with a triangulation approach to analyze and understand the complexities of the municipality's health needs and type of intervention needed.

THE HEALTH STATUS OF THE COMMUNITY

The main causes of morbidity in children are upper respiratory tract infections, acute diarrheal diseases, and parasitic diseases. In young adults the main causes of morbidity are communicable diseases and noncommunicable conditions. The main communicable diseases are intestinal parasitism, upper respiratory tract infections, and vectorborne diseases such as dengue fever and leishmaniasis. Arterial hypertension, chronic obstructive pulmonary diseases, and diabetes mellitus are among the most frequent reasons for consultation in the adult population. The main cause of mortality is cardiovascular diseases. Waterborne diseases have decreased because of improved drinking water quality, better sanitation, and enhanced health habits.

The Role of Universidad del Rosario

To build a new space for field practice and education and extend the activities of Universidad del Rosario for the development of a new Colombia, a partnership with the local government was created. This endeavor offered the opportunity for students to acquire competencies for their future performance as professionals. The purpose of the partnership was to develop a methodology (that could eventually be replicable) that promotes a healthy environment and strengthens actions to improve the quality of life and community participation. It is expected that this will trigger the nation's development, fomented by local governments. The university and the municipality signed a formal agreement of mutual cooperation within the health and other sectors to work with the available resources in the development of a Healthy Municipality through an adaptation of the COPC approach.

Medical students performed the fieldwork in their last semester (16–18 students per semester). Prior to their fieldwork they reviewed the literature on Healthy Municipalities and COPC. Together with an instructor from the School of Medicine and the mayor of Nocaima and his staff, they were in the field each Friday during the whole semester. The work was done in teams of two or three students and with the participation of an instructor from the university, municipality agents, community leaders, and lay members of the community.

A process of *veredas* (division and organization of the municipality's inhabitants by sidewalks) meetings were held with the participation of the municipal authorities, community members, and the university. A consensus was reached about priorities for Nocaima. Four axes of action were decided: employment generation, a healthy and useful school initiative, comprehensive human development, and basic care plan support. From 2000 to 2009, 276 medical students in their last semester did their fieldwork in Nocaima, and their final presentations were shared with the mayor, municipal workers, and the community.

THE INTERVENTION PROGRAM

Several activities were implemented to address the needs of the community, including employment generation, the Healthy and Useful Schools Initiative, a comprehensive human development program and a basic care plan support for the population.

Employment Generation

A total of 308 *enramadas* (sugar cane mills) are run by families that own a small plot of land on which they also live. On Fridays, the transformation of cane into blocks of panela takes place, following a 100-year-old tradition. The countryside product is sold to intermediate merchants and taken to the cities. The producers in Nocaima compete with the Valle del Cauca Plains, where the process is strongly industrialized and done in the *latifundio* (a big, privately owned land area). The Nocaima community has asked for an alternative means of earning their family income using their land and manpower. People in the rural areas want to continue to use their soil and land but must obtain a fair reimbursement for their efforts to satisfy their families' basic needs. From 2007 to 2009, the program received aid and support from the Universidad del Rosario business administration faculty to take over the leadership of this axis while continuing to cooperate in the fieldwork. It is useful for students in the medical field to learn about the intersectoral and multidisciplinary approach and the creation of teamwork settings to build social development.

Healthy and Useful Schools Initiative

The Healthy and Useful Schools Initiative (HUSI) was initiated by the Pan American Health Organization (PAHO) in the American Region. The purpose of the HUSI was to develop or strengthen the health services' and education systems' capacity so they could work together to design, develop, implement, sustain, and evaluate their Health-Promoting Schools.

The local community was concerned about working men and women leaving the countryside for the cities and abandoning their land plots. There was a sense of ownership, and it was thought that it could be developed through the HUSI. The 19 urban and rural schools (about 2700 children and 76 teachers) have been covered by the HMM. Medical students carried out an assessment of the community's attitudes and expectations toward the schools. During these years children have been screened for growth and development. Additionally, workshops on healthy nutrition and lifestyles and the implementation of the scholar vegetable garden have occurred. All of this has connected the health sector to the educational sector as an ally for social development. It has stimulated teachers and children to create change and be more proactive in improving their behaviors. Thus children, who are future adult citizens, grow up making decisions that benefit their communities, the environment, and their own lives.

Comprehensive Human Development

The comprehensive human development initiative proposes primary and secondary prevention to deal with community-identified problems, such as early adolescent pregnancy, alcoholism and drug addiction among children and young adults, intrafamily violence, and inadequate use of spare time. As a result, cultural opportunities, recreation, and sports have been created and put into action, taking into account the growth and development stages of individuals. Three youth talent festivals, with the participation of urban and rural citizens, have been held.

Basic Care Plan Support

Nocaima supports and follows selected areas of national guidelines of the basic care plan, especially in rural areas. Some of the activities were related to tap water standards. A literature review was done, and a checklist for observations related to drinking water standards was used in visits and surveillance of water sources and plants. As a consequence, between 2001 and 2003 there was an improvement of the infrastructure, which brought about a decline in the incidence of waterborne diseases. Additionally, there were activities related to garbage handling and disposal. Basic knowledge was provided about prevalent endemic illnesses and vectorborne diseases, such as cutaneous leishmaniasis and dengue fever. Additional knowledge was provided about hypertension and diabetes, and there was also an improvement in the delivery of health services at the town's health center, according to national standards.

COMMUNITY PARTICIPATION AND INTERSECTORAL COOPERATION

As previously discussed, programs were planned and implemented with the active participation of community members and representatives of the local authorities in a continuous consultation throughout the whole process. This contributed to the sustainability of the program and the development of the community.

LESSONS LEARNED

- The partnership between the local government, the community, and the university is successful. A healthy municipality has to have political commitment and be supported by local institutions and community members. University students and the faculty reinforce the selected tasks to be carried out by the community leaders and members.
- The HMM significantly increased the degree of intersectoral collaboration among multiple stakeholders. A particular success is the role of the municipality in the management and delivery of public health services. Positive political and organizational support was found to be a critical factor in the success of strategic planning and implementation of programs, reexamination of the strategy, and renewed planning. The outcome of the HMM has not yet been examined due to a lack of financial and human resources.
- The program is sustainable. After 8 years the program has prevailed, even with instability within the local government, which had three mayoral administrations during the program.

- A joint economic assessment performed by community leaders, rural teachers, and students and business administration faculty from the Universidad del Rosario has shown the viability and efficiency of the partnership and identified an opportunity for its continuation.
- The program can be replicated and adapted to other local realities. A current project is replicating the Nocaima experience in Las Mercedes county. The proposal is to develop a Comprehensive Dimensional Farm/Pilot Model[13] in a grammar and high school located in a rural area.[8] This may be managed by an intersectoral committee with a strong link between education–health and local production, with a partnership between the public and private sector. The main goal is that community members living on land plots will continue working the land, which in turn would provide enough income as an incentive to remain in the area.

- The university's social responsibility mission is being tested through the work in Nocaima. The role of the university in extending their work in the communities and working with community members and governance can be an example for other universities to follow. This approach could offer new and innovative opportunities for the development of a community health curriculum. The curriculum would be developed to create professionals and work in and with communities to promote healthy environments and lifestyles and improve the quality of life, alongside the curative and rehabilitative tasks of medical care.

ACKNOWLEDGMENTS

To the people and municipality authorities of Nocaima and to X Semester Medical students for their participation in the Healthy Municipalities Movement in Nocaima.

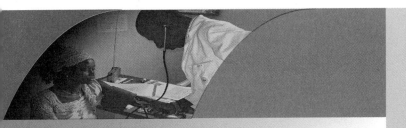

Discussion Questions

- Can the healthy communities approach be applicable to large communities (more than 50,000 inhabitants)?

- Does a university need to have a role in society beyond its educational role?

- What principles of COPC did you identify in this case?

- What else would you include in the process?

REFERENCES

1. Organización Panamericana de la Salud, Información de la Salud y Análisis. *Situación de la Salud en las Américas. Indicadores Básicos 2008.* Washington, DC: Pan American Health Organization; 2008.

2. *El conflicto, callejón con salida: Informe nacional de Desarrollo Humano para Colombia, 2003.* Bogotá, Colombia: UNDP; 2003 www.pnud.org/indh2003. http//www.cepur.org/biblioteral/pdf/8562.pdf. Accessed May 2010.

3. Arquidiócesis de Bogotá. *Desplazados por violencia y conflicto social en Bogotá.* Arquidiócesis de Bogotá, Bogotá,1997.

4. Latorre ML. Indicadores de Seguimiento al Sector Salud en Colombia. Así Vamos en Salud. Diciembre 15, 2008.

5. Muertes Violentas en Colombia, Instituto Nacional de Medicina Legal. Bogota. Septiembre, 2009.

6. Le Quid. Atlas Economique Mondial 2007 du Nouvel Observateur, Paris, 2007. http://www.studentsoftheworld.info/country_information.php?Pays=COL. Accessed April 2010.

7. Seguimiento al Sector Salud en Colombia. Así Vamos en Salud. Indicadores de Financiamiento. Julio 13, 2009. www.asivamosensalud.org. Accessed August 2009.

8. Alvarado R, Garzón A, Monroy J, Guarín D. Serie Salud Rosarista. Documentos de Investigación. Facultad de Medicina. No. 1. ISSN 1692-7753. Trabajo y Cultura por un Municipio Saludable: El Caso de Nocaima, Cundinamarca. Mayo 2003.

9. Flores F. Estadísticas Vitales de Nocaima. Oficina de Planeación Municipal, Nocaima, Cundinamarca Febrero, 2009.

10. Villamizar D, Angarita MA, Castaño N, Mejía MG. Grupo Apoyo al Plan de Atención Básica (PAB). X Semestre Universidad del Rosario, (Internal document) Mayo 11, 2006.

11. Gofin J, Gofin R. Community-oriented primary care: a public health model in primary care. *Revista Panam Salud Pública.* 2007;21:177–184.

12. Abramson JH, Abramson ZH. *Research Methods in Community Medicine.* 6th ed. West Sussix, England: Wiley & Sons; 2008.

13. Rosas Roa A. Granja Integral Dimensional. Rojas Eberhard Ediciones Ltda. Bogotá. 2002.

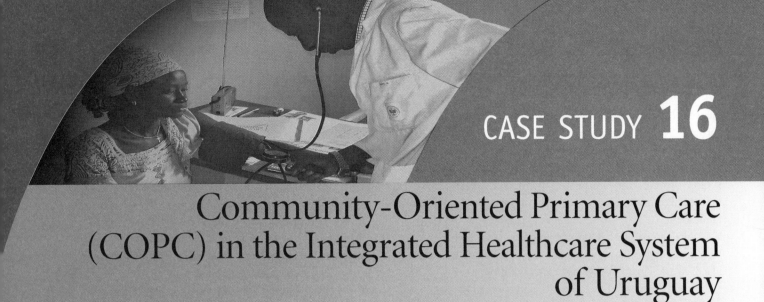

CASE STUDY **16**

Community-Oriented Primary Care (COPC) in the Integrated Healthcare System of Uruguay

Ramiro Draper, Serafín Alonso, Karina Sosa, Patricia Rambao, Nancy Acosta, Claudia López, Silvia Sica, Mónica Arroyo, and Irina Giacosa

BACKGROUND

Uruguay is a country of 3.5 million inhabitants, situated between Argentina and Brazil.[1] With the advent of the first democratically elected socialist government on March 1, 2005, the healthcare system was defined by the government as one of the priority reforms.[2] Within this reform process, the country started to move from a traditional curative model to an integral model based on primary health care. These changes were brought about by pressing the ethical need to achieve social equity, universality, and access to services for all the country's people based on social solidarity. To start this process, a territorial division of the country into health regions, zones, and areas was established.

In 2006, the Ministry of Public Health (MoPH) invited experts[a] to offer the first capacity-building course, a workshop on community-oriented primary care (COPC), aimed at the 22 regional health coordinators and other 15 healthcare professionals working in the health teams in the capital city, Montevideo. Since then, this strategy has been incorporated as the standard practice of teams working at the first level of care across Uruguay. In this case study, we will describe the experience of developing COPC in Villa Aeroparque.

Aeroparque is a small township (*villa* in Spanish) considered to be a health area by the MoPH. It has well-defined geographic limits and is located in a suburban area of the Departamento of Canelones,[3] 26 kilometers away from the capital city. The community, established in 1971, consists of 4934 people according to the 2004 census.[4] The streets are paved with gravel, and only the main road has lighting. There are abundant green spaces. Transportation is scarce and irregular. Practically all adults have mobile phones.

The houses are mostly made of concrete blocks with tin roofs, having either concrete or earth floors with few rooms, with high rates of cohabitation and shared sleeping arrangements. Most houses have drinking water and electricity. Sanitary disposal is precarious; in many cases sewage is dumped directly onto the ground or into streams by means of gutters. There is a good garbage collection service. A 250-square-meter community hall was built in which an Education and Cultural Center is now being set up. Multifunction sport grounds were also built. All this development was carried out within the framework of the government's Program for Irregular Settlements.[5] There are small family-run grocery shops; there is no pharmacy, bookstore, library, or public offices. A community policeman works during school hours.

Villa Aeroparque has two private kindergartens and two public schools with approximately 900 students. Only about 40% of young people have access to secondary education because they have to travel to distant education centers; the nearest is located 2.5 kilometers away. There is also a Center for the Integrated Care of the Family,[6] which provides comprehensive care for 126 children aged 0–3 years. The center supervises their development and provides early stimulation. Extracurricular activities include a club for children aged 6–12 years (77 children) and workshops for adolescents (computers, music, and crafts).

Regarding community organization, there are neighborhood and school development committees and a health committee (the members are health center's users). These are called

---

[a]Professor Jaime Gofin and Professor Rosa Gofin.

Network of Social Organizations of Aeroparque (Red de Organizaciones Sociales de Aeroparque [R.O.S.A.]). There is a soup kitchen run by local people where children are given free breakfast or afternoon tea from Monday through Saturday. There are several Christian churches, but only two of them have an important social commitment, particularly working with children and adolescents.

Villa Aeroparque has a young population (see Table C16-1); 51% are younger than age 19 years, and only 4% are older than age 65 years. The men-to-women ratio is 1.2:1.

Twenty percent of the population lives under the extreme poverty line.[4] Workers are low-skilled laborers (men are engaged in construction work, gardening, and security companies; women are domestic workers either in private households or in cleaning services). In 2005, the unemployment rate reached approximately 15%. Nearly 80% of the adult population has no secondary education.

Health Services

The only healthcare service is the Policlínica Aeroparque (Health Center Aeroparque), a public service provided by the State Health Services Administration (Administración de Servicios de Salud del Estado [ASSE]) within the sphere of the MoPH that started to operate in January 2007. This center provides medical care for residents without health insurance—approximately 3000 people. ASSE gave priority to this service in view of the joint report presented by the Coordination Committee of the Departamento of Canelones and the Health Committee of Villa Aeroparque, and a pilot project was initiated. The health team consists of two general practitioners, a community pediatrician, a gynecologist, a dentist, a nutritionist, a nurse and two nurse assistants, a psychologist, a social worker, a social and educational agent, an administrative assistant, and a cleaning assistant.

The community pediatrician is defined as the professional who, after having been allocated an area of activity, becomes involved in the area with humility, respect, and dedication, showing social solidarity. The pediatrician reaches out to meet children in all environments, which is essential to achieve better compliance with checkups, treatments, and other health center activities. The role of the pediatrician implies that this doctor is just another person in the community with specific knowledge.

The health center provides comprehensive care, including curative, promotive, and preventive care for people through the life cycle, such as vaccination, Papanicolaou tests, and family planning. It also provides laboratory and pharmacy services. Aeroparque also has folk healers who are not part of the health center. The nearest health services at the secondary level of care are located more than 5 kilometers away.

The health team works in coordination with different institutions in the area, highlighting schools, the local Council (representatives of the Municipality of Canelones), the Ministry of Social Development (Ministerio de Desarrollo Social [MIDES]), the Honorary Commission to Fight Cancer (Comisión Honoraria de Lucha Contra el Cáncer [CHLCC]), non-governmental organizations (NGOs) that deal with legal counseling, and the local community police.

THE HEALTH STATUS OF THE COMMUNITY

Following preparatory workshops, the community diagnosis was carried out in 2007 by members of the health team, community leaders, and school teachers. The following social, economic, development, and infrastructure problems were identified, as well as the lack of basic healthcare services:

- domestic violence, undocumented people, and legal problems
- cohabitation with domestic animals
- deterioration of streets, lack of public lighting, and insecurity
- regressive illiteracy
- school failure and adolescent issues (lack of training and work habits, immaturity in facing life projects, addictions, pregnancy)

TABLE C16-1 Distribution of the Population by Age and Sex

	Total	0–3	4–5	6–14	15–19	20–24	25–29	30–49	50–64	65–79	80+
Males	2245	197	106	504	237	195	168	528	226	71	13
Females	2689	195	118	939	208	180	193	550	189	83	34
Total	4934	392	224	1443	445	375	361	1078	415	154	47

Source: National Institute of Statistics (INE).[4]

- poor registration of clinic users and record keeping
- lack of pediatric, gynecologic, dental, and psychosocial care
- poor control of high blood pressure and diabetes, poor eating habits

Prioritization of Actions

Although a prioritization process was carried out following the method of the Pan American Health Organization (PAHO)[7] and COPC,[8] the programs that were originally given priority were those developed by the MoPH.[2] The dynamics of teamwork within a community with multiple existing deficiencies led the team to progressively address all the problems that were mainly of a social nature, as identified in and by the community, in parallel to the problems prioritized by the MoPH at the central level.

THE INTERVENTION PROGRAM

The intervention program addressed the needs of children, women, and specifically noncommunicable diseases and psychosocial problems.

Child Healthcare Program

The program addressed the health of 0–2 year olds and school children.

Objectives

The objectives of the child healthcare program were prevention of infant morbidity and mortality through routine surveillance; promotion of breastfeeding; early diagnosis of vision problems and learning and psychomotor disorders; immunizations; and improvement of oral health.

Activities

The health center provided care according to appointments and daily demand. At education centers, activities included anthropometric controls, immunizations, vision screening, and oral health examinations. Together with the child psychiatrist, psychologist, and social worker, an approach was developed to address behavioral problems, learning disorders, and violence. All the information, including the WHO growth charts,[9] was recorded on a work sheet designed by the health team.

Activities at households included outreach to children whose parents, because of cultural neglect or some other reason, were reluctant to receive professional medical care. The work at the street level was a fundamental instrument for the professional team and the involvement of the community. It contributed to reaching 100% of the children, as planned.

Results

Regarding children aged 0–2 years, there were 65 births in 2008; 86% were of normal birth weight, 63% were exclusively breastfed for 6 months, and 100% were immunized. The risk of overweight was 17%, overweight was 10%, and 5% experienced stunted growth.

Regarding the health of schoolchildren aged 4–12 years, there were 528 children covered by ASSE (the remaining 500 children were covered by private insurance), and all of them were immunized. Anthropometric data showed the following: 3.3% and 1.1% were stunted and wasted, respectively; 14.8% were at risk of overweight; and 5.3% and 0.9% were overweight and obese, respectively. A positive vision screening was found in 14% of the children. To address oral health, a dental room was set up in one of the schools in which all first graders were treated and taught to brush their teeth (toothbrushes and toothpaste were given to all the children). Children in the sixth grade were given the Atraumatic Restorative Treatment (ART) of the PAHO program.[10]

Women's Health Program

This program addressed the reproductive needs of women, with special attention to adolescents, and the early detection of selected malignancies.

Objectives

The objectives of the women's health program were to improve perinatal outcomes through adequate prenatal care; perform early diagnosis of uterine cervical cancer for 100% of women within the first year after they became sexually active; perform early diagnosis of breast cancer through breast self-examination, breast exams during consultations, and mammography for all women at risk; and prevent unwanted pregnancies and repeated adolescent pregnancies.

Activities

A network of agents (health center team, community agents, and female patients themselves) was set up that reached 100% of pregnant women who used ASSE, as planned (approximately 60% of all pregnant women in Villa Aeroparque).

Results

In 2007, 90 pregnant adolescents (aged 10–19 years) were reached; in 2008, 83 pregnant women were reached (33% of the total pregnant women). A high pregnancy rate is common in this kind of population where adolescents have no alternative life project but maternity. Antenatal care and care of women who just gave birth started at an increasingly early period, achieved by phone calls and home visits. All pregnant women were referred for dental care.

In 2007, when the service was started, very few women had undergone any medical examinations in their lifetime. An educational effort was started to highlight the importance of preventive exams, and rapid progress was made. In 2007, 274 Papanicolaou tests were carried out, and another 127 were performed in 2008. Four cases of low-grade intraepithelial lesions (LSIL) and two cases of high-grade squamous intraepithelial lesions (HSIL) were detected, which were referred and treated. In 2008, 40 mammograms were performed in 1 day by a mobile mammography unit sent by the Honorary Commission to Fight Cancer; others were done at a reference center. One case of advanced-stage breast cancer was detected. From 2007 to 2008, 371 women consulted the community doctor for family planning, 85 women had IUDs inserted by a gynecologist, and 123 women remained under periodic supervision.

To prevent repeated adolescent pregnancies, education is being provided to adolescent girls and their partners by a multidisciplinary team made up of a gynecologist, general practitioner, social and educational agent, psychologist, and nursing staff.

Noncommunicable Chronic Diseases Program

Noncommunicable chronic diseases, mainly cardiovascular diseases, hypertension, and diabetes, have being identified as priorities by the MoPH.

Objectives

The objectives of the noncommunicable chronic diseases program were to reach 100% of diagnosed diabetics, hypertensives, and dyslipidemic patients; to control glycated Hb values inferior to 8 in the first year of care of diabetic patients; to control hypertension levels to less than 135/80; to control LDL levels to under 130 mg/dl among dyslipidemic patients; to identify metabolic syndromes in cardiac patients; to improve dietary practices and compliance with pharmacologic treatment; and to stop tobacco addiction.

Activities

In early 2008, audits of 1225 medical records were done for patients who met the following criteria: older than age 15 years, users of ASSE, and consultations sought in 2007. Cardiovascular risk factors were evaluated, including tobacco addiction, diabetes, high blood pressure, and overweight or obesity; dyslipidemias were not analyzed because of the lack of laboratory data.

Results

Twenty-three percent of patients smoked, 8% were overweight or obese, 17% were hypertensive, and 3.8% were diabetic.

Seventy-five percent of patients had poorly treated glycemia and blood pressure values. Priority was given to the group of patients with greater cardiovascular risk, that is, diabetic, obese, and hypertensive patients and those who had already experienced a cardiovascular event. The team considered it a priority to launch a health education program, working with mutual aid groups and including the participation of the families of health center users so that the participants could share experiences and knowledge, help one another, spread information, and improve or adopt a healthy lifestyle. Likewise, activities to encourage self-esteem and a sense of belonging, as well as enriching and entertaining activities, were used.

Psychosocial Care

In addition of taking care of diseases and health behaviors, the psychosocial needs of the population were taken care of.

Social Service

The identified social and infrastructure problems—local identity, social security, rights, domestic violence, food insecurity, projects for recreational areas, roads, internal shelters and public lighting, and compliance with traffic rules—were addressed through the R.O.S.A. network. In 2007, a strong collaboration with the Ministry of Social Development[11] was developed to issue identification for adults and minors who had no identity papers (approximately 20% of the population), which prevented them from having access to the Social Emergency programs implemented by the government.

Psychological Service

The health center has a psychologist who works 24 hours a week, distributed between community and clinic hours. The request for psychological care is mostly focused on children who experience problems at school, such as poor performance and high repetition rates. Another psychologist works as a social and educational agent,[12] a role that is devoted to individual work with pregnant and puerperal adolescents. They supervise and counsel the adolescents on their development and motivate them to continue their studies to improve their chances of entering the labor market. Other tasks are devoted to all adolescents, such as addressing their comprehensive health care, sexual and reproductive rights, and life projects. This work is carried out through workshops that take place at area schools. A Network for the Prevention of Toxic Substances is being set up jointly with local people. This network operates by means of youth workshops.

The adult population is referred to the psychological service for domestic violence, sexual abuse, distress, depression, noncompliance with doctors' treatments, and tobacco and other addictions.

COMMUNITY PARTICIPATION AND INTERSECTORAL COOPERATION

Communication among local people is very difficult and rife with conflict. Those who participate have multiple interests, and it is not always clear whether they represent or act on behalf of a group or simply for their own interest.

From the beginning of the Aeroparque experience, the team developed actions to promote its integration with other institutions, such as joining the R.O.S.A. network and encouraging the continual participation of local people.

With this strategy and a major partnership with the school system, it was possible to enhance child care, carry out promotional activities with both children and their families, and develop activities for adolescents. A high coverage of pregnant women and health promotion among adults with cardiovascular risk was achieved.

LESSONS LEARNED

- The role of the community pediatrician as a provider of individual and community care goes beyond the usual role of a community pediatrician whose duty is to work in a specific area.
- A data collection work sheet is an effective follow-up tool in preventive and curative activities.
- Community participation has been a key tool in reaching pregnant women and children. The task of earning community confidence has been accomplished through work outside the walls of the healthcare center. These activities developed at the street level and in environments where daily community activities are carried out. They are invaluable for the community's health care and promotion of health.

ACKNOWLEDGMENTS

To Verónica Rodríguez and Rossana García, nursing assistants; Claudia Mederos, DDM; Leticia Arbelo, Lic. Nutr.; and Manuel Alonso, Teresa Nuñez, and Susana Barate, members of the Aeroparque team. This case study was translated from Spanish by Patricia Draper.

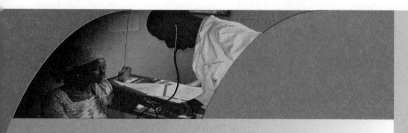

Discussion Questions

- How can health priorities that are decided at the central level be reconciled with local priorities?

- What community-oriented work methods can be carried out in communities with poor resources and an abundance of health problems?

- Is a national health policy necessary to develop a COPC approach at the local level?

- What attitudes are required from healthcare professionals who participate in community COPC work?

- What needs to be done in a population like Aeroparque to assure sustainability and continuity in the work initiated in schools to allow adolescents to overcome their poor family environment?

REFERENCES

1. Portal del Estado Uruguayo (Web site of the Uruguayan State.) www.uruguay.gub.uy. Accessed May 2009.

2. Ministerio de Salud Pública (Ministry of Public Health). www.msp.gub.uy. Accessed May 2009.

3. Municipality of Canelones. www.imcanelones.gub.uy. Accessed May 2009.

4. Instituto Nacional de Estadísticas (INE, National Institute of Statistics). 2004 census. www.ine.gub.uy. Accessed May 2009.

5. Programa Integral de Asentamientos Irregulares (PIAI, Program for Irregular Settlements). www.piai.gub.uy. Accessed May 2009.

6. Centro de Atención Integral Familiar (CAIF, Center for Integrated Care of the Family). www.caif.gub.uy. Accessed May 2009.

7. Ahumada J, Arreaza A, Durán H, Pizzi M, Sarué E, Testa M. *Health Planning, Problems of Concept and Method*. Washington, DC: Pan American Health Organization; 1965. Scientific publication No. 111. www.paho.org. Accessed May 2009.

8. Gofin J, Gofin R. Atención primaria orientada a la comunidad: un modelo de salud pública en la atención primaria. *Rev Panam Salud Pública/Pan Am J Public Health*. 2007;21:177–184.

9. World Health Organization. The WHO child growth standards. http://www.who.int/childgrowth/standards/en/. Accessed May 2009.

10. Práctica de Restauración Atraumática (PRAT) para la Caries Dental Una Iniciativa Global (1998–2000)—Centro Colaborador OMS Escuela Odontológica de la Universidad de Nijmegen. 2001. http://new.paho.org/hq/index.php?option=com_docman&task=doc_details&gid=683&Itemid=1335. Accessed August 2009.

11. Ministerio de Desarrollo Social (Ministry of Social Development). Emergency plan, 2005. www.mides.gub.uy. Accessed May 2009.

12. Ministerio de Desarrollo Social (Ministry of Social Development). INFAMILIA. www.infamilia.gub.uy. Accessed May 2009.

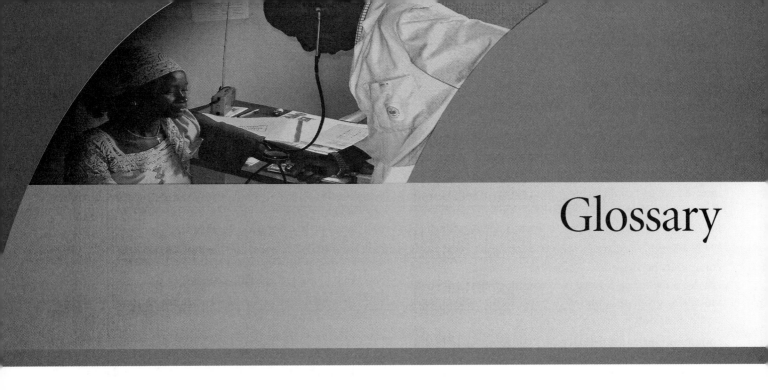

Glossary

behavioral change interventions A type of community intervention strategy usually guided by theory and models explaining behaviors and what influences them.

capacity building An activity that assures a trained workforce based on appropriate competencies that address health literacy, cultural competence, behavioral science and methodology, inequities and inequalities, and team building. Capacity building in COPC and COPH can best be realized by interprofessional training where the different disciplines involved in community health care share the same learning space, which should be community based.

community For health care purposes, a community could be defined geographically; as people registered in a health service, or special groups such as children in schools, workers in a factory, or refugees or other groups.

community diagnosis In both COPC and COPH, information about the community's health problems and their determinants and consequences that characterizes the community and its health status. Just as a diagnosis of a patient's state of health is a prerequisite for good clinical care, so a community diagnosis, leading to a needs assessment, provides a basis for the care of a community.

community health The collective expression of the health of individuals and groups in a defined community. It is determined by the interaction of personal and family characteristics, the social, cultural, and physical environments, and health services and the influence of societal, political, and globalization factors.

community health care Care that is provided to a community as a whole or any of its subgroups. This care includes the as-

sessment of health needs and prevention, promotion, treatment, and rehabilitation, and it is provided by health services or other health-related organizations.

community health intervention Interventions that deal with the health–ill health continuum through organized and systematic actions directed to maintain, promote, or restore health in a defined community.

community health measurement The use of indicators that reflect a community's state of health. Indicators such as infant mortality and maternal mortality reflect not only the health status of a specific group, but also of the total population. Health indicators draw attention to overall socioeconomic conditions and the community's quality of and access to medical care.

community health program Interventions designed to deal with a community's main health problems. It is an organized and integrated set of activities and services that are carried out in a predetermined sequence. The program may focus on a single problem or on a community syndrome of associated problems that are causally interrelated or have shared or related causes.

community healthcare practice Population-based healthcare practice that deals with the natural history of a disease, from its origins to its manifestation to its outcome. It integrates preventive and health promotion activities in conjunction with the care of the sick and their rehabilitation for a defined community. The two main approaches of delivering community health care are community-oriented primary care (COPC) and community-oriented public health (COPH).

community intervention setting The site or space where interventions take place. The site can be extended to diverse locations depending on the program that is developed and the degree of cooperation among the different organizations that take part in the program.

community involvement   A community's participation in an intervention that could include observing, complying with the program, or fully partnering with the healthcare team, depending on the organization of the community and its willingness to participate.

community participation   Community participation in health are the activities performed by community members (individuals or groups) intended to improve the community's health, their health care, or organization of health services.

community-oriented primary care   An approach of healthcare delivery that is characterized by integration of primary care and public health. It addresses the identified needs of all members (both healthy and sick) of a defined community through health intervention programs in primary care with the collaboration of other health-related sectors. It includes health promotion activities, provision of preventive care, and treatment and rehabilitation and involves the community in its care.

community-oriented primary care steps   The six steps are the components of a cyclic process in the development of community-oriented primary care: (1) definition and characterization of the community; (2) prioritization; (3) detailed assessment of the prioritized condition; (4) planning and implementation of the intervention program; (5) evaluation; and (6) reassessment carried out at the end of the process to decide on a renewal appraisal of new priorities. The steps are sequential and can overlap.

community-oriented public health   The discipline that applies population health principles in the context of the community's health. It deals with the identification and analysis of the health status and its determinants in a particular community, group of communities, or geographic region. It is followed by interventions addressing the community's health needs and their determinants through promotion and prevention actions through multidisciplinary and intersectoral cooperation. The interventions are carried out in different settings where people live, study, work, receive care, or spend their leisure time. Community-oriented public health reinforces the social justice and social accountability dimensions of public health.

community-oriented public health functions   A set of actions, which are the responsibility of local health departments or health agencies, that are carried out to improve, promote, protect, and restore the health of the community through col-

lective action. These actions can be delivered by institutions other than (or in cooperation with) health agencies, such as social services, housing departments, or police and fire departments, among others.

community-oriented public health services   Community-oriented public health services that are delivered by health departments or public health agencies. Within their roles of policy development and implementation and their capabilities for priority identification and setting health goals, health departments can provide the leadership, resources, incentives, and direction for local communities to address their priority health issues.

community syndrome   The coprevalence and the interaction of different health conditions, behaviors, somatic and psychological characteristics, as well as their shared determinants.

COPC   Community-oriented primary care.

COPH   Community-oriented public health.

culturally sensitive intervention   The language and content of the intervention respect the community makeup or different groups within a heterogeneous community.

definition and characterization of a community   The definition of a community is based on one of the principles of COPC—to know who the primary care service is responsible for and who the COPC program will be developed for. The characterization of the community entails knowing about its physical and sociodemographic characteristics, its resources and assets, and its health status.

detailed assessment   The measurement of the size and distribution of the health problem, according to relevant sociodemographic variables, and its determinants at each stage of its natural history.

determinants of community health   The personal and family characteristics, the social, cultural, and physical environments, and health services and the influence of societal, political, and globalization factors.

epidemiology   The basic science of community health care. The study of the distribution and determinants of health-related states or events in a specific population or populations and the application of this study to the control of health problems.

evaluation   An assessment that provides information about an intervention program's achievements. It provides the healthcare team and the community with empirical evidence regarding the program's degree of effectiveness. An evaluation also provides information on what worked and what did not, and it analyzes the extent of resource utilization and whether the resources were used efficiently; consequently, it indicates the need for continuation or modification of the program. Evaluations are an integral part of the intervention and should planned at the outset of the program.

evidence-based community health care It is an intervention in community health care that had been shown in properly designed evaluations to be effective. The best evidence is provided by a randomized controlled program intervention trial.

fragmentation of health services Having multiple healthcare providers for different health needs, as opposed to receiving overall health care at one location.

health According to the World Health Organization, "a state of complete physical, mental and social well-being and not merely the absence of disease or infirmity."

health indicators Health indicators are measurements that reflect a community's state of health.

healthcare team A group of healthcare professionals that is responsible for health assessments at the individual, family, and community levels. The healthcare team takes responsibility for the health care of all members of the community, whether geographically or otherwise defined. The team can include family doctors, pediatricians, nurses, a health educator, and others.

identification of health needs at the community level The evaluation of healthcare needs of a community that are identified through information provided by the community members, beyond individual consultations and by quantitative and qualitative surveys. It includes not only physical health, but also mental and emotional health and behaviors and their sociocultural, environmental, and biological determinants.

integration It includes the coordination or blending of processes or structures or activities in a unified whole. Care that is provided to a community as a whole or any of its subgroups, that includes prevention, promotion, treatment, and rehabilitation.

integration in community health care In COPC, an encounter between primary care and public health. COPC is integrative in purpose (protect and maintain health at the individual and community level), in content (carry out activities of health promotion, prevention, and treatment), and in process (carry out primary care and public health functions by the same team or service).

integration of health services A reorientation of the existing organizational, functional, and professional tasks that requires coordination between institutions and local health teams.

monitoring The follow up on how the process of a program is implemented according to the preestablished set of activities.

natural history of diseases The course of a disease from onset to its outcome. The stages involved are the pathological onset, presymptomatic stage, manifestation of the condition, and outcome (recovery, disability, or death). It can be applied to communicable and noncommunicable diseases and also adapted to the evolution of health behaviors.

needs assessment The gathering of available and new information on the community's health status and its determinants. In community health care, two different approaches may be taken: comprehensive health needs assessment or selective health needs assessment.

planning community interventions An organized and systematic process that includes various steps: (1) conducting an assessment of the community's health status, its determinants, and the resources available, including a process of prioritizing the health conditions that need to be dealt with among all competing problems; (2) selecting an effective and adequate intervention; (3) planning the intervention and its implementation in the community; and (4) evaluating the intervention to assess its affect on the community health status and the process of the program.

population-based public health It addresses public health activities to populations regardless of community boundaries.

primary care The point of entrance to healthcare services directly accessible to the public. Primary care is characterized by being the first contact with the services; practiced not only for individual care but in the context of family and community; accessibility, coordination, continuity, accountability, and comprehensiveness.

primary health care "The co-prevalence and the interaction of different health conditions, behaviors, somatic and psychological characteristics, as well as their shared determinants. The essential health care made universally accessible to individuals and families in the community by means acceptable to them, through their full participation and a cost that the community and country can afford. It forms an integral part both of the country health system of which it is the nucleus and of the overall social and economic development of the community." WHO, Alma Ata 1978.

prioritization A process that aims to select a specific health condition, problem, set of related problems, or health behaviors, according to specific criteria that are deemed to take precedence among others.

program review An evaluation that asks, How well is this program working? A before and after survey is usually performed.

program trial An evaluation that asks, How effective is this program? To appraise whether the program outcome is due to the specific intervention and not extraneous factors. It requires an experimental or quasiexperimental design that requires a control group.

public health The process of mobilizing local, state, national, and international resources to insure the conditions in which people can be healthy.

surveillance The ongoing identifcation and assessment of changes in the health status of the population and the demographic characteristics of the population.

sustainability The establishment of a managerial process to ensure that the services and activities have enough material and human resources to function over the long term. Sustainability is also achieved when the community has access to the knowledge, skills, and resources needed to conduct effective health promotion programs.

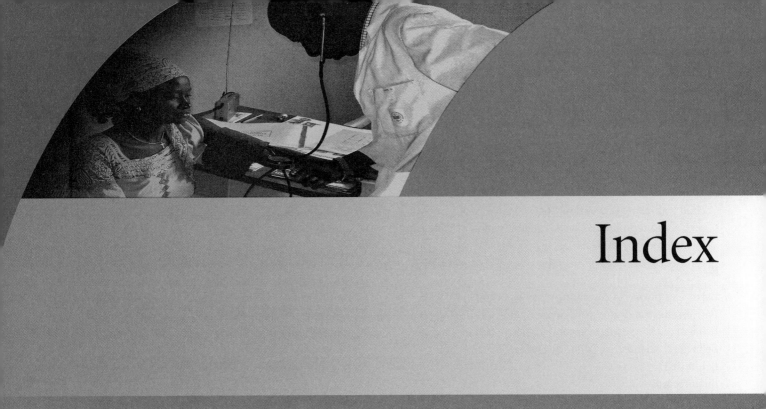

Index